Managing the Global Health Response to Epidemics

Recent epidemics have prompted large-scale international interventions, aimed at mitigating the spread of disease in a globalized world. During a crisis, however, global health actions – including planning and organizing, communicating about risk, and cost–benefit evaluations – aren't usually part of a single, integrated global response. Arguing that an uncoordinated approach can be challenged by local conditions and expectations, generating a wide range of resistance and difficulties, this volume provides important insights for future outbreak management and global health governance.

Drawing on experiences with A(H1N1) and Ebola virus disease, the book is divided into three parts looking at how responses to global health crises have developed, lessons learned from particular pandemics and the ethical implications of our management of them. Individual chapters focus on, among other issues, financing, cost–benefit analysis, matrix management, risk communication and organizational strategies.

Taking a social science perspective, this valuable book outlines the current state of global health emergency responses and explores ways in which they can be improved. It is a useful read for academics and practitioners interested in global health, the sociology of health and illness, health economics and emergency management.

Mathilde Bourrier is Professor in the Department of Sociology, University of Geneva, Switzerland.

Nathalie Brender is Associate Professor in the Geneva School of Business Administration, HES-SO University of Applied Sciences and Arts Western Switzerland.

Claudine Burton-Jeangros is Professor in the Department of Sociology, University of Geneva, Switzerland.

Routledge Studies in Public Health

Available titles include:

www.routledge.com/Routledge-Studies-in-Public-Health/book-series/RSPH

Managing the Global Health Response to Epidemics

Social Science Perspectives

Edited by Mathilde Bourrier, Nathalie Brender and Claudine Burton-Jeangros

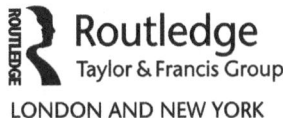

Routledge
Taylor & Francis Group

LONDON AND NEW YORK

First published 2019
by Routledge
4 Park Square, Milton Park, Abingdon, Oxon OX14 4RN
605 Third Avenue, New York, NY 10017

First issued in paperback 2023

Routledge is an imprint of the Taylor & Francis Group, an informa business

British Library Cataloguing-in-Publication Data
A catalogue record for this book is available from the British Library

Library of Congress Cataloging-in-Publication Data
Names: Bourrier, Mathilde, 1966– editor. | Brender, Nathalie, editor.
| Burton-Jeangros, Claudine, editor.
Title: Managing the global health response to epidemics : social
science perspectives / edited by Mathilde Bourrier, Nathalie
Brender, and Claudine Burton-Jeangros.
Description: Abingdon, Oxon ; New York, NY : Routledge, 2019. |
Includes bibliographical references and index.
Identifiers: LCCN 2018039387 | ISBN 9781138578999 (hardback) |
ISBN 9781351263047 (ebook)
Subjects: | MESH: Epidemics–prevention & control | Communicable
Diseases–epidemiology | Communicable Disease Control–organization
& administration | Global Health
Classification: LCC RA651 | NLM WA 105 | DDC 614.4–dc23
LC record available at https://lccn.loc.gov/2018039387

ISBN: 978-1-03-257018-1 (pbk)
ISBN: 978-1-138-57899-9 (hbk)
ISBN: 978-1-351-26304-7 (ebk)

DOI: 10.4324/9781351263047

Typeset in Baskerville
by Wearset Ltd, Boldon, Tyne and Wear

Publisher's Note
The publisher has gone to great lengths to ensure the quality of this reprint but points out
that some imperfections in the original copies may be apparent.

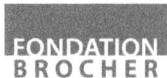

The Brocher foundation mission is to encourage a research on the ethical, legal and social
implications of new medical technologies. Its main activities are to host visiting researchers
and to organize symposia, workshops and summer or winter academies. More information
on the Brocher foundation program is available at www.brocher.ch

Contents

Contributors

Loïs Bastide is Assistant Professor of Sociology at the University of French Polynesia, and a research associate at the Institute for Sociological Research, University of Geneva.

Mathilde Bourrier is Professor of Sociology in the Department of Sociology, University of Geneva. She works on the social construction of safety, focusing on the conditions under which organizational reliability can be achieved and sustained. She is especially interested in organizational design and resources allocation during severe and challenging conditions in high-hazard organizations.

Nathalie Brender is Associate Professor of Risk Management, Corporate Finance and Accounting in the Geneva School of Business Administration, HES-SO University of Applied Sciences and Arts Western Switzerland. Her research in risk governance in health addresses the relationship between risk assessment and the management of the response.

Claudine Burton-Jeangros is Professor in Sociology at the University of Geneva. Her research in sociology of health and medicine covers health inequalities and meanings attached to risk.

Philippe Calain is a medical doctor specialized in infectious diseases and tropical medicine. He received a doctorate in biology in 1995. In 2006 he joined the headquarters of MSF Switzerland, where he is currently Director of Research at the Research Unit on Humanitarian Stakes and Practices (UREPH). His current areas of interest include humanitarian ethics, public health ethics, the governance of global health, and extractive industries.

Alexandrine Dupras has had varied professional experiences in the international development and humanitarian sectors. Before undertaking her current position with Oxfam in Jordan in early 2018, she worked for a year at the headquarters of the International Committee of the Red Cross in cooperation and capacity building.

Ann Keller is Associate Professor of Health Policy at the University of California, Berkeley School of Public Health. Keller studies the role of expertise in public decision-making, focusing on how expert systems are designed in the public sector and how expertise is maintained in contested political domains.

David Maradan is an economist specializing in cost-benefit and cost-effectiveness analysis. He is a lecturer at the Geneva School of Business Administration, HES-SO University of Applied Sciences and Arts Western Switzerland, the University of Fribourg and the Swiss Distance University.

Aude Parfaite is a research assistant at Geneva Canton Hospital (HUG) and a PhD candidate in sociology at the University of Geneva.

Hélène Pasquini-Descomps has over ten years' professional experience working in investment banking and asset management in Japan, the United States and Switzerland. She is also a lecturer in market and corporate finance.

Marc Poncin is a researcher and humanitarianism expert with Médecins Sans Frontières (MSF). He also served as Deputy Director General and Head of Programs of the Swiss branch of MSF.

Acknowledgments

This book would not have been possible without the help of decisive persons and supportive institutions. We wish to thank the Swiss National Science Foundation for its support over a course of four years (2013–2017). We wish to thank the Geneva School of Business Administration for its support in organizing a first workshop in June 2014, at the onset of the empirical fieldwork. The Swiss Brocher Foundation helped us structure this book project by allowing us to organize a two-day workshop in their premises by Lake Geneva in Hermance in November 2016. We wish to thank WHO experts for their support, especially Sylvie Briand, Nahoko Shindo, Gaya Gamewhage and Albena Arnaudova for their willingness to engage with social scientists, despite their constant mobilization on urgent matters and lack of time and the level of anxiety that they were encountering throughout the course of the project. We also would like to thank Marsha Vanderford for her help in setting up the US Centers for Disease Control and Prevention visit in the summer of 2015. We are also grateful to Max Hardiman, Raymond Hutubessy and Thomas Vogel for their support, particularly in approaching the economic questions from different angles. We hope that this volume can remain a marker of our collaboration. We deeply thank our research partners, Hitoshi Oshitani, Chris Ansell and Ann Keller, for their participation and willingness to share their knowledge, both scientific and practical. We met more than 100 people along this journey, and cannot name them all. But we wish to convey special thanks to Philippe Calain, Aude Thorel, and Anne Perrocheau. They helped us maintain our drive and vigilance throughout this long and demanding research endeavor. We would like to thank our students, undergraduates and graduates, who helped us sometimes directly, as research interns, and sometimes indirectly, as benevolent students in our classes, sympathetic to our outbreak examples. And a special thanks to our colleagues, in our own institutions or at a distance, who showed an interest in our global health research.

Geneva, December 21, 2018

Introduction

Mathilde Bourrier, Nathalie Brender and
Claudine Burton-Jeangros

Conducting fieldwork in the Global Health System, and making sense of its functioning, values, cultures, practices, goals, interests and controversies have been difficult. Despite the wide spectrum of publications on the subject and the select and numerous outlets where topics of global health are discussed, one feels both inspired and overwhelmed by constant new literature landing on one's desk, and starved of analytical information and empirical studies based on insiders' views. Anthropologist Theresa MacPhail expressed in her book something similar to our deep feeling: "Adding to the project's complexity was the fact that no study quite as large or as interdisciplinary had ever been attempted. We were in uncharted research territory" (MacPhail, 2014, 12). There is a puzzling lack of views from within. Not that experts commenting each day on the global health developments are not insiders, to the contrary. However, it is worth noticing that there are very few perspectives that attempt to describe their actual work, their daily activities and their compromises in the making. This is a very prolific milieu, when its goals, objectives, visions, failures, reforms and grand plans are considered. Interestingly, it often leaves out of the picture the petty bargains, transaction costs but also innovative adjustments made daily in the corridors of public health institutions, or close to interventions in the field. Hence, the conditions under which global health practices are decided upon, designed and carried away remain under-researched.

This book hopes to unveil some of the internal dynamics of global health, in light of two major recent crises: the A(H1N1) pandemic between 2009 and 2010 and the 2014 Ebola epidemic. Our hope is that readers of this volume will discover analytical frames and plural accounts doing justice to some of the various levels at which managing global epidemics is done today. The two very different crises are somehow from opposite ends of the epidemiological and preparedness spectrum, as we will demonstrate. This polarity allows us to examine the Global Health System in two contrasting modes of functioning: a well-prepared-for epidemic versus an unexpected outbreak – albeit, ruthless surprises, varied controversies and similar difficulties in contextualizing chosen public health interventions lie at the core of both responses.

Social sciences perspective and epidemics

For a long time, a social sciences perspective in international and global health has been restricted to the field of medical anthropology. This often meant the point of view of physicians holding a degree in anthropology (e.g. Paul Farmer, Vinh-Kim Nguyen or Didier Fassin) was integrated in order to tackle the complex nexus of questions revolving around illness and culture. On the epidemics front, anthropologists have long been very active. Questions regarding contagion, chains of transmission, inequalities and social apprehension of phenomena pertaining to uncertainty, disease and death are all of great scientific interest to anthropologists. However, their concrete implication in outbreak response only began to have effect, and moderately so, at the end of the 1990s. It started with a number of collaborations and recommendations aiming at modifying the design of outbreak responses. A number of publications (see Hewlett & Hewlett, 2008; Brunnquell et al., 2007; Epelboin et al., 2007; Leach & Hewlett, 2010) attest to this effort to introduce the "anthropological piece" (in the words of one informant at US CDCs in August 2015) as an integral part of a comprehensive global response. Briefly, the general idea behind this was to design public health interventions more sensitive to social contexts.

More recently, social sciences were further invited to contribute to epidemics responses through the lens of risk communication. At the beginning of the twenty-first century, energy and resources devoted to all-hazards preparedness brought under the spotlight research from communication sciences. Numerous institutions and initiatives tried to summarize existing knowledge and develop best practices guidelines in terms of communicating risks to the public. Public health interventions during epidemics might encompass a vast arsenal of measures, ranging from vaccination campaigns, social distancing measures, nursing barriers, to quarantines or containments. The social acceptance of these diverse interventions is, however, intrinsically linked to the trust that public health agents are inspiring in the targeted populations. In the early 2000s, the risk communication component made its entry to a fully developed outbreak response in an attempt to gain large public support for public health measures. In a document prepared for the "WHO Consultation on the Public Health Research Agenda for Influenza" in November 2009, risk and crisis communication in the context of public health was included along with "modern tools for early detection and disease monitoring/surveillance" and "the role of mathematical modelling in public health decision making". These three sub-themes had little in common; however, from the WHO's perspective they represented new fields, worth exploring in the hope that they would provide further tools to strengthen outbreak responses. Today, and after the 2014 Ebola epidemic, risk communication further gained its credentials and became the new talking point.

While there have been attempts to include more social sciences scholars in responses to SARS, H5N1 and A(H1N1) outbreaks, the majority of experts deployed in the field have a medical background. Most of them are epidemiologists, public health or infection control specialists, clinicians or virologists. A minor proportion of logistics and finance personnel and psychologists, mostly active in communication activities, were integrated in the teams (Brender, 2014).

The anthropological piece and the risk communication component have both been integrated as plug-in modular sets of guidelines, now considered as useful to the more traditional pillars of an outbreak response, coming from biomedical sciences mainly. They are understood as enabling conditions, helping a biomedical response to be more easily accepted by the public and more effective in the end. The period under study in this book marks a transition. Anthropological knowledge and risk communication precepts have made their full entry in the agenda of the global health response to epidemics. The expectations are high as Chapter 4, by Claudine Burton-Jeangros, will show, while the implementation of risk communication guidelines remains challenging in several respects.

As far as economics are concerned in the context of epidemics, a series of observations can be made. The perception of the benefits and costs constitutes a central dimension of risk assessment, both in the sociology of risk (Renn, 2008) and risk management standards (ISO, 2018) and techniques (ISO, 2009). However, if money is the talk of the town, or rather its lack thereof, one cannot say that economics are considered as being one of the pillars of any public health intervention during an epidemic. The other way to say it is that public health measures are usually not decided with cost and benefit data in hand. When cost-utility information is available, it is often fragmented, not comparable and not analyzed in relation to a pandemic severity (Pasquini-Descomps et al., 2017). Costs issues might be investigated after the crisis, but rarely in hindsight (see Brender et al., Chapter 7), probably also due to the fact that cost does not represent a constraint in high-income countries and its discussion is even considered unethical when human lives are at stake. Indeed, an outbreak's extra budget remains marginal in comparison to national health budgets (see Pasquini-Descomps et al., Chapter 8, for an analysis of a pandemic's financial costs).

Paradoxically, the same is true with the organizational aspects of responses to outbreaks. At first sight, a flu pandemic as well as a filovirus outbreak response, or any kind of outbreak response for that matter, are all about designing a proper organization capable of pulling forces towards containing the epidemic. Vast and constant organizational adjustments, the development of new options, improvised lines of command, the allocation of resources, tasks sharing and reporting mechanisms were all part of both the A(H1N1) pandemic and the 2014 Ebola epidemic throughout. At all levels of their respective responses, locally, nationally and internationally, they were decided with little consideration for what organization sciences have to say about managing high-hazard activities, with the exception of CDCs, which have used incident command systems for quite some time. Moreover, how to account for the transnationalization of international authority over health issues, currently established, maintained and exercised through transnational networks of a wide range of actors, remains a puzzle. This has implications for any kind of public health intervention on the ground. As Chapter 9, by Mathilde Bourrier, will introduce, urges towards more central leadership and clear lines of command and control are contradicted by the current flat and dispersed organizational state of the global health field. Injecting more resilient thinking throughout the Global Health System might represent a way forward, under the conditions of a clear move towards the decentralization of power and resorting to diverse sources of expertise.

The purpose of the book

This book embraces a social sciences perspective at large. It is not necessarily limited to risk communication issues, although those are very important. Nor does it further develop the albeit essential anthropological knowledge base because it is already quite substantial. What it does is explore recurrent challenges that a comparison between the A(H1N1) pandemic and the 2014 Ebola epidemic have brought to light. It aims at telling a complex story – one of managing global epidemics. It connects problems seen from different angles. First, managing epidemics is a transboundary and transnational problem. Second, it mobilizes actors, organizations and resources in different loci, within and outside the Global Health System, locally, nationally and internationally. Third, it sets in motion concepts, frameworks, historically charged actions (coercive measures like quarantines and isolation for example) and others more recently founded (around the preparedness arsenal). Fourth, it triggers controversies of all kinds, and following some of them proved to be an invaluable heuristic to avoid cognitive overflow syndrome and/or simply drowning in the prolific scientific literature and institutional documentation around contemporary global health issues.

This book demonstrates that managing epidemics through public health interventions has in fact a fragile social acceptance. Despite potentially powerful biomedical measures, always in development (treatments, vaccines), and centuries-old public health measures (quarantines, isolation, contact tracing, bans, social distancing measures), on which public health interventions rely most of the time, they remain contested outside (i.e. in the public) as well as inside public health institutions. The A(H1N1) pandemic and 2014 Ebola epidemic are both marked by major controversies. As other scholars have described, medical uncertainties, ambiguous results, challenging evaluations of risk constantly provoke internal debates within public health institutions. We were also struck by the constant internal professional controversies. And we could only witness that some of these debates are virally reaching out to the public, enrolling various and diverse segments of the population, through media (of all types), whistle blowers (of all kinds) and advocacy groups (of all origins). What is interesting about epidemics is that, with the strategies put in place to contain them, they almost instantly reveal the social fabric of any society or group.

Few questions preoccupy our leaders more than how we organize and face complex risk issues pertaining to global health matters, environmental and industrial disasters and humanitarian crises. Current thinking emphasizes that these crises need to be taken care of urgently, as events unfold. However, they also require medium and long-term solutions; their management is therefore a long-term project. Large epidemic outbreaks clearly constitute crises that call for multi-dimensional and multi-scale responses. Addressing them brings to the forefront issues pertaining to human health, zoonoses, environmental issues, social inequalities, political imbalance and the economic divide between high, middle and low-income countries. Fighting deadly epidemics has preoccupied kingdoms, national states and international institutions for centuries. Their potential to cross borders and destabilize entire regions are notorious. The International Health Regulations (IHR) revised in 2005 and finally implemented in 2007 are a tribute to and a legacy of this long-term international commitment, binding 196 Members States under the stewardship of the World Health Organization. The IHR define the rights and obligations of countries to report public health events, and establish a number of procedures that the WHO and its Member States must follow in order to secure global health. One of the famous instruments is the declaration by the WHO of a Public Health Event of International Importance (PHEIC). Such a declaration signals that the health issue at stake is beyond the capacity of a single country and needs to be tackled through a broader framework of response. Both the 2014 Ebola epidemic and the A(H1N1) pandemic gained the status of PHEIC.

The story behind the book

Our journey navigating global health waters during the two recent major epidemics of our times started as a collective project entitled "Unraveling lessons learned from A(H1N1)", supported by the Swiss National Science Foundation, from 2013 to 2017. The three editors of this book, sociologists Mathilde Bourrier and Claudine Burton-Jeangros and international relations and risk management expert Nathalie Brender, joined forces to develop a project that initially aimed at exploring the complex relationships that occurred between organizational patterns, risk communication issues and economical decisions during the A(H1N1) pandemic, examined in retrospect. Questions about risk management strategy from the vantage point of organizational processes, risk communication and costs incurred had at the time almost never been addressed within a multidisciplinary framework. Furthermore, these three aspects – organizing, communicating and costing – of the response were affected by harsh controversies during and after the pandemic A(H1N1), particularly in Europe.

The project aimed at analyzing the policy makers', public officials' and experts' responses in three countries (Switzerland, USA and Japan) in relation to the WHO's frameworks. It intended to explain how organizational mitigation strategies, risk communication and cost–benefit analysis should be closely intertwined. We hypothesized at the time that planning and developing organizational responses during acute crises needed to be articulated with a corresponding risk communication strategy that would not only report on the intrinsic difficulties of planning, deciding and organizing for such events but also mirror the organizational design of the response that had been chosen. Similarly, we envisioned that organizational responses should aim at offering an economic evaluation of the costs incurred and seek to look for large support in affected communities for these cost allocations. We argued beforehand that because these three aspects (organizing, communicating and costing) were usually addressed separately, social controversies were able to gain momentum to destabilize whatever "reasonable" (in the sense of reasonable buy-in) decisions were made earlier by public health agencies in relation to these issues.

Retrospectively, the three of us had a keen interest in recurrent controversies that plagued any epidemic we had read about. We hoped that we could make sense of these incessant debates and see whether they could be curtailed if the interaction between organization, money and communication was designed or thought through differently. Before starting our empirical fieldwork, we convened a first workshop on June 26–27, 2014, with the support of the Geneva School of Business Administration (HEG Geneva), with whom Nathalie Brender and her colleagues, David Maradan and Hélène Pasquini-Descomps, were affiliated. We were looking for some feedback on our future fieldwork strategies. In particular, advice from our international colleagues in the United States and Japan proved to be essential in the pursuit of feasible and sound data collection.

However, by the time we started our fieldwork, the 2014 Ebola epidemic started in Guinea, Sierra Leone and Liberia. Although our informants in different settings had accepted revisiting the A(H1N1) pandemic with us, Ebola was on the lips and minds of many. We decided to add the case of Ebola, because it was difficult to avoid when knocking at our WHO informants' doors in Geneva. It was impossible to ignore this excruciating tragedy, happening far from Geneva but at the same time shaking the heart of the Global Health System. One of its main institutions, namely the World Health Organization was Geneva-based. Also, the Swiss section of Médecins Sans Frontières was the first to sound the alarm from their

Guéckédou base in Guinea, where the epidemic is thought to have started. During the fall season of 2014, our project changed name and became: "Unraveling Lessons Learned from the A(H1N1) Pandemic to the 2014 Ebola Epidemic".

This book is a testament to the progression we made between 2013 and 2018, navigating between the A(H1N1) pandemic recollections of local, national and international actors, who were active during the pandemic and collecting active actors' narratives in the midst of their response to the 2014 Ebola epidemic. Sometimes, not always, they were the same actors. The world they described to us was chaotic and a lot of the time they unveiled deeply pressing and puzzling challenges. Interestingly, both crises have very different profiles and comparing them might lead to gross misunderstandings. The A(H1N1) pandemic first hit the Americas and soon the European continent and then reached the rest of the world. Pandemic influenza was a much feared epidemic, which had attracted for a long time a lot of resources, and against which preparedness efforts had been structured by international institutions. Even if the origin (Mexico) and the subtype (swine flu) came as a surprise, public health experts and epidemiologists suspected that a pandemic might break out at anytime. In a sense, the level of readiness was high. Ebola virus disease, although well-known, feared and seen as a text-book Emergent Infectious Disease, had so far mainly concerned African countries and had been spatially confined. The level of investment, in terms of medical treatments, vaccines, subject matter experts or preparedness plans had never reached the level attained by the flu. It had been kept minimal and the disease mainly interested some medical army labs for counterterrorism purposes (for more details on both crises, see Bourrier, Chapter 3). Despite extremely different profiles, these two major episodes shook the global health world. They prompted numerous internal and public controversies pertaining to the three cornerstones of our initial research design: (1) the type of public health interventions and the very organizational strategies within the response at all levels; (2) the risk communication strategies towards the public and their operationalization at all levels; (3) the costs and financial issues related to the national and international responses.

A team effort

We enriched our team with the participation of economist David Maradan, socio-anthropologist Loïs Bastide, in a post-doc position at the time, and Hélène Pasquini-Descomps, a PhD candidate in management. The six of us have contributed different chapters to this book. They reflect our initial scientific joint interests in this project, later expanded through new opportunities that emerged in relation to the Ebola outbreak. For example, Loïs Bastide and Claudine Burton-Jeangros embarked on a research-action when they were asked to debrief Ebola deployees of the WHO Emergency

Communication Network upon their return to Geneva (see Bastide, Chapter 5).

From the beginning we were also able to count on precious partners in our research. This is true for political scientist Ann Keller, who contributed Chapter 1, drawing on her own former research on outbreak responses (Keller et al., 2012) and transboundary crises (Ansell et al., 2010). Political scientist Chris Ansell has been a companion from the beginning as well as a pioneer in this kind of research (Ansell et al., 2012; Ansell & Keller, 2014). Hitochi Oshitani, professor of virology, and an eminent expert on outbreak responses was also involved from the beginning, and proved to be an invaluable guide to Japan's public health institutions.

Along the way, we met different colleagues and experts, whose knowledge proved to be essential to the development of our thinking. Philippe Calain is one of them, and we are happy that he accepted our request for a new version of an earlier chapter he wrote with Marc Poncin on the ethical puzzles that the 2014 Ebola epidemic generated. While teaching our regular classes at the University of Geneva, our project also caught the attention of various undergraduate and graduate students. For example, Mariama Diallo, a sociology Bachelor's degree student of Guinean origin, decided to embark on a journey back home to collect youth voices regarding the Ebola outbreak. Another student, Alexandrine Dupras, who was studying for a public management Master's degree at the University of Geneva at the time, contributed a chapter (see Dupras, Chapter 6) to the book based on her internship at the WHO. Kayla Jenni, studying for a Master's degree in standardization, social regulation and sustainable development at the University of Geneva, and Béatrice Nass, studying for a Master's in peace research in international politics at the Eberhard-Karls University in Germany, spending a semester abroad at the University of Geneva, helped Loïs Bastide and Claudine Burton-Jeangros in their examination of risk communication strategies. Finally, Aude Parfaite, a research assistant in the intensive care unit at the Geneva University Hospitals of Canton Geneva, and a sociologist by training, got the assignment from her management to evaluate the hospital's crisis management during the singular care of an Ebola-infected Cuban doctor, medically evacuated from Liberia in November 2014. Her observations provided material for her chapter in this book (see Parfaite, Chapter 10).

Different social sciences disciplines are thus represented in this volume. A core set of sociology (sociology of health; sociology of risk; sociology of organizations and work), economics and risk management formed the first building block. We then added the political science perspective, as well as that of ethics. International public health knowledge and expertise in outbreak management were later sought to enrich our own initial perspective.

We were fortunate enough to develop the project for this book with the support and under the auspices of the Brocher Foundation, in Hermance

Switzerland, during a decisive workshop on November 8–10, 2016. Members of the core team, along with colleagues and experts with whom we had been closely associated throughout the project, presented first drafts, sharing findings and doubts. Discussions and feedback on this preliminary material proved crucial for the preparation of this volume, which not only includes chapters from the initial team but also rallies colleagues met along the way.

Our multifaceted methodology

The initial team embarked on this journey with a research design both precise and flexible. This was a wise choice because the road turned out to be bumpy. First, as mentioned earlier, when the empirical fieldwork phase started in the summer of 2014, Ebola struck, leaving the informants we had planned to contact more eager to speak about Ebola than to reflect on the outdated pandemic flu. We decided to follow different courses in parallel, especially because depending on the research angles (organizational strategies, risk communication, costs issues), different research strategies had to be put in place. We had initially planned to examine pandemic response in retrospect, at the international level from the WHO's perspective, at the national level from Japan's, the United States' and Switzerland's perspectives, and at the local level from the Geneva canton's perspective. We rapidly decided that the US perspective would only be tackled through the position of the Centers for Disease Control and Prevention, which certainly does not cover the entire institutional apparatus of the United States, where flu pandemic is concerned. However, even if limited, fieldwork at US CDCs certainly gave us a good window of opportunity to approach one of the major clearing houses of the Global Health System.

Of course, the Geneva location helped us tremendously. Blaise Lempen (2010) coined the expression describing Geneva as "the Laboratory of the 21st century". The WHO is based in Geneva, so we could meet with different kinds of people, not all located in Geneva, but present because they were traveling to and/or from headquarters. Therefore, Geneva can certainly be envisioned as a Mecca for global health matters. It is unquestionably one of the main power centers of the Global Health System. The *Directory of Geneva Global Health Actors* (2018)[1] in its third revision, conceived by the Global Health Centre, a Geneva-based think tank, attests that fifteen out of twenty of the world's most important Global Health Actors have a solid presence in Geneva, which is thus labeled the "Global Health Capital".

We also used the Geneva case as a local generic model in the context of the A(H1N1) pandemic and to a lesser extent in the 2014 Ebola case. The strategies that local authorities displayed while unfolding their pandemic plans can be considered as a proxy and emblematic of many strategies developed locally in high-income countries (Europe and the United States essentially). The failure of vaccination campaigns, the difficulty to adjust the pandemic plan, and the disappointing coordination between police forces and public health authorities have all been singled out in various countries (Barrelet et al., 2013).

We adopted hybrid data collection, mixing semi-direct interviews, extensive document analysis, financial data and especially budgets, and some observations during specific sessions, expert meetings and public presentations. As will be explained below, conducting ethnographic observations, as we had planned to do, remained difficult.

Interviewing on and off the record

Members of the team responsible for examining organizational questions and risk communication issues (Mathilde Bourrier; Claudine Burton-Jeangros; Loïs Bastide) addressed both crises with interviewees – first at the international level at the World Health Organization in Geneva, then at the national level in Switzerland and in Japan; and at the local level in the Canton of Geneva. We also interviewed experts in outbreak responses for both crises at the US Centers for Disease Control and Prevention in Atlanta. We added interviews with Médecins Sans Frontières (MSF) experts working for the Swiss Section in Geneva to cover the Ebola outbreak. Members responsible for investigating the costs topic (Nathalie Brender; David Maradan; Hélène Pasquini-Descomps) addressed the A(H1N1) pandemic with interviewees at the WHO, at the national level in Switzerland and in Japan, and at the local level in the Canton of Geneva, as well as at the US Centers for Disease Control and Prevention in Atlanta. They did not include Ebola in their research design, except for the Cuban patient hosted in the Geneva canton, because events were unfolding and data were lacking.

More than 100 interviews were conducted over the 2014–2016 period. They covered our three initial research pillars as follows, with some participants covering more than one topic: (1) organization issues (sixty-one interviews); (2) risk communication issues (thirty-eight interviews); and (3) costing issues (twenty interviews). Forty-three interviews were conducted at the WHO, from September 2014 and throughout 2015, mainly with experts from the former Pandemic and Epidemic Disease Department and the Communications Department. Some were affiliated with the Global Outbreak Alert and Response Network, and WHO-CHOICE. At the US CDCs, twenty-three interviews were conducted in August 2015, mainly with staff delegated to the Emergency Operations Center and the Joint Information Center. In Switzerland, during 2015, twenty-one interviews were conducted at both the federal and local levels, with experts from the Swiss Federal Office of Public Health (FOPH) in Bern, from the Department of Health at the state level in the Geneva and Vaud Cantons, from Geneva University

Hospitals (HUGs), Geneva Police Department and media. In Japan, in March 2015 and July 2016, eighteen respondents were interviewed, ranging from the Office for Pandemic Influenza and New Infectious Diseases Preparedness and Response (an office dependent on the prime minister services, precisely at the cabinet secretariat) at the national level, the Ministry of Health, Labour and Welfare, including experts from the National Institute of Infectious Diseases, to experts from the Mitsubishi Research Institute, who helped in designing risk communication campaigns during the A(H1N1) pandemic. We also met local health authorities at Kawasaki City. In addition, five experts from MSF were interviewed upon their return from West Africa in 2015.

Some interviews were recorded, but due to the pressures our informants were experiencing, we sometimes decided to only take notes. This was especially so while investigating the Ebola case, where our informants were totally immersed in daily struggles and sometimes manifested their discomfort over talking to us. The majority of recorded interviews were transcribed and coded using Atlas Ti. The interviews were semi-structured, open-ended and face-to-face. Public health experts, civil servants and responders with a primary role during the A(H1N1) pandemic and 2014 Ebola epidemic were sought at local, national, federal and international levels. We granted anonymity to all concerned due to the sensitivity of the issues, especially in the Ebola case. Consequently, we choose not to refer explicitly to their titles or positions.

Collecting published and grey literature

Important documentation was collected for the project. On one hand, we identified the scientific literature related to the two epidemics, more specifically in the social sciences (anthropology, sociology and economics). On the other hand, we collected the institutional documents prepared before, during and after the A(H1N1) pandemic and 2014 Ebola epidemic. As a starting point, a review of pandemic plans and audit reports that flourished after the termination of the A(H1N1) pandemic in 2010 was done and proved to be very useful. Over 2000 documents were thus archived and shared using the Open Source reference manager software Zotero. The volume of this documentation exceeds our capacity to treat it and there is no doubt that further research can be done using this database. Not surprisingly, the WHO comes out as one of the main producers of documents (300) along with American institutions such as CDCs, the US National Institutes of Health, the Homeland Security Department and the Department of Health and Human Services, which contributed to more than 400 documents in our database. We also collected 130 documents in Switzerland, and seventeen in Japan. Twenty-four documents were issued by Médecins Sans Frontières. There is an imbalance in terms of documents concerning both crises: we collected 261 documents regarding the A(H1N1) pandemic and 596 concerning the 2014 Ebola epidemic. The 2014 Ebola epidemic was unfolding when we started our data collection and it generated important coverage, while understandably, the A(H1N1) pandemic was fading away, attracting less coverage from the media or from any other source. It is also certain that we, ourselves, were so immersed in trying to make sense of the Ebola crisis, that we became biased and paid more attention to that than to the flu pandemic. However, this is not true for all members of the team, as for example our colleagues studying costs issues had decided not to examine the Ebola crisis because of a lack of access to any meaningful data for their calculations.

It is important to note that the grey literature is an important part of the data collection here. Many institutions within the Global Health System are publishing recommendations, action plans, roadmaps, expert points of view, audit reports, lessons-learned reports and guidelines. This is obviously true for the WHO and for CDCs, which are major clearing houses of the Global Health System. But this is also true for numerous institutions like European CDCs, MSF or prominent research institutions that produce academic as well as think tank publications to shed light on specific global health policy issues. Most of these documents are available on their respective websites. They can be categorized as first-tier grey literature in the typology of Adams and colleagues (2016). Occasionally, we also were recipients of concept notes, presentations or videos, deemed second-tier grey literature. Without conducting a systematic analysis of the volume of media coverage or of the media content, we also collected some news articles. We did not include emails, tweets, blogs or letters (i.e. third-tier grey literature) that were privately sent to us as material for analysis.

Observing the Global Health System's practices

As expected, it has not been easy gathering information on daily negotiations and decisions. Experts we had planned to interview, in various points of the Global Health System, starting with the WHO, as much as they were willing to revisit with us, at a distance, the pandemic episode of 2009–2010 and its aftermath, were rapidly mobilized as part of the international outbreak response to Ebola. Facing pressures and tensions, experts became too busy and unwilling to share information with outsiders, even if well introduced. Gatekeepers also played a role. Despite our efforts, we could not access the WHO's Ebola Response Team and the physical locations of various task forces. We therefore had to use the following strategies to stay connected as much as we could to the theater of operations.

Embedding interns

Loïs Bastide and Claudine Burton-Jeangros were asked in 2015 by the WHO Department of Communications to collect and analyze accounts from deployees in risk communication activities returning from West Africa. These accounts were collected by Loïs Bastide, accompanied by two Master's degree students who were granted intern status within the WHO for four months. Mathilde Bourrier worked with an intern, in order to better understand the benefits and the limitations of a matrix structure in the context of the Ebola outbreak response, and in the context of outbreak responses more broadly. Two chapters in this volume – Loïs Bastide's (Chapter 5) on the functioning of the Emergency Communications Network and Alexandrine Dupras' (Chapter 6) on the Ebola matrix structure – draw on their experiences during these placements. They also provided other chapters with background information.

Making use of invitations to expert consultations conferences

During the period we were also invited to sit as observers and sometimes talk as participants at different expert meetings, forums and workshops. Due to the specific location of Geneva, as a global health hub, and the WHO's home-town, frequent academic or public policy events are organized around global health topics. They proved to be useful to better understand the contours of the debate. They also offered some contextual knowledge of where lines of fracture were lying or heading to. This is especially true of the meetings to which we were invited, usually by WHO secretariat members.

Of notable importance were different consultations: the "WHO Emergency Communication Network training" on March 27–29, 2015; the "WHO Emergency Risk Communications (ERC) for Outbreak and Health emergencies workshop" on November 24–25, 2015; the "WHO Informal Consultation on Anticipating emerging infectious disease epidemics", on December 2, 2015; the "RICE Project workshop" on December 3–5, 2015; the "WHO Public Health Research Agenda for Influenza", on December 6–8, 2016; the "Risk communication guideline development group" on June 22–23, 2015 and February 16–17, 2017. Attending these meetings has proven to be of great value in order to contextualize the debates arising from managing the 2014 Ebola crisis and epidemics more broadly at the international level. They gave materiality to the ethereal notion of global health. Researchers can learn a great deal by attending such events, where formal presentations increase the generation of knowledge and where some conversations in the hallways are always possible. These conferences and consultations can certainly be considered as elite events. Their importance for negotiating accesses should be acknowledged (Sampson & Turgo, 2018), but in our case not overstated.

In addition, we were invited to other types of functions (Swiss MSF Assembly on May 9, 2015 for example), or several panels, as speakers or participants (Ebodakar organized in May 2015 in Dakar, where Loïs Bastide was able to join in) in academic settings (e.g. Swiss Sociological Congress in June 2015 in Lausanne; French-speaking international sociological association in July 2016 in Montreal). Nathalie Brender, David Maradan and Hélène Pasquini-Descomps were also invited to present their work on economic considerations on A(H1N1) influenza pandemic risk management at the 5th International Disaster and Risk Conference IDRC in 2014, and at the International Health Congress in Oxford in 2017.

Accessing global health institutions

While being granted recurrent and regular access to the WHO's premises was difficult, despite having members of the WHO inside our project from the beginning, accessing US CDCs was possible under a very strict regimen (for more information, see Bourrier, 2017). If, in retrospect, we could analyze our access to the WHO as having been informal and guarded in some respects, our access to US CDCs proved to be more formal yet in the end accepted. This very access was facilitated by risk communication expert Marsha Vanderford, at the time Associate Director for Communications for the Center for Global Health at the US Centers for Disease Control and Prevention and soon to move to the Geneva WHO headquarters to become Director of Communications. Then, and from a different angle, it was negotiated under the auspices of the University of California at Berkeley, through its Internal Review Board, thanks to our colleague and partner Ann Keller. In parallel, we filed the paperwork to obtain security clearance granted by the Security Department of the US CDCs. Although telling the story of this step-by-step process to gain access could be worth an entire chapter, we restrict ourselves here to the following observations. Access to the CDCs, although controlled and restricted, allowed us to make contact with informants, willing to speak freely with us, on the basis that we were cleared, both scientifically and security wise. Providing a letter of consent to each informant was considered proof of trust. And the fact that our research partner, Ann Keller, had done research with and on the CDCs prior to 2015 was of considerable help. We were escorted at all times, and had to live with a lot of restrictions: for example, we were not supposed to station at the Emergency Operations Center (EOC) and only walked through once by accident; we were not allowed to interview people who were still "active" at the EOC. Despite these restrictions, in the end we collected a lot of decisive material.

Similarly, accessing Japanese institutions was facilitated by our research partner, Hitoshi Oshitani, who helped Mathilde Bourrier in March 2015 in organizing a small interview campaign under very strict time constraints in Japan. In 2016, he also helped Hélène Pasquini-Descomps to gain access to costing information. Without that introduction, and with no prior knowledge of Japan, nor linguistic skills, it would have been almost impossible to meet with public health experts.

Limitations

Despite this extensive data collection, under the conditions we just specified, limitations were encountered. First, to understand the management of global epidemics the researcher is confronted with the intricacies of the Global Health System. Despite the ideal location that Geneva undoubtedly represents, the ramifications and the complexities that the system entails remain a research puzzle. Second, obtaining financial data represented a challenge in itself. Reconstituting the different cost elements, particularly in federal systems, and converting them to comparable standards with other countries was even more difficult considering the fact that cost information was often partial, prepared ad hoc and considered as not important, or even unethical when human lives are at stake. Third, following actors during their daily activities poses some challenges to the qualitative methodologies that some of us in the team routinely use. Here again, we could open up debates on researching this kind of network of organizations. Such debates are worth conducting; however, we restrict the point here to one single comment. The main reason for adopting a hybrid data collection approach – mixing analysis of documents, semi-structured interviews, and observations, shadowing actors during meetings or routine work activities – revolves around the issue of contextualization. Stress, burden, points of convergence and divergence, policy issues, ethical dilemmas, political considerations, technical puzzles, and last but not least scientific uncertainties constitute the bread and butter of global health experts. They are regularly criticized for their lack of foresight. They frequently take the blame for their decisions. Hence, it is of crucial importance to be able to examine and understand their working environments. Social scientists are equipped to take into account the social production of knowledge, expertise and decisions. Their studies aim at providing contextual elements to decisions and actions that might otherwise be interpreted too narrowly and fail to explain what others might see as irrational, foolish, political or bureaucratic. It is hoped that in the future members of the numerous institutional arenas invested in global health issues will be convinced that global health is not only a topic and a banner under which different institutions rally. Global health is a social production, as worth examining as any other social activity. Investigating working practices and decision-making processes should improve our understanding of how and why managing global epidemics remains a heavily contested social activity.

Plan of the book

This volume is divided in three parts. In the first part "Setting the stage", three chapters introduce readers to the socio-history of epidemic responses. In Chapter 1, "The challenges of building pandemic response systems based on unique cases: 2003 SARS, 2009 A(H1N1) and 2014 Ebola epidemic", Ann Keller introduces a wide array of preoccupations triggered by the building of response capacities in very limited and rare cases. In Chapter 2, "The future strikes back: global public health crises and the rise of preparedness", Loïs Bastide, revisiting the socio-history of preparedness, introduces the reader to the dynamics that have shaped the organizational philosophy of global health responses over the last two decades.

In the second part "Lessons learned from the A(H1N1) pandemic and 2014 Ebola virus disease: a multidisciplinary point of view", seven chapters have been collected to present the specificities of both crises. In Chapter 3, "Comparing the 2009 A(H1N1) pandemic and 2014 Ebola virus disease: of viruses, surprises in outbreak responses and global health work", Mathilde Bourrier compares both crises, unfolding radical differences and also pointing towards intriguing continuity between the two. Claudine Burton-Jeangros, in Chapter 4, "Epidemics and risk communication: why are lessons not learned?", takes stock of the important material developed to guide communication between institutions and the public in outbreak contexts while revealing persistent difficulties in the application of such guidelines. Loïs Bastide, in Chapter 5, "Emergency capabilities: deploying the WHO's communication in West Africa during the 2014 Ebola epidemic", examines the specific case of the Emergency Communication Network, operating during the 2014 Ebola epidemic from the WHO's headquarters. The chapter brings to the foreground the extreme difficulties that first-line responders were encountering and how they managed to make use of a formal/informal professional network to support their adaptive strategies. In Chapter 6, "The use of matrix structure in epidemic management", Alexandrine Dupras revisits how, to what extent and to what benefit matrix management was applied within the WHO during the Ebola outbreak. In Chapter 7, "Shaping A(H1N1) pandemic response: money will follow", Nathalie Brender, David Maradan and Hélène Pasquini-Descomps explore how costs and benefits were taken into account when decision makers selected and implemented mitigation strategies against the A(H1N1) pandemic. In Chapter 8, "Financing the crisis: public expenditure on the A(H1N1) influenza pandemic in Switzerland, Japan and the United States", the same team reviews the public expenditure strategies that Switzerland, Japan and the US displayed to cover for A(H1N1) pandemic costs and puts them in perspective with regard to national public health budgets. Finally, Mathilde Bourrier, in Chapter 9, "The organizational puzzle of the Global Health System: insights from high reliability organizations theory", reframes the organizational puzzles of the Global Health System from the standpoint of the high-reliability theory. The aim is to seek alternatives to the dominant thinking based on structural reforms of the Global Health System.

In the third part, "Complementing views: double standard in ethics and care", two chapters offer a different angle on the understanding and functioning of crucial parts of the system. Aude Parfaite, in Chapter 10, "Scarcity in the midst of abundance: the case of the medical evacuation of the Cuban patient in Geneva, Switzerland", gives a vivid account of organizational challenges that a well-resourced hospital had to face when a medically evacuated Cuban doctor infected with Ebola virus was offered treatment. In Chapter 11, Philippe Calain and Marc Poncin provide a new version of their article "Reaching out to Ebola victims: coercion, persuasion or an appeal for self-sacrifice?", first published in *Social Science and Medicine*. This chapter places readers alongside humanitarian responders and Ebola victims. It exposes dilemmas that the current public health interventions doctrine and namely coercive measures have generated.

At the end of this journey, the general conclusion, "Global health revisited", underlines some transversal issues in the book, with a focus on the recurrent controversies emerging from the combined analyses of the A(H1N1) pandemic and 2014 Ebola virus disease. Considering the contrasting scales and disciplinary perspectives, persistent debates are clearly worth emphasizing. While they suggest that some lessons are difficult to learn, we will discuss how social sciences expertise could and should be taken more seriously in order to improve the management of future global outbreaks.

Note

1 The distribution of Geneva global health actors is: 60 percent come from NGOs or IOs, 16 percent from the UN system, 5 percent from the private sector, and 6 percent from academia. For further details, see www.graduateinstitute.ch/globalhealth/directory-geneva.

References

Adams, R. J., Smart, P., & Huff, A. S. (2017). Shades of grey: guidelines for working with the grey literature in systematic reviews for management and organizational studies. *International Journal of Management Reviews*, 19(4), 432–454.

Ansell, C., & Keller, A. (2014). *Adapting the Incident Command Model for Knowledge-Based Crises: The Case of the Centers for Disease Control and Prevention.* IBM Center for the Business of Government.

Ansell, C., Boin, A., & Keller, A. (2010). Managing transboundary crises: identifying the building blocks of an effective response system. *Journal of Contingencies and Crisis Management*, 18(4), 195–207.

Ansell, C., Sondorp, E., & Stevens, R. H. (2012). The promise and challenge of global network governance: the Global Outbreak Alert and Response Network.

Global Governance: A Review of Multilateralism and International Organizations, 18*(3)*, 317–337.

Barrelet, C., Bourrier, M., Burton-Jeangros, C., & Schindler, M. (2013). Unresolved issues in risk communication research: the case of the H1N1 pandemic (2009–2011). *Influenza and Other Respiratory Viruses*, 7*(suppl. 2)*, 1–6.

Bourrier, M. (2017). Conditions d'accès et production de connaissances organisa-tionnelles. *Revue d'anthropologie des connaissances*, 11*(4)*, 521–547.

Brender, N. (2014). *Global Risk Governance in Health*. London: Palgrave Macmillan.

Brunnquell, F., Epelboin, A., & Formenty, P. (2007). Ebola: no laughing matter / Ebola: ce n'est pas une maladie pour rire. DVD. Capa Télévisions.

Epelboin, A., Formenty, P., Anoko, J., & Allarangar, Y. (2007). Humanisation and informed consent for people and populations during responses to VHF in central Africa (2003–2008). *Humanitarian Borders*, 25–37.

Hewlett, B. S., & Hewlett, B. L. (2008). *Ebola, Culture and Politics: The Anthropology of an Emerging Disease*. Belmont, CA: Cengage Learning.

International Organization for Standardization (ISO). (2009), IEC 31010:2009 Risk management – Risk assessment techniques.

International Organization for Standardization (ISO). (2018), ISO 31000:2018 Risk management – Guidelines.

Keller, A. C., Ansell, C. K., Reingold, A. L., Bourrier, M., Hunter, M. D., Burrowes, S., & MacPhail, T. M. (2012). Improving pandemic response: a sensemaking per-spective on the spring 2009 H1N1 pandemic. *Risk, Hazards & Crisis in Public Policy*, 3*(2)*, 1–37.

Leach, M., & Hewlett, B. S. (2010). Hemorrhagic fevers: narratives, politics and pathways, in Dry, S., & Leach, M. (eds), *Epidemics: Science, Governance and Social Justice*. London: Earthscan.

Lempen, B. (2010). *Genève, Laboratoire du XXIe siècle*. Geneva: Georg Editeur.

MacPhail, T. (2014). *The Viral Network: A Pathography of the H1N1 Influenza Pan-demic*. Ithaca, NY: Cornell University Press.

Pasquini-Descomps, H., Brender, N., & Maradan, D. (2017). Value for money in H1N1 influenza: a systematic review of the cost-effectiveness of pandemic inter-ventions. *Value in Health*, 20*(6)*, 819–827.

Renn, O. (2008). *Risk Governance: Coping with Uncertainty in a Complex World*. London: Earthscan.

Sampson, H., & Turgo, N. N. (2018). Finding the way into a global industry: The usefulness of elite events to social science researchers. *Journal of Organizational Ethnography*, 7*(1)*, 2–15.

Part I

Setting the stage

1 The challenges of building pandemic response systems based on unique cases

2003 SARS, 2009 A(H1N1) and 2014 Ebola epidemic

Ann Keller

Introduction[1]

A growing body of research on crisis response attempts to identify the cognitive and organizational challenges involved in managing a crisis in an effort to prepare organizations for the decisions, processes, coordination and logistical feats necessary to limit its negative effects (e.g., Ansell, Boin, & Keller, 2010; Christensen, Lægreid, & Rykkja, 2016; Comfort 2007; Lagadec, 2009; LaPorte, 2007; Moynihan, 2012; Nohrstedt & Weible, 2010; and 't Hart, 2013). Apparent successes in preventing crises – e.g., the low failure rates of high-reliability organizations (LaPorte & Consolini, 1991; LaPorte, 1996) or the use of incident command systems in firefighting (Bigley & Roberts, 2001; Comfort, 2007; Lutz & Lindell, 2008; and Moynihan, 2009) – create both the imperative and the challenge of trying to improve capacity in other domains. Though countries tolerate endemic disease by engaging in incremental, long-term public health campaigns, unpredictable outbreaks of severe diseases prompt resource intensive, concentrated responses. Professionals engage in planning and post hoc evaluation of such events in order to draw lessons that might improve future performance. Two significant challenges emerge from this orientation. First, public health agencies charged with leading outbreak response efforts must transform their organizations from a routine-operations mode into that of emergency response. Second, organization leaders face pressure to develop expertise in responding to short-lived, infrequent events.

The most obvious approach to improve organizational performance, trial and error learning, is not available for health crises that are infrequent and distinct. Because of the lack of opportunity to make use of trial and error learning, organizations with the responsibility to respond to crises must find other means of developing what might stand in for experience. One mechanism is to review a recent crisis in order to draw from it lessons that might help responders improve their performance or, perhaps, limit the number of failures when responding to the next epidemic or pandemic. In this chapter, I examine whether efforts at generating lessons learned from isolated and infrequent events is likely to improve performance in future crises.

This exercise arises from the observation that, when examining three crises – 2003 SARS, 2009 A(H1N1) and 2014 Ebola together – the lessons drawn, respectively, from each begin to look less certain The difficulty in drawing lessons, I argue, stems from the nature of the problems themselves. Sudden outbreaks of deadly diseases create an imperative for rapid and effective response. Yet these health events exhibit properties of "wicked" (Rittel & Webber, 1973) and "unruly" problems (Ansell, 2016) where response efforts can become a source of surprising dynamics. Challenges arise from: (1) the novelty of pathogens and the unpredictability of even known pathogens; (2) surprises arising from geography and scale; and (3) difficulties stemming from the distributed nature of response, which involves predicting the behavior of autonomous actors, including both individuals and organizations. The intersections of these three sources of uncertainty can produce unique dynamics that may not repeat in future crises. By failing to note the deep and persistent sources of uncertainty inherent in responding to acute public health crises, lessons learned tend to presume uncertainties can be resolved quickly in order to roll out appropriately scaled response. An alternate approach would be to build response efforts around persistent uncertainty, surprise and contingency in ways that support responders in poorly understood and dynamic response environments.

Theoretical framework

While learning in the simplest organizational settings can occur through trial and error, many organizations, owing to the nature of their tasks, have difficulty making causal inferences that allow for simple learning (Wilson, 1989). Moreover, as Argyris and Schön point out, trial and error learning represents single-loop learning – i.e., learning directly about the actions and theory used to accomplish an organizational task or goal (1978). A focus on single-loop learning can inhibit double-loop learning where the organization shows a willingness to question values and assumptions related to the goal itself. Learning from isolated events should pose even greater challenges for learning. This can stem from the infrequency of events that allow organizations to drift away from practices deemed necessary following a major organizational failure (Mahler & Cassamayou, 2009). Analyses that point to forces inhibiting the application of learning in organizations over time presume that organization leaders correctly identified sources of organizational failure in the first place.

When it comes to learning from "unruly" events, the challenges for learning may be even more formidable. For instance, even when the same infectious agent is driving an outbreak, outbreaks can display remarkably unique dynamics. While responders may gain valuable experience during a crisis, the learning may not be particularly useful for the next. Even more frustrating, past experience can prove to be *misleading* in that novel aspects of a current outbreak may be discounted. This occurs when confirmation bias encourages responders to identify expected rather than unexpected patterns during a crisis and fail to note atypical signals. Errors, while clear in hindsight, are incredibly hard to identify during a crisis as responders attempt to characterize events using partial, uncertain and error-prone data to understand their circumstances (Keller et al., 2012).

Drawing lessons from such events is also challenging given that, during any event, officials engage in multiple activities to change the course of an epidemic or pandemic. Moreover, even without intervention, pandemics are often self-limiting; one cannot claim with confidence that public health intervention stemmed the tide of a given outbreak. Even if the outcome is a clear success or failure, quite rare in and of itself, it is impossible, with precision to determine whether one or some combination of interventions made a difference. While there are occasional natural experiments that shed light on the effectiveness of some intervention, even comparative learning can be challenging. For example, countries select intervention strategies not simply for technical reasons, but also for cultural and political reasons (Baekkeskov, 2016; Connor, 2016; MacPhail, 2014). Thus, analysts need to treat differences in outcomes in light of substantial socio-geographical differences across cases. While those who study crisis response might think of response options as discrete and portable entitles, responses can often not be abstracted from the socio-political contexts in which they are used.

Some of the difficulty in learning from epidemic/pandemic crises stems from the nature of the public health emergencies themselves: they express many features of both "wicked" and "unruly" problems. Difficulties addressing wicked problems stem from complexities with problem uniqueness and problem formulation. If problems are unique, performance cannot be improved through trial and error learning. Challenges involved in formulating a problem make it difficult to assess what "state" has occurred and what responses might be appropriate or even when a response has been successful (Rittel & Webber, 1973). Unruly problems highlight how temporal complexities add mounting challenges to response efforts (Ansell, 2016). Unruly problems manifest unevenly over time and space and can produce surprising discontinuities or crescive dynamics where incremental change in the problem fails to generate alarm until the problem has grown past the point of manageable intervention. They can produce vicious cycles where feedbacks aggravate the original problem. Moreover, a response to an unruly problem can, itself, generate new and unexpected dynamics.

Many of these characteristics identified by wicked and unruly problems arise during health crises. Specifically, a disease outbreak can cross geographical and sectoral boundaries, requiring communication and coordination between actors and organizations that may not have a history of routine interactions. Thus, they force experimentation with novel organizational networks and processes (Ansell, Boin, & Keller, 2010). Where these can produce surprising successes, they are also likely to generate unpredictable failures. Health crises can attack the very organizational apparatus that is supposed to contain them in that healthcare workers are often at higher risk than the general population during an outbreak. This can create a vicious cycle in that, once a healthcare system is overwhelmed, it may become a source of transmission rather than a site for outbreak control.

Disease outbreaks can exhibit temporal surprises including sudden shifts in state or sense-making hurdles associated with crescive problems. An example of the former occurred when SARS, though generating cases within China for weeks, suddenly appeared across continents after several travelers contracted the disease from a single doctor staying in a hotel in Hong Kong. Difficulties in recognizing crescive problems dogged the early days of the response to Ebola 2014. Officials, fully aware of ongoing transmission in three countries, assumed existing response efforts would soon reduce the number of new infections. The realization that the opposite was occurring – an outbreak spiraling towards epidemic – came weeks after a stepped-up response could have kept the outbreak within the scope of prior Ebola events. In addition, the very same disease agent can have dramatically different expressions across geographic settings. How cases of Ebola spread in West Africa versus their very limited spread in the United States and Europe demonstrates a quite predictable difference in the socio-geography of an outbreak. Rich countries with vast resources are not likely to experience sustained transmission. However, this is not just an issue of low versus high-income settings. For example, concurrent with the 2014 epidemic in West Africa, the Democratic Republic of Congo experienced an outbreak that spread across several villages and totaled sixty-six cases.[2] The relatively small size of this outbreak in the Democratic Republic of Congo cannot be attributed to differences in resources across the four countries.[3] Thus, one needs more than a level of development to explain why an outbreak of Ebola in similarly poor countries in Africa grew to almost seventy times the size of the next largest epidemic.

The behavior and beliefs of citizens who are at risk of infection produce a significant source of uncertainty and surprise. Another stems from response systems themselves. Responders, who face especially challenging dynamics involved in understanding the nature of the outbreak, are also required to carry out response at incredibly high levels of performance. For example, managing infection control practices for highly infectious and virulent diseases in hospital settings requires that organizations and their workforces transform their performance from routine to high-reliability operations.[4] These transformations, if they are to be successful, need to take place within hours as an infected patient who arrives in an emergency department can put other patients and the healthcare work-force at risk. Public health workers who conduct contact tracing – finding all potential contacts with someone during a suspected period of conta-gion – can allow new transmission chains if they fail to identify a single contact. While studies of high-reliability organizations demonstrate that nearly failure-free performance is possible, the organizations that are able to produce such levels of performance are not creating the conditions for that performance in a matter of days (LaPorte & Consolini, 1991).

If all healthcare facilities could manage such transformations, then public health guidance establishing an appropriate standard of care might be sufficient to prepare hospitals to recognize and successfully manage an influx of suspected cases. However, many hospitals struggle, even when guidance is available, to put recommendations into practice.[5] Public health officials, if they could predict which hospitals needed support, might be able to concentrate support resources in the right place at the right time. Yet, it is not clear, at the outset, which hospitals will falter. For example, at the outset of SARS, one might not have predicted, that among the hardest hit cities, Toronto would have one of the highest rates of trans-mission to healthcare workers relative to the number of suspected and confirmed SARS cases.[6] Events in Dallas during 2014 Ebola demonstrated a similar dynamic: a hospital in a rich country, even after they knew they were managing a patient with laboratory-confirmed Ebola, still failed to institute high-reliability operations, leading to infection of two healthcare workers. These cases illustrate that infectious agents are not the only vari-able in an epidemic that can be unpredictable. All of the following produce sources of uncertainty for those trying to orchestrate effective response: patients, families of patients, communities, healthcare workers, journalists and the media. Moreover, interactions between these actors produce additional sources of uncertainty.

In spite of these hurdles to successful analysis from one or a handful of cases, the post-crisis literature attempts to identify points of failure and success and draw lessons from rare and unique cases. This chapter will provide a high-level overview of 2003 SARS, 2009 A(H1N1) and 2014 Ebola and review the "lessons" drawn from each case. From there the chapter will discuss the extent to which those lessons might have con-tributed to success or failure in subsequent events, recognizing that firm conclusions, even when comparing across events, are likely to be elusive. This chapter does not aim to come to definitive conclusions. At the same time, the chapter picks very distinct international health events. To the extent that comparison of such dissimilar cases suggests common patterns across all three, one might examine those features as candidates for crisis learning.[7] The chapter concludes with a discussion of how, in light of the difficulty of learning from rare events, response efforts might contend more directly with uncertainty and contingency in order to improve the pace of learning within a given event.

Data for this analysis comes from reviews of published and unpublished accounts of these events as well as from interviews and participant observation conducted during the 2009 A(H1N1) pandemic and from interviews with responders involved in Ebola 2014.[8] Though each of these health crises is an outbreak that crossed international borders and stimulated significant international response efforts, the three events are dissimilar in many respects. SARS was a novel pathogen, while A(H1N1) and Ebola were not. SARS and Ebola produced outbreaks that did not reach the level of global pandemic, while A(H1N1) did. A(H1N1) proved to be a relatively mild infectious agent, whereas SARS and Ebola were, respectively, considerably more virulent. SARS outbreaks occurred in cities with relatively well-functioning public health and healthcare systems, whereas Ebola occurred in weak states with incredibly fragile public health and healthcare systems. The dissimilarity of the cases can produce insights if the comparison generates insights that appear to hold across cases. At the same time, the dissimilarity in cases can also mask the extent to which purportedly similar events can produce surprising dynamics.

Background

SARS 2003: impressive response or luck?

The outbreaks of SARS in the fall of 2002 in China first appeared on the international stage on February 10, 2003 when an international disease surveillance organization alerted public health officials to stories about a respiratory illness spreading in China (Heymann & Rodier, 2004).[9] Though the disease was spreading in China beginning in November 2002, Chinese authorities began reporting cases of atypical pneumonia to the WHO in February of 2003 (Heymann & Rodier, 2004).[10] On February 21, a doctor who had treated patients in China traveled to Hong Kong and transmitted the infection to sixteen additional people who spread the disease to Singapore, Vietnam and Canada (Heymann & Rodier, 2004; Cheng et al., 2013). The WHO began its own investigation of the disease in response to reports of cases in both Hong Kong and Hanoi, leading to the WHO's first and second global alerts on March 12 and 15, respectively. The second alert provided an early case definition, indicated that healthcare workers were at risk, and provided advice to travelers to raise awareness about symptoms and potential exposure (Heymann & Rodier, 2004). Over the following weeks, the WHOs travel alerts included recommendations for screening of passengers at airports before boarding planes and, controversially, advice against travel to the most affected cities (Paquin, 2007).

Using its Global Outbreak and Response Network, the WHO sent teams to support municipal-level response in China, Hong Kong, Hanoi and Singapore (Mackenzie et al., 2014). While Canadian officials were in touch with counterparts at the WHO, Toronto did not receive a GOARN team to support the Canadian response. In partnership with GOARN, the WHO also created three virtual networks to support the response (Heymann & Rodier, 2004; Mackenzie et al., 2004). The first was a team of scientists who collaborated, apparently without regard for whom would receive credit, on the discovery of the causative agent. The second and third virtual networks collaborated to collect, analyze and disseminate information about the clinical support of patients with the infection and about the epidemiology of the disease, for example, whether the infection was airborne or spread through droplets.

The hardest hit cities employed a number of public health interventions including: (1) isolation and support of suspected patients; (2) contact tracing and monitoring and even quarantine of patient contacts; (3) negative pressure rooms and barrier nursing to protect healthcare workers from infection; (4) hospital closures of all non-essential services; (5) school closures; and (6) public health information to the general public about recognizing symptoms and relevant precautions (Cheng et al., 2013). In Hong Kong, Hanoi and Singapore, these measures or some subset of them led to a steady decrease in the number of cases. Moreover, the travel measures may have limited spread to other cities. Toronto, however, stands out in that after declaring its outbreak contained in April 2003, it experienced a second wave of cases and transmission lasting until July (NACSPH, 2003; Low, 2004).

A(H1N1) 2009: why all the fuss?

In April of 2009, public health officials in Mexico, through existing influenza surveillance, noticed an uptick in what they thought was seasonal influenza. The severity of illness and the timing were notable in that seasonal influenza should be ending in April, not getting worse. Laboratory tests suggested a novel influenza, prompting officials in Mexico to send laboratory samples to a laboratory in Canada that, on April 23, confirmed the results (Mexico Ministry of Health, 2009). Around the same time, public health officials in the United States picked up a case of swine flu and, on April 13, sent the evidence to the CDC for confirmation. Days later, CDC officials then confirmed a second case of swine flu through routine influenza surveillance (Ginsberg et al., 2009). While it is common for a swine flu case to occur once every one to two years, such cases typically occur when the infected person has had contact with pigs and leads to no sustained human transmission (CDC, 2009a). That neither of the lab-confirmed cases had had any contact with pigs and that two cases had no relationship to one another suggested the presence of a novel influenza with sustained human-to-human transmission (Ansell et al., 2009). Upon confirmation on novel influenza, officials from Mexico and the United States independently made use of the apparatus put in place by the WHO in the wake of SARS. On April 24, each country made reports of a "public health emergency of international concern" prompting the WHO to declare an outbreak of novel influenza in Mexico and the United States (Neumann & Kawaoka, 2011).

Response to the novel influenza grew out of WHO efforts in the preceding years to build an international system to respond to pandemic influenza (Katz 2009; Wilson, Brownstein, & Fidler, 2010). The WHO initiated this effort after the experience with SARS and in light of concerns about the H5N1 virus mutating to allow for sustained human-to-human transmission (Webby and Webster, 2003). The WHO led a successful effort to revise the IHR so that countries were required to report any outbreaks that might have international ramifications, build up their basic public health capacity in surveillance and outbreak responses (Gostin, 2009; Katz, 2009). In addition, the WHO encouraged countries to engage in pandemic influenza preparedness. For its part, the WHO committed to creating a pandemic alert system in which the WHO could announce pandemic "phases", which, ideally, would indicate to countries that they should initiate response actions planned in accordance with that "phase".[11] Countries drew up response plans with the 2018 influenza and fears of a potential H5N1 pandemic in mind. As a result, planned response to pandemic phases – which tracked spread of disease, not its severity – assumed that any pandemic would warrant costly and disruptive measures (Keller et al., 2012).

Once public health officials sounded the alarm for 2009 A(H1N1), countries began to review and implement their pre-planned response efforts as the WHO announced one pandemic phase level after another. Countries with sufficient resources stepped up surveillance, began counting cases to track the spread of the disease, and issued guidance about intervention measures to communities with active cases. However, as experts began to debate whether the novel influenza was severe or mild, public officials struggled with whether disruptive public interventions were warranted (Ansell et al., 2009). For example, the CDC first recommended school closures in counties with confirmed cases and then revised that recommendation, asking local jurisdictions to decide for themselves whether to pursue school closure as a measure to slow transmission (CDC, 2009b). In their revised guidance, the CDC refers to the US National Strategy for pandemic influenza that suggested school closures as a measure that could slow transmission if implemented early (CDC, 2009b). Replicating their role from SARS, the WHO mobilized a GOARN team of influenza experts who traveled to Mexico to aid their response (Katz, 2009). However, once there the team struggled to find a role.

In April 2009, vaccine manufacturers began vaccine development in order to meet an expected fall wave of the pandemic in the northern hemisphere. Countries in the southern hemisphere grappled with the disease without an available vaccine (Ansell et al., 2009). Notably, many countries, in their pandemic influenza plans, tied contracts with vaccine manufacturers to WHO-declared phases (Godlee, 2010). Such contracts were triggered when the WHO announced a pandemic influenza (phase 6) on June 11, 2009 (Godlee, 2010).

Growing public mistrust marred the subsequent roll out of vaccination in northern countries. In many countries, the public alleged that vaccine companies influenced the WHO to exaggerate the severity of the pandemic in order to generate profits rather than basing their recommendations purely on public health standards. Studies following the pandemic suggest that a lack of trust in the vaccine or in the need for vaccination contributed to low vaccination rates (Brien, Kwong, & Buckeridge, 2012; Han et al., 2016). In countries where mistrust of public health officials and the vaccine was not widespread, the delay in availability of the vaccine produced a mismatch in demand for an availability of vaccine (Falco, 2009).

Many OECD countries who had committed to sharing vaccine stocks with low-income countries delivered no shipments of vaccine until the pandemic was almost complete, demonstrating the weakness of such mechanisms in creating more equitable global distributions of vaccines across countries (Kumar et al., 2012). At the end of the pandemic, death tolls were similar to seasonal influenza, leading to criticism that the level of response was too extreme given the pandemic's severity (Godlee, 2010). Subsequent investigation into potential conflicts of interest among those serving on the WHO's influence vaccination advisory board put the WHO on the defensive, both for its pandemic phase alert system and for its role in promoting widespread vaccination against the novel influenza (Cohen & Carter, 2010; Godlee, 2010).

Ebola 2014: failing by the book

Ebola emerged in Guinea in December 2013 with the likely index case resulting from a child living in a remote part of the country who may have come into contact with infected bats (WHO, 2015; Coltart et al., 2017). Healthcare workers treating the family members and traditional healers infected during this early phase of the outbreak suspected cholera (WHO, 2015). In March, the ongoing chain of transmission raised alarm at the Ministry of Health who contacted their counterparts at the WHO regional office (WHO, 2015; Coltart et al., 2017). Health officials in Guinea sent blood samples from an infected patient to Lyon France, which confirmed the most virulent form of Ebola (Baize et al., 2014; WHO, 2015). The laboratory-confirmed case in a country that had never had an Ebola outbreak prompted the WHO to send a GOARN team of experienced Ebola experts to Guinea to aid with coordinating the response in Guinea (WHO, 2014). Following the laboratory confirmation, Médecins Sans Frontières (MSF) set up three Ebola treatment units (ETU) in Guinea, using its experience and established apparatus for supporting patients and limiting spread of infection to healthcare workers. The WHO alerted neighboring countries and received reports of suspected cases from both Sierra Leone and Liberia. However, in both countries, the suspected cases were linked to cases in Guinea. Moreover, after the initial reports of suspected cases from Sierra Leone and Liberia, both countries revised downward their total suspected and confirmed cases and reported no new cases between April 6 and May 25.[12] On May 18, 2014, the WHO reported that, for more than three weeks, five out of the six prefectures in Guinea had reported no new cases. Moreover, with no new cases reported in Liberia and Sierra Leone since April 9, the WHO projected the "EVD outbreak could be declared over [in these two countries] on 22 May 2014".[13] Though MSF continued to run ETUs in Guinea and a handful of international NGOs were active in supporting response efforts in Liberia, including an ETU set up by Samaritan's Purse, teams participating in the GOARN deployment to Guinea returned to their home countries in the latter part of May under the assumption that the outbreak had already run its course.[14]

In hindsight, situation reports were picking up only a fraction of the actual numbers of new cases. The error likely stemmed from a lack of surveillance capacity and a lack of trust among citizens in the region's governments and healthcare systems. While the official international response mounted by GOARN was winding down in Guinea, cases were spreading rapidly in all three affected countries.

As early as April 2014, MSF and the WHO began to publicly disagree about the nature of the crisis. As MSF tried to raise the sense of urgency to bring more resources to the response, Gregory Hartl, a WHO spokesperson, reassured the press that the outbreak was small relative to past outbreaks and was well in hand (UNOG, 2014). Hartl went further by tweeting that MSF should not "exaggerate" the nature of the crisis (Fletcher, 2015). By early June, MSF wrote a formal letter insisting that the international response was woefully inadequate given the scale of transmission (Interview, August 2015). At the time, MSF was the only organization on the ground with substantial experience with Ebola. In spite of that unique position – both past and current experience with the ongoing outbreak – MSF was not able to raise the level of alarm or cast doubt on the view that the current response was sufficient. The first inkling in the formal case counts that the outbreak was not nearing its end came when Sierra Leone declared six new cases on May 25. The WHO responded by sending six international experts as well as releasing emergency funds and supplies.[15] It was not until mid-July, however, when the CDC sent its own team of responders to Liberia (Dahl et al., 2016), that MSF's warning began to gain official currency.[16]

The US CDC initially approached Liberia's request for assistance the way it would have approached past outbreaks of Ebola; it sent a team of seven people to Liberia (Dahl et al., 2016). Once in Liberia, the team quickly began to appreciate the unprecedented scale of the crisis. The death toll among Liberian healthcare workers, seventy-nine, had cut significantly into the country's sparse healthcare workforce and led many remaining healthcare workers to stay away from hospitals struggling to treat sick patients. As cases mounted in all three countries, mistrust of the government or of responders sparked community resistance and even violence directed at healthcare facilities and personnel (Wilkinson & Fairhead, 2017; WHO, 2015). Moreover, neither Sierra Leone nor Liberia had sufficient laboratory capacity to keep up with the increasing number of suspected cases, transport capacity to move suspected patients from the community to treatment centers, nor the human and information infrastructures necessary to carry out contact tracing that would allow for monitoring and rapid isolation of potentially infected contacts who developed symptoms. Under these conditions, the number of cases rapidly stripped the capacity of existing treatment units, creating international headlines as patients died outside ETUs already stretched beyond capacity.

Lacking fully functioning healthcare and public health systems and, at the worst part of the epidemic, experiencing hundreds of new cases each week,[17] all three countries required massive influxes of personnel, equipment and public health expertise. While many healthcare workers volunteered to travel to affected regions to help with response efforts, visa issues often delayed their arrival (Interviews, August 2015). Moreover, the initial pool of healthcare workers willing to volunteer was insufficient. Reports of attacks on clinics, a lack of training to prepare for work in ETUs, and concerns about access to healthcare all likely stemmed the initial supply of volunteers (Interviews, August 2015). While money from donor countries poured in, a lack of personnel hampered the response. Moreover, the normal mode of response to an Ebola outbreak starting with pitch perfect contact tracing was not available given the relative scale of cases to infrastructure (Interviews, August 2015). Policy and healthcare delivery missteps in each country created public mistrust of official messages requiring responders to come up with new approaches for interacting with communities where people might be infected (Bell et al., 2016; WHO, 2015).

Public health officials not only failed to predict and detect the rapid increase in cases; they also failed to predict the sudden decline in numbers of new cases. In September, model predictions conducted by the WHO and the CDC predicted, respectively 20,000 and 500,000 additional cases, with the CDC's worst-case scenario reaching over 1 million additional cases (Meltzer et al., 2014). Though CDC Director Frieden predicted that ongoing response efforts would prevent this worst-case scenario (Grady, 2014), the United States continued to pour additional resources into the response, particularly in Liberia where the US Army constructed eleven additional Ebola treatment units. These units, however, ended up treating only twenty-eight patients (Onishi, 2015).

Though transmission would continue in all three countries well into 2015, the pace of new infections fell in line with past Ebola outbreaks where smaller teams had the capacity to identify new cases, transport patients into well-functioning treatment centers, and conduct contact tracing to prevent further spread into the community. Public messaging and citizen response to the crisis also stemmed the pace of infection as citizens mounted community efforts to reduce transmission (WHO, 2015). Moreover, both the WHO and NIH launched vaccine trials in 2015 with the WHO's ring approach studies suggesting the vaccine may be 100 percent effective against Ebola (Henao-Restrepo et al., 2017). While survivors in all three countries continue to cope with the aftermath, both social and medical, of their infections, officials reported the last cases connected to the epidemic in June 2016.

Lessons learned

Lessons learned from SARS tend to focus on the relatively successful international response coordinated by the WHO or on the less successful experience in Toronto (Table 1.1). The WHO gained confidence that it could play a central role as a clearing house for collecting, evaluating and disseminating information on the causative agent, clinical practices and the epidemiology of the novel agent and that, through GOARN, would supply valuable support to the most impacted cities. The WHO also points to its travel advisories and airport screenings as helping to limit the number of cases reaching new countries and quickly identifying those patients who did carry the infection to new locations. China is cast as a negative example in that earlier reporting to the WHO might have activated this response earlier and limited the total number of infections. Reviews of the experience in Toronto focus on the need for a stronger public health infrastructure in Canada and call for a greater emphasis on planning and emergency preparedness. Reviews cite a lack of pre-existing plans for managing an outbreak of a novel infectious disease (NACSPH, 2003; Hawryluck, Lapinsky, & Stewart, 2005; Campbell, 2006) and the absence of any pre-planned emergency response structure that could help coordinate response (NACSPH, 2003; Koplan et al., 2013; Hawryluck, Lapinsky, & Stewart, 2005).

The revised International Health Regulations (IHR) can be understood as an embodiment of the lessons learned from SARS. The IHR includes a mechanism for countries to officially report to the WHO diseases of international concern (Plotkin et al., 2007). Moreover, the IHR requires the WHO to collect and disseminate relevant information about an outbreak, casting the organization as a clearing house for vetted information about an outbreak (Drazen, 2003; WHO, 2003). Recognizing that international information sharing is predicated on good information about an outbreak, the IHR includes provisions for member countries to develop minimum core public health capacities including surveillance, response and sufficient laboratory testing. Based on the role the WHO played in recommending airport screening, the revised IHR tries to limit ineffective travel and trade restrictions and encourages countries to follow evidence-based WHO recommendations.

Table 1.1 2003 SARS lessons learned

Lessons	Sources
Importance of early detection	WHO, 2003; Cheng et al., 2013
Need to create norm of openness; information sharing	US GAO, 2004; Hawryluck, Lapinsky, & Stewart, 2005; WHO, 2003;
Need for preparedness plans including plans for surge capacity and case-reporting procedures	NACSPH, 2003; Hawryluck, Lapinsky, & Stewart, 2005; Campbell, 2006
Create an emergency response structure (ICS or something similar) to guide response and manage coordination and communication	NACSPH, 2003; Koplan et al., 2013; Hawryluck, Lapinsky, & Stewart, 2005
Develop surveillance capacity	NACSPH, 2003; Koplan et al., 2013
Create infection control capacity (protocols, worker training, independent safety inspections)	WHO, 2003; Hawryluck, Lapinsky, & Stewart, 2005; Campbell, 2006; Cheng et al., 2013; Koplan et al., 2013
Increase laboratory capacity	NACSPH, 2003; Campbell, 2006; Cheng et al., 2013; Koplan et al., 2013
Use of traditional public health methods (surveillance, contact tracing, isolation and quarantine)	Drazen, 2003; WHO, 2003; Cheng et al., 2013; Koplan et al., 2013
Coordination between animal and human health surveillance	Cheng et al., 2013; Koplan et al., 2013
Risk assessment and risk communication to frontline healthcare workers	Campbell, 2006
Risk assessment and risk communication to public	NACSPH, 2003; WHO, 2003; Koplan et al., 2013; Hawryluck, Lapinsky, & Stewart, 2005
Use of global alert to signal need for increased local vigilance	WHO, 2003
Airport screening	WHO, 2003
National public health institute or other centralized public health agency	NACSPH, 2003; Koplan et al., 2013
Plans to manage patients and close contacts facing morbidity and mortality	Hawryluck, Lapinsky, & Stewart, 2005
Creation of mobile education teams who can support clinics/hospitals treating suspected patients; GOARN effectiveness	US GAO, 2004; Hawryluck, Lapinsky, & Stewart, 2005; WHO, 2003;
Support healthcare workers under stress	Hawryluck, Lapinsky, & Stewart, 2005
Invest in public health personnel, capacity	NACSPH, 2003; Campbell, 2006
Invest in healthcare workforce	Ontario Nurses Association, 2018
Use precautionary principal in healthcare settings when managing patients with novel infectious agent	Campbell, 2006; Ontario Nurses Association, 2018
Strengthen collaboration between public health and private healthcare systems	NACSPH, 2003; Campbell, 2006
International collaboration for rapid creation of evidence base that can be disseminated to sites managing outbreak	Drazen, 2003; WHO, 2003
The WHO acting as clearing house for information supports local response efforts	WHO, 2003

Additional lessons include the potential conflict that can emerge between officials and the healthcare workforce asked to put themselves at risk during an outbreak, and between officials and the public. Some reviews emphasize the need for training for healthcare workers in proper infection control (WHO, 2003; Hawryluck, Lapinsky, & Stewart, 2005; Campbell, 2006; Cheng et al., 2013; Koplan et al., 2013) and better risk communication to healthcare workers or the public (Campbell, 2006). Studies also endorse the idea that teams of well-informed experts, like GOARN, can support local response efforts (US GAO, 2004; Hawryluck, Lapinsky, & Stewart, 2005; WHO, 2003). In additional some researchers go beyond a focus on infection control and discuss the need to support healthcare workers, patients, family members and close contacts, all of whom can experience high levels of stress or trauma during an outbreak (Hawryluck, Lapinsky, & Stewart, 2005).

A specially convened advisory committee in Canada points to the lack of centralized coordination from the federal government, a lack of general public health infrastructure, poor coordination between the federal, provincial and municipal levels, and a lack of protocols for information sharing between the public and private sectors. In making recommendations for improvements, the report offers as an instructive model the US Centers for Disease Control and Prevention, citing its ability to coordinate action across levels of government as well as with private sector responders (NACSPH, 2003).

Lessons from A(H1N1) are as varied as the countries that mounted a pandemic response (Table 1.2). Both Mexico and the US were prompt in sharing with the WHO their discovery of novel influenza cases. This put the revised IHR and its associated reporting mechanisms in a positive light (Gostin, 2009; Katz, 2009).[18] At the same time, several note inherent weaknesses in the IHR, like an inability to penalize countries that do not create minimum core capacity, report outbreaks to the WHO, and/or impose counter-productive travel and trade restrictions (Fidler, 2009; Fineberg, 2014; Gostin, 2009; Katz, 2009; Wilson, Brownstein, & Fidler, 2010).

Analysts direct much of their criticism regarding the response to the WHO. First, its alert system indicated the spread of infection, but not its severity, cuing a level of alarm that was, perhaps, unwarranted (Bethge, Elger, & Glusing, 2010). Reviews of the response call for incorporating disease severity into WHO alerts (Fidler, 2009; Fineberg, 2014) and recommend revisiting the links between IHR functions, WHO alerts, and pandemic response plans (Fineberg, 2014; Godlee, 2010). Second, the WHO received heavy criticism for conflicts of interest on its vaccine advisory committee (Cohen & Carter, 2010: Godlee, 2010). Some view the effort to roll out vaccines as problematic, citing the amount of public expenditure (Godlee, 2010), the timing of vaccine rollout (Falco, 2009; Neumann & Kawaoka, 2011), or the lack of effective sharing from rich to poor countries (Fidler, 2010). Views towards national vaccination efforts are not

Table 1.2 2009 A(H1N1) lessons learned

Lessons	Sources
Improve ability of member countries to meet IHR minimum core public health capacities	Fidler, 2009; Fineberg, 2014; Gostin, 2009; Wilson, Brownstein, & Fidler, 2010
Increase compliance with IHR provisions (esp. regarding travel and trade)	Fidler, 2009; Fineberg, 2014; Gostin, 2009; Katz, 2009; Wilson, Brownstein, & Fidler, 2010
Improve WHO capacity for sustained response (personnel and/or budget)	Fineberg, 2014
Develop means to assess the severity of an outbreak/epidemic/pandemic	Fidler, 2009; Fineberg, 2014
Encourage advanced agreements for vaccine distribution and delivery	Fineberg, 2014
Reach agreement on virus and vaccine sharing from poor to rich countries	Fidler, 2009; Fineberg, 2014; Gostin, 2009
Improve research on influenza	Fineberg, 2014
Improve communication (within the WHO and from the WHO to member countries)	Fineberg, 2014
Revisit selection of and role of Emergency Committee under IHR	Fidler, 2009; Fineberg, 2014; Wilson, Brownstein, & Fidler, 2010
IHR supports information sharing (early report, use of national focal points, WHO communication back to member countries)	Fineberg, 2014; Fidler, 2009; Gostin, 2009; Katz, 2009; Wilson, Brownstein, & Fidler, 2010
Focal points are effective	Wilson, Brownstein, & Fidler, 2010
The WHO is able to integrate information from countries and NGOs	Wilson, Brownstein, & Fidler, 2010
Potential for the WHO to use PHEIC for more types of events where international mobilization could aid response	Wilson, Brownstein, & Fidler, 2010
Improve technologies for faster and greater volume vaccine production	Falco, 2009; Neumann & Kawaoaka, 2011
International support for country response was effective (personnel or provision of antivirals)	Katz, 2009; Fineberg, 2014
The WHO lack ability to enforce reporting requirements under IHR	Gostin, 2009
Positive role of influenza planning/ preparedness	Fidler, 2009; Fineberg, 2014
Problems related to linking pandemic response plans to WHO phase level declarations	Fineberg, 2014; Godlee, 2010
Need for better information sharing between animal and human health surveillance	Fidler, 2009
Revise the WHO vaccine advisory committee selection, conflicts of interest	Cohen & Carter, 2010; Fineberg, 2014; Godlee, 2010

uniform, however. For instance, the United States anchors higher rates of seasonal influenza vaccination among healthcare workers and pregnant women to the successful outreach to these two groups during 2009 A(H1N1) (Interview, August 2015; Kerr, Van Bennekom, & Mitchell, 2016).

Because of public mistrust of the vaccine and resistance against vaccination, many have called for revised standards for vaccine advisory committee members to guard against real or apparent conflicts of interest (Cohen & Carter, 2010; Fineberg, 2014; Godlee, 2010). Relatedly, many reports emphasize the need for public health officials to improve communication strategies in an effort to build trust between officials and the public during an outbreak (Fineberg, 2010; Leung & Nicoll, 2010). In spite of problems related to vaccination and the issue with communication about the pandemic's severity, some experts involved in the response felt the effort to mobilize both vaccination and treatment provided a valuable opportunity to see how pandemic response systems actually work and helped officials identify remaining gaps in such systems (Ansell et al., 2009).

Lessons from 2014 Ebola center on the failure of WHO member countries to fulfill their obligations under the 2005 revised IHR (Table 1.3). This includes building basic surveillance and response capacity, but also the requirement that member countries not impose unnecessary trade and travel sanctions on countries experiencing an outbreak (Bell et al., 2016; Gates, 2015; Moon et al., 2015; WHO, 2015; WHO Ebola Interim Assessment Panel, 2015). Similar to SARS, critics note a lack of transparency on the part of countries experiencing an outbreak. However, unlike SARS, where WHO leadership pressured China to share information about its outbreak, critics charge that the WHO under Margaret Chan failed to play this leadership role (Cheng & Satter, 2015).

Ebola 2014 also raised questions about the WHO's lack of operational capacity beyond small-scale GOARN deployments (Moon et al., 2015; WHO Ebola Interim Assessment Panel, 2015). Thus, what gets billed as a success during SARS – the WHO's role in convening experts and collecting and disseminating information rapidly to cities managing the crisis – is cast as a failure during 2014. Moreover, even its role as a clearing house for accurate and supporting technical information looks like a failure in this case in that the organization was extremely slow to recognize that cases were mounting when, if containment was working, they should have been falling. Many analyses treat this as evidence of insufficient use of IHR mechanisms and a lack of resources and independence on the part of the WHO (Moon et al., 2015; WHO Ebola Interim Assessment Panel, 2015). The WHO itself, in its review of the epidemic (WHO, 2015), implies the need for more caution with respect to formal data collection by noting how such pre-planned mechanisms can fail. For instance, they recount "blind spots" created when communities mistrusted responders attempting to find new cases (WHO, 2015). Some reviews point to the need to be able to assess country-level preparedness which, if done well, could help establish levels of confidence given to formally collected data (Bell et al., 2016; WHO, 2015). Mistrust between the public and those carrying out response efforts demonstrate the need for culturally appropriate and

Table 1.3 2014 Ebola lessons learned

Lessons	Sources
Host country should treat discovery of cases as an emergency; vigilance should be maintained even when cases apparently decline	WHO, 2015
Healthcare workers trained in infection control	Bell et al., 2016; Médecins Sans Frontières, 2017; Hewlett et al., 2015; WHO, 2015
Support healthcare workers with information, training, pay and address stress and exhaustion	WHO, 2015; Hewlett et al., 2015
Plan for establishing isolation wards	WHO, 2015
Consider population mobility and dynamics with respect to mobility during course of outbreak	WHO, 2015
Expect responders not to be trusted; approach communities assuming the need to be transparent and build trust (e.g. bring treatment/response to communities with cases increases transparency of response efforts and builds trust)	WHO, 2015
Develop core public health capacities as outlined in IHR including funding for poor countries to meet IHR requirements (surveillance, healthcare infrastructure and personnel, response capacity, transportation, communication, lab capacity)	Bell et al., 2016; Gates, 2015; Moon et al., 2015; WHO, 2015; WHO Ebola Interim Assessment Panel, 2015
Plan for community engagement; transparency in response	Gates, 2015; Hewlett et al., 2015; WHO, 2015; WHO Ebola Interim Assessment Panel, 2015
Recognize logistical hurdles/complexity involved in coordinating response when cases are geographically dispersed	WHO, 2015
Evaluate blind spots in characterizing understanding of an outbreak	WHO, 2015
Consider that increasing response capacity can increase ability to see the extent of an outbreak (capacity leads to insight, not insight first, and then an argument for increasing capacity)	WHO, 2015
Rapid response teams useful in slowing transmission chains	Bell et al., 2016; WHO, 2015
Develop pillars of Ebola response: lab, treatment beds, contact tracing, burial, community engagement, country leadership	Bell et al., 2016; WHO, 2015
Understand country-level preparedness	Bell et al., 2016; WHO, 2015
Prep hospital team that is prepared to manage high-risk patients	Hewlett et al., 2015
Maintain transparency with staff, patients and community	Hewlett et al., 2015
Create safety culture in Ebola treatment units	Hewlett et al., 2015

continued

Table 1.3 Continued

Lessons	Sources
Use Emergency Operations Center, Incident Management System to coordinate response efforts and include an Ethics Unit within EOC	Bell et al., 2016
Increase ability of international actors to mobilize personnel for response	Gates, 2015
Increase capacity to conduct research during an outbreak	Gates, 2015; Moon et al., 2015; WHO Ebola Interim Assessment Panel, 2015
Rely on computer models to guide response efforts	Gates, 2015
Incorporate cell phone and internet data to track spread of cases	Gates, 2015
Make use of military for rapid creation of new capacity (e.g., transportation, communication, treatment centers, etc.)	Bell et al., 2016; Gates, 2015
Implement airport screening to slow spread of cases to new countries	Bell et al., 2016
Create response teams that can train providers lacking Ebola experience	Bell et al., 2016
Increase authority of the WHO over member countries with respect to outbreak reporting	Moon et al., 2015; WHO Ebola Interim Assessment Panel, 2015
Increase WHO outbreak response capacity (e.g., new unit, budget, staff, surge capacity)	Moon et al., 2015; WHO Ebola Interim Assessment Panel, 2015
Create financial incentives/penalties for compliance/lack of compliance with the IHR	WHO Ebola Interim Assessment Panel, 2015
Integrate humanitarian and health capacities within the UN	Moon et al., 2015; WHO Ebola Interim Assessment Panel, 2015
Create system of intermediate alerts when circumstances may not warrant full PHEIC	WHO Ebola Interim Assessment Panel, 2015

sensitive messaging and interactions with communities hit by the disease, leading some analyses to conclude that community engagement is one of the pillars of an effective Ebola response (Bell et al., 2016; WHO, 2015). Health officials' interactions with people in affected communities gave rise to another repeat lesson: those trying to help will not necessarily be accepted as such by communities experiencing a health event (see Bastide, Chapter 2).

The epidemic demonstrated the importance of experience and/or training in managing patients with Ebola. Even well-resourced, private sector hospitals in rich countries failed to mount effective infection control (Bell et al., 2016). While some point to CDC guidance as insufficient (McNeil, 2014), others argue that Dallas Presbyterian failed to train its nursing staff to successfully care for a patient with Ebola (Mohan, Susma, & Hennessy-Fiske, 2014). After two healthcare workers in Dallas contracted Ebola, the CDC revised its approach and insisted that patients would be routed to one of three biocontainment facilities, two of which had successfully treated infected healthcare providers intentionally evacuated from West Africa to the United States.[19] Next, they sent a team of CDC experts to hospitals around the country to create a longer list of approved hospitals they deemed prepared to treat Ebola patients. This effort replaced their initial approach – providing general guidance that assumed any hospitals where a patient presented with Ebola would treat that patient.[20]

Taking a comparative perspective

In looking at these experiences together, several lessons drawn from individual instances begin to look shaky. For instance, while officials in Canada pointed to the United States as having a stronger public health infrastructure and better communication between public health actors and the private healthcare system (NACSPH, 2003), the US experience with its first imported case of Ebola suggests that Canada's confidence in the US capacity may have been misplaced. While the CDC may have a more systematic way to communicate with local and state health departments as well as private sector providers, that did not prevent a series of missteps between CDC and its counterparts in Texas. For example, when public health officials suspected that Thomas Duncan might have Ebola, CDC officials recommended against testing for Ebola given the patient's report that he had no contact with anyone who was infected. When monitoring the healthcare workers who had treated Thomas Duncan, CDC allowed one to board a plane in spite of a slightly elevated fever. The infected healthcare worker began to exhibit symptoms later the same day. In both instances, CDC officials were following carefully crafted guidance about how to manage patients with suspected infection and known contacts. However, in retrospect, their adherence to the guidance looks overly formulaic and rigid. Casting a slightly more precautionary stance around these early potential cases, while inappropriate for settings with sustained transmission because of the likelihood of generating problematic false positives, might have been warranted as public health officials and healthcare workers grappled with their first domestically discovered cases.[21] This raises a question about when confusion about how to respond stems from lack of well-functioning communication infrastructure or from a more fundamental problem, i.e., not actually knowing how best to respond.

In examining all three cases, SARS stands out for the level of community compliance with officially recommended public health measures. The extent of public rejection of public health interventions in both A(H1N1) and Ebola demonstrate that citizens, in any country, are likely to form their own narratives about the nature of the threat and the acceptability of official response and that citizens in every country across SES-levels are subject to non-scientific ways of explaining their experiences. Lessons drawn from Ebola tend to be cast in terms of the need for anthropologists to accompany epidemiologists into the field to find better ways to engage with local communities. Yet the cultural divides between those managing response and citizens, clearly exposed during Ebola, are equally present during A(H1N1) where officials in one's own country led the response. In fact, the experience during Ebola demonstrates that citizens and response officials did find ways to interact and cooperate in supporting response, whereas citizens in many OECD countries never shed their presumption of a profit motive on the part of public health officials recommending vaccination.

Looking across cases, one begins to detect a faith in the IHR system that is, perhaps, not yet warranted. International collaboration during SARS with the WHO acting as a central node and clearing house provides an example of a well-functioning international response. Based on the assumption that more transparency from China would have allowed this system to be mobilized earlier would have stemmed the tide of the outbreak. A(H1N1) provides a story of early detection, but notes that, by not communicating about severity, the WHO sent the wrong signals about the scale of response each country might undertake. During 2014 Ebola, Guinea reported the first laboratory-confirmed case to the WHO. Moreover, the severity of the outbreak, as measured by the number of infected patients who died from the disease, was known as soon as the laboratory confirmed the strain of Ebola circulating in Guinea. Thus, even with early reporting and a clear view of the disease severity, it is clear that responders still did not know what they were trying to confront in West Africa. Of course, almost every analysis of the 2014 Ebola crisis points to the problem of countries not meeting their requirements for minimum core public health capacities under the IHR. Without surveillance, laboratory and treatment capacity, it is difficult to "see" what is happening. Very few analyses of these events cast doubt on the IHR system as a functional tool for helping recognize and respond to international public health emergencies. Faith in the IHR likely stems from its promise to provide a system of early reporting and information sharing. However, given our present configuration where poor countries lack the resources to meet the minimum core public health capacities, case reporting and information sharing may be a source of error.

A second source of error – one that has institutional expression in the IHR – is more subtle. Specifically, there may be a bias where public health officials associate expanding transmission with unsuspecting public and healthcare systems. Thus, if an outbreak is recognized and a response is underway, one presumes that officials are able to adequately characterize the course of the outbreak. If such a bias exists, it may be hard to detect insufficiency of an initiated response in that no response achieves effectiveness immediately. There may be considerable ambiguity involved with allowing a current response effort a few more days, or even weeks, to show results versus rejecting that effort as insufficient.

Furthermore, if officials do not characterize an outbreak correctly at the outset, response efforts, improperly scaled, can magnify the initial error. One part of the WHO's review of their experience with Ebola hints at this problem. They write that they began to discover they were wrong about the scale of the epidemic when, upon building new treatment centers, beds filled with new patients essentially overnight (WHO, 2015). This suggests that the scale of the international response, which was far too small, created an impression of less transmission than was actually occurring. This turns the temporal logic of the IHR on its head. If early alert and case counting is supposed to guide response, but accurate case counting depends on a response that is appropriately scaled, early case counting may be a source of considerable error. Few lessons learned adequately address how the international community should respond in the face of significant uncertainty and contingency.

Discussion

In setting out these three fairly dissimilar cases of epidemic/pandemic response to assess how their treatment together might shift what we take as lessons from each event, one needs to be cautious that the number of cases, from a statistical standpoint, is far too low to generate strong conclusions. At the same time, the comparison may offer ideas for ways to improve sensitivity to the persistent challenges associated with identification of non-routine health threats likely to cross international borders.

One interesting pattern is the extent to which surprise emerges in the cases where public health officials had more directly relevant past experience to draw on. SARS, the novel infectious agent, produced the fewest course corrections. This could be a function of the fact that the disease was traveling quickly and, with its dramatic fatality ratio, elicited enough fear to support major public health interventions. However, for both 2009 A(H1N1) and 2014 Ebola, public health officials struggled to launch appropriately scaled response. Many post hoc analyses respond to this by calling for earlier circulation of reliable information. If such reliable information is only produced in the process of trying to respond and learning what is and is not working, more attention needs to go to how to support learning in the early phases of response.

Given that the revised IHR identified a lack of healthcare and public health infrastructure as a major source of risk in terms of the potential for international spread of infectious disease, one might argue that Ebola 2014 was no surprise at all. At the same time, predictions about how such an outbreak might escalate stemmed from a presumption that transmission would occur before public health officials knew an outbreak was underway. Had lead public health agencies believed that they could miss significant and ongoing transmission *after* they knew about an outbreak and while response was underway, one would have seen very different behaviors from lead public health agencies like the WHO and the CDC. First, these organizations would have been more likely to accept MSF's account as valid. Unfortunately, the number of cases captured in official reporting suggested an outbreak consistent with the scale of past Ebola outbreaks, perhaps increasing confidence in the formal account.

A second potential insight is that sources of failure, obvious in hindsight, are hard to predict when planning for future crises, even though this is precisely what planners are trying to do. Though the SARS experience triggered concerns about novel influenza, none of the planning included the contingency of a less-than-severe pandemic. Efforts to create a better global system of disease detection and response were based on assuming a worst-case scenario of an infectious agent taking hold in a country with limited surveillance and response capacity. Though the WHO had reasonable assessments of those countries that were not meeting the basic public health and health system capacities outlined in the 2005 IHR (WHO, 2013; Fineberg, 2010), response planners failed to predict how a lack of operational response capacity within the WHO might play out if a severe outbreak hit a setting with a weak health system. In fact, one review of A(H1N1) that *did* identify the need for a global public health workforce characterized the WHO as well-suited to respond to outbreaks of hemorrhagic fever in Africa:

> [T]he WHO is better designed to respond to focal, short-term emergencies, such as investigating an outbreak of hemorrhagic fever in sub Saharan Africa, or to manage a multiyear, steady state disease-control program than to mount and sustain the kind of intensive, global response that is required to deal with a rapidly unfolding pandemic.
>
> (Fineberg, 2010, 1339)

This passage illustrates the conceptual ordering that placed A(H1N1) in one category – the potential for pandemic spread – and hemorrhagic fever in another – severe, but also localized. Fineberg, like many others, failed to conceive of hemorrhagic fever as the infectious agent that would, because of sheer numbers of cases and geographic spread, demonstrate the weakness stemming from the WHO's lack of operational and surge capacity. We are now attuned to the fact that pandemics can be mild even while they are spreading globally and that severe diseases that tend to stay localized can spiral out of control. At the same time, this analysis suggests that this new awareness is unlikely to help us predict how the next international health crisis will challenge our current systems of response.

A third insight one might draw from this comparison is that it is difficult to separate response efforts from the particular social geographies in which those responses are carried out. The variation in public acceptance of vaccination campaigns across countries during A(H1N1) demonstrates that the success of a vaccination intervention is not only dependent on the effectiveness of the vaccine once administered. Whereas contact tracing is the *sina qua non* of controlling an Ebola outbreak, myriad factors shape the conditions under which contact tracing can be carried out. This led to an interesting implicit linguistic debate within the CDC (Interviews, August 2015). One responder took issue with colleagues' claims that "there was no contact tracing" being carried out in West Africa during the summer of 2014. This responder argued, to the contrary, that responders were conducting contact tracing and offered considerable evidence in support of that conclusion. In spite of this, many at CDC continued to characterize the early days of the response as not including contact tracing. This argument about the presence/absence of contact tracing demonstrates the cognitive dissonance that "failed contact tracing" generated for those with past Ebola outbreak experience. Before 2014 Ebola, there was no such thing. This suggests the need for a reorientation in thinking about interventions. School closures, airport screenings, contact tracing, vaccination campaigns are not tools with inherent levels of effectiveness. They operate successfully, unsuccessfully, or somewhere in between based on a host of factors that are unpredictable and turbulent in each setting where they are applied.

Conclusion

The exercise of trying to draw lessons across three dissimilar international public health crises is not intended to generate firm conclusions about how to revise and improve future response actions. At the same time, this analysis argues for an analytic reorientation that considers response actions in light of the social geographies in which those responses are carried out and that presumes early response efforts will be fraught with uncertainty and contingency, in spite of and some times because of the structures put in place in advance to manage crises. It is obvious, after Ebola 2014, that a single disease agent can create remarkably disparate outcomes depending on a host of social, economic and geographic factors. This can lead to large errors in prediction when drawing on an existing base of experience. Such outcomes, instead of being treated as a result of mismanagement, should be expected as part of confronting unruly problems.

While public health experts might want to create an "evidence base" that allows them to draw on past experiences of success to guide future response efforts, an evidence base is not a substitute for the negotiation between officials and citizens in determining the collective action or inaction that will define response efforts during a crisis. In this sense, the nature of a crisis is and must be socially constructed as officials and communities come to grips with each new event. Current response efforts attempt to tie pre-planned response actions to future scenarios according to predictable variation in scope and severity. Unfortunately, variability in how communities experiencing a significant health event view that event is often left out of this equation. Familiar killers like seasonal influenza or malaria create higher annual mortality than outbreaks like Ebola or SARS without generating commensurate calls for intervention. Thus, requests for the public to engage in intervention efforts are likely to be tested against the public's view of the scale of the event itself. A review of these three dissimilar events suggests that there may be turbulence in how officials and communities come to understand an event and that that turbulence may extend well into the crisis.

Given the potential for outbreaks to create surprising social and geographic dynamics, it may be that apparently "successful interventions" should have the status of hypotheses when applied to new events or even during a single event across time and space. With such an approach, those guiding response efforts should not lose the confidence to try an apparently successful intervention. Instead, these might be launched with a more careful statement about the predicted results of an intervention and with a need to identify, a priori, the kinds of data and feedback that would lead responders to consider a change in course. Such an approach would also adjust the emphasis put on detection as the most important contingency in managing public health crises. While the first step in assessing whether an outbreak has the potential to reach crisis proportions is to identify the outbreak, myriad opportunities for surprise and missteps continue well into the course of the crisis. Mounting an appropriately scaled response at the outset may be less important than staying attuned to deviations in expected outcomes over the course of the event.

Notes

1 Funding supporting interviews and participant observation of the 2009 A(H1N1) pandemic comes from the United States National Science Foundation (SES-0826995). Funding for interviews related to the 2014 Ebola epidemic come from the Swiss National Science Foundation. I would like to thank individuals involved in one or more of the responses to the outbreaks described here for taking the time to share their insights about response efforts and for their dedication in trying to resolve such outbreaks quickly and effectively. I would also like to thank Dr. Mathilde Bourrier for her insightful comments and guidance on a draft of this chapter which helped to sharpen the analysis and improve the clarity of the argument.
2 Data for number of cases associated with distinct outbreaks of Ebola come from the Centers for Disease Control and Prevention Outbreak Chronology: Ebola Virus Disease. www.cdc.gov/vhf/ebola/outbreaks/history/chronology.html (Accessed February 27, 2018).
3 The four affected countries achieve similar scores on human development (United Nations Development Program, 2015).
4 See Parfaite (Chapter 10) on the Geneva Canton Hospital's experience.
5 For example, during the first known outbreak of SARS, the WHO alerted the international community about the outbreak and its spread outside of China before any cases arrived in the United States. The United States may appear to be an example of high-level performance in treating patients with SARS (seventy-four suspected and eight confirmed cases) in that no healthcare workers in the US contracted the disease. However, in spite of their heightened

awareness of the spreading outbreaks, a survey of healthcare workers who treated probable and confirmed cases revealed that lapses in infection control were common. For example, 44 percent of the healthcare workers surveyed reported interacting with suspected cases without the use of protective masks (Park et al., 2004).

6 Data on the number of SARS infections among healthcare workers by city from 2002 to 2003 are available at: www.who.int/csr/sars/country/table2004_04_21/en/ (Accessed May 24, 2018).

7 This approach draws on John Stuart Mill's Method of Similarity that examines dissimilar cases in order to rule out variables that might, otherwise, in a single case study, be associated with an outcome of interest (Mill, 1974).

8 Funding supporting interviews and participant observation of the 2009 A(H1N1) pandemic comes from the United States National Science Foundation (SES-0826995). Funding for interviews related to the 2014 Ebola epidemic come from the Swiss National Science Foundation.

9 The Canadian national public health agency, Health Canada, created the Global Public Health Intelligence Network (GPHIN) to track global news wires and websites for information that might be connected to an emerging outbreak (Health Canada, 2015).

10 For a timeline of the emergence of SARS, see the WHO website: www.who.int/csr/don/2003_07_04/en/ (Accessed May 9, 2018). Note that Heymann and Rodier's report (2004) indicates that GPHIN first picked up news reports of cases of atypical pneumonia on February 10 and claims that China's report to the WHO of a disease outbreak occurred one day later. The current timeline listed here gives February 10 as the first date of report by Chinese officials to the WHO and lists February 24 as the date when GPHIN picked up media stories about a spreading disease.

11 See the WHO guidance, which recommends linking national level responses to WHO-declared pandemic phases: *WHO Global Influenza Preparedness Plan: The Role of WHO and Recommendations for National Measures before and during Pandemics*, World Health Organization. 2005 (WHO/CDS/CSR/GIP/2005.5).

12 Data come from the WHO's April 2014 Ebola Situation Reports that are no longer publicly available. These data are available from the author upon request.

13 Data come from the WHO's May 2014 Ebola Situation Reports that are no longer publicly available. These data are available from the author upon request.

14 According to situation reports published by CDC during the outbreak, a team of five people from CDC joined the GOARN deployment in Guinea (reported March 31, 2014). That number grew to seven in early May. However, by May 27, 2014, with the optimistic forecast by the WHO that the outbreak was coming under control, CDC ended its deployment (reported May 27, 2014). CDC situation reports from the outbreak are no longer publicly available, but are available from the author upon request.

15 Data come from the WHO's May 2014 Ebola Situation Reports that are no longer publicly available. These data are available from the author upon request.

16 Written accounts and interviews indicate that Liberia formally reached out to the United States to request support, however, none of these accounts provides the specific date of the request.

17 For data and graphs showing the weekly increases in cases in each country, see: www.cdc.gov/vhf/ebola/outbreaks/2014-west-africa/cumulative-cases-graphs.html (Accessed: March 1, 2018).

18 Condon and Sinha (2009) are more guarded about the effectiveness of reporting under the IHR. They note that Mexico reported all suspected cases while

the United States reported only laboratory-confirmed cases. They argue that this created a misperception on the part of the international community that the epidemic started in Mexico and was more severe there. Many countries applied more severe restrictions to Mexico than the United States. Condon and Sinha anticipate that Mexico's experience, in spite of its exemplary reporting, might encourage countries not to be as transparent.

19 The biocontainment facilities were Emory University Hospital in Atlanta, Nebraska Medical Center in Omaha and the National Institutes of Health in Bethesda. While all three treated patients with no transmission to healthcare workers, the NIH did not receive a patient with Ebola until March 2015.

20 For more information on the CDC's tiered approach instituted after transmission to healthcare workers at Dallas Presbyterian, see the CDC's website: www.cdc.gov/vhf/ebola/healthcare-us/preparing/assessment-hospitals.html.

21 One review of the SARS experience does suggest a precautionary approach when recommending personal protective equipment for healthcare workers (Campbell, 2006). While a more precautionary approach might have stemmed the scale of transmission during 2014 Ebola, the experience with A(H1N1) suggests that officials who recommend a precautionary approach will not necessarily have those recommendations readily accepted.

References

Ansell, C. (2016). Unruly Problems, in Ansell, C. & Ogard, M. (eds), *Governance in Turbulent Times*. Oxford: Oxford University Press, pp. 159–180.

Ansell, C., Boin, A., & Keller, A. (2010). Managing Transboundary Crises: Identifying the Building Blocks of an Effective Response System. *Journal of Contingencies and Crisis Management*, 18: 195–207. doi:10.1111/j.1468-5973.2010.00620.x.

Ansell, C., Keller, A., & Reingold, A. et al. (2009). Workshop Minutes, Global Infectious Disease Response Workshop on H1N1, July 19–21, Berkeley, California.

Argyris, C., & Schön, D. (1978). *Organizational Learning: A Theory of Action Perspective*. Reading, MA: Addison Wesley.

Baekkeskov, E. (2016). Same Threat, Different Responses: Experts Steering Politicians and Stakeholders in 2009 A (H1N1) Vaccination Policy-making. *Public Administration*, 94: 299–315. doi:10.1111/padm.12244.

Baize, S., Pannetier, D., Oestereich, L. et al. (2014). Emergence of Zaire Ebola Virus Disease in Guinea. *New England Journal of Medicine*, 371(15): 1418–1425. doi:10.1056/NEJMoa1404505.

Bell, B., Damon, I., Jernigan, D. et al. (2016). Overview, Control Strategies, and Lessons Learned in the CDC Response to the 2014–2016 Ebola Epidemic. *MMWR Supplements*, 65(3): 4–11. doi:10.15585/mmwr.su6503a2.

Bethge, P., Elger, K., & Glusing, J. (2010). Reconstruction of a Mass Hysteria: The Swine Flu Panic of 2009. *Speigel Online*, 12 March. Available at: www.spiegel.de/international/world/reconstruction-of-a-mass-hysteria-the-swine-flu-panic-of-2009-a-682613.html (Accessed: May 14, 2018).

Bigley, G. A., & Roberts, K. H. (2001). The Incident Command System: High-Reliability Organizing for Complex and Volatile Task Environments. *Academy of Management Journal*, 44(6): 1281–1299. doi:10.2307/3069401.

Brien, S., Kwong, J. C., & Buckeridge, D. L. (2012). The Determinants of 2009 Pandemic A/H1N1 Influenza Vaccination: A Systematic Review. *Vaccine*, 30(7): 1255–1264. doi:10.1016/j.vaccine.2011.12.089.

Campbell, A. (2006). The SARS Commission – Final Report. Available at: www.archives.gov.on.ca/en/e_records/sars/report/index.html (Accessed: May 8, 2018).

CDC (Centers for Disease Control and Prevention). (2009a). Swine Influenza A (H1N1) Infection in Two Children – Southern California, March–April 2009. *Morbidity and Mortality Weekly Report*, 58(15): 400–402.

CDC (Centers for Disease Control and Prevention). (2009b). Change in CDC's School and Childcare Closure Guidance. Media Statement (May 5, 2009). Available at: www.cdc.gov/media/pressrel/2009/s090505.htm (Accessed: May 11, 2018).

Cheng, M., & Satter, R. (2015). Emails Show the World Health Organization Intentionally Delayed Calling Ebola a Public Health Emergency. *Business Insider*, March 20.

Cheng, V., Chan, J., To, K., & Yuen, K. (2013). Clinical Management and Infection Control of SARS: Lessons Learned. *Antiviral Research*, 100(2): 407–419. doi:10.1016/J.ANTI VIRAL.2013.08.016.

Christensen, T., Lægreid, P., & Rykkja, L. (2016). Organizing for Crisis Management: Building Governance Capacity and Legitimacy. *Public Administration Review*, 76(6): 887–897.

Cohen, D., & Carter, P. (2010). Conflicts of Interest: WHO and the Pandemic Flu "Conspiracies", *BMJ (Clinical research ed.)*, 340: c2912. doi:10.1136/bmj.c2912.

Coltart, C., Lindsey, B., Ghinai, I., Johnson, A., & Heymann, D. (2017). The Ebola Outbreak, 2013–2016: Old Lessons for New Epidemics. *Philosophical Transactions of the Royal Society of London*, 372(1721).

Comfort, L. (2007). Crisis Management in Hindsight: Cognition, Communication, Coordination, and Control. *Public Administration Review* 67: 189–197.

Condon, B. J., & Sinha, T. (2009). Chronicle of a Pandemic Foretold: Lessons from the 2009 Influenza Epidemic (May 3, 2009).

Connor, M. (2016). Clinical Management of Ebola Virus Disease in Resource-Rich Settings, in Evans, M., Smith, T., & Majumder, M. (eds), *Ebola's Message: Public Health and Medicine in the Twenty-first Century*. Cambridge, MA: The MIT Press, pp. 31–44.

Dahl, B. A., Kinzer, M. H., Raghunathan, P. L. et al. (2016). CDC's Response to the 2014–2016 Ebola Epidemic: Guinea, Liberia, and Sierra Leone. *Morbidity and Mortality Weekly Report*, Supplements, 65(3): 12–20.

Drazen, J. M. (2003). SARS: Looking Back over the First 100 Days. *New England Journal of Medicine*, 349(4): 319–320. doi:10.1056/NEJMp038118.

Falco, M. (2009). CDC: Production of H1N1 Flu Vaccine Lagging. *CNN*, October 16.

Fidler, D. P. (2009). H1N1 after Action Review: Learning from the Unexpected, the Success and the Fear. *Future Microbiology*, 4(7): 767–769. doi:10.2217/fmb.09.54.

Fidler, D. P. (2010). Negotiating Equitable Access to Influenza Vaccines: Global Health Diplomacy and the Controversies Surrounding Avian Influenza H5N1 and Pandemic Influenza H1N1. *PLoS Medicine*, 7(5): e1000247. doi:10.1371/journal.pmed.1000247.

Fineberg, H. (2010). Pandemic Preparedness and Response: Lessons from the H1N1 Influenza of 2009. *New England Journal of Medicine*, 370, 14: 1335–1342.

Fineberg, H. V. (2014). Pandemic Preparedness and Response: Lessons from the H1N1 Influenza of 2009. *New England Journal of Medicine*, 370(14): 1335–1342. doi:10.1056/NEJMra1208802.

Fletcher, M. (2015). Médecins Sans Frontières: The Organisation at the Heart of the Ebola Outbreak. *Telegraph*, April 18.

Gates, B. (2015). The Next Epidemic: Lessons from Ebola. *New England Journal of Medicine*, 372(15): 1381–1384. doi:10.1056/NEJMp1502918.

Ginsberg, M., Hopkins, J., Maroufi, A. et al. (2009). Swine Influenza A (H1N1) Infection in Two Children – Southern California, March–April 2009. *Morbidity and Mortality Weekly Report*, 58(15): 400–402. Available at: www.cdc.gov/mmwr/preview/mmwrhtml/mm5815a5.htm (Accessed: May 10, 2018).

Godlee, F. (2010). Conflicts of Interest and Pandemic Flu. *BMJ (Clinical research ed.)*, 340: c2947. doi:10.1136/BMJ.C2947.

Gostin, L. O. (2009). Influenza A (H1N1) and Pandemic Preparedness under the Rule of International Law. *Journal of the American Medical Association*, 301(22): 2376–2378.

Grady, D. (2014). Ebola Cases Could Reach 1.4 Million within Four Months, C.D.C. Estimates. *New York Times*, September 23.

Han, Y., Michie, S., Potts, H., & Rubin, G. (2016). Predictors of Influenza Vaccine Uptake during the 2009/10 Influenza A H1N1v ("Swine Flu") Pandemic: Results from Five National Surveys in the United Kingdom. *Preventive Medicine*, 84: 57–61. doi:10.1016/j.ypmed.2015.12.018.

Hawryluck, L., Lapinsky, S. E., & Stewart, T. E. (2005). Clinical review: SARS – lessons in disaster management. *Critical Care*, 9(4): 384–289. doi:10.1186/cc3041.

Health Canada. (2015). Big Data and the Global Public Health Intelligence Network (GPHIN) – CCDR: Volume 41 (September 3). Canada Communicable Disease Report CCDR.

Henao-Restrepo, A., Camacho, A., Longini, I. et al. (2017). Efficacy and Effectiveness of an rVSV-vectored Vaccine in Preventing Ebola Virus Disease: Final Results from the Guinea Ring Vaccination, Open-label, Cluster-randomised Trial (Ebola Ça Suffit!). *Lancet*, 389(10068): 505–518.

Hewlett, A., Varkey, J., Smith, P., & Ribner, B. (2015). Ebola Virus Disease: Preparedness and Infection Control Lessons Learned from Two Biocontainment Units. *Current Opinion in Infectious Diseases*, 28(4): 343–348. doi:10.1097/QCO.0000000000000176.

Heymann, D. L., & Rodier, G. (2004). SARS: Lessons from a New Disease, in Learning from SARS: Preparing for the Next Disease Outbreak: Workshop Summary. National Academies Press (US). Available at: www.ncbi.nlm.nih.gov/books/NBK92444/ (Accessed: May 9, 2018).

Katz, R. (2009). Use of Revised International Health Regulations during Influenza A (H1N1) Epidemic, 2009. *Emerging Infectious Diseases*, 15: 1165–1170.

Keller, A., Ansell, C., Reingold, A. et al. (2012). Improving Pandemic Response: A Sensemaking Perspective on the Spring 2009 A (H1N1) Pandemic. *Risk, Hazards & Crisis in Public Policy* 3: 1–37. doi:10.1515/1944-4079.1101.

Kerr, S., Van Bennekom, C. M., & Mitchell, A. A. (2016). Influenza Vaccination Coverage during Pregnancy: Selected Sites, United States, 2005–06 through 2013–14 Influenza Vaccine Seasons. *Morbidity and Mortality Weekly Report*, 65(48): 1370–1373. doi:10.15585/mmwr.mm6548a3.

Koplan, J. P., Butler-Jones, D., Tsang, T., & Yu, W. (2013). Public Health Lessons from Severe Acute Respiratory Syndrome a Decade Later, *Emerging Infectious Diseases*, 19(6): 861–863. doi:10.3201/eid1906.121426.

Kumar, S., Quinn, S. C., Kim, K. H., & Hilyard, K. M. (2012). US Public Support for Vaccine Donation to Poorer Countries in the 2009 A (H1N1) Pandemic. *PLoS ONE*, 7(3): e33025. https://doi.org/10.1371/journal.pone.0033025.

Lagadec, P. (2009). A New Cosmology of Risks and Crises: Time for a Radical Shift in Paradigm and Practice. *Review of Policy Research*, 26(4): 473–486.

LaPorte, T. R. (1996). High Reliability Organizations: Unlikely, Demanding and at Risk. *Journal of Contingencies and Crisis Management*, 4: 60–71. doi:10.1111/j.1468-5973.1996.tb00078.x.

LaPorte, T. (2007). Critical Infrastructure in the Face of a Predatory Future: Preparing for Untoward Surprise. *Journal of Contingencies and Crisis Management*, 15(1): 60–64.

LaPorte, T. R., & Consolini, P. M. (1991). Working in Practice but Not in Theory: Theoretical Challenges of "High-reliability Organizations". *Journal of Public Administration Research and Theory*, 1 (January): 19–48.

Leung, G., & Nicoll, A. (2010). Reflections on Pandemic (H1N1) 2009 and the International Response. *PLoS Med*, 7(10): e1000346.

Low, D. E. (2004). SARS: Lessons from Toronto, in *Learning from SARS: Preparing for the Next Disease Outbreak: Workshop Summary*. Washington, DC: National Academies Press (US). Available at: www.ncbi.nlm.nih.gov/books/NBK92467/ (Accessed: May 8, 2018).

Lutz, L. D., & Lindell, M. K. (2008). Incident Command System as a Response Model within Emergency Operation Centers during Hurricane Rita. *Journal of Contingencies and Crisis Management*, 16(3): 122–134. doi:10.1111/j.1468-5973.2008.00541.x.

MacPhail, T. (2014). *The Viral Network: A Pathography of the H1N1 Influenza Pandemic*. Ithaca, NY: Cornell University Press.

Mackenzie, J. S., Drury, P., Arthur, R. et al. (2014). The Global Outbreak Alert and Response Network. *Global Public Health*, 9(9): 1023–1039. doi:10.1080/17441692.2014.951870.

Mackenzie, J. S., Drury, P., Ellis, A., Grein, T., Leitmeyer, K. C., Mardel, S., & Ryan, M. (2004). The WHO Response to SARS and Preparations for the Future, in S. Knobler, A. Mahmoud, S. Lemon, A. Mack, L. Sivitz, & K. Oberholtzer (eds), *Learning from SARS: Preparing for the Next Disease Outbreak – Workshop Summary*. Washington, DC: The National Academies Press, pp. 42–50.

Mahler, J. G., & Casamayou, M. H. (2009). *Organizational Learning at NASA: The Challenger and Columbia Accidents*. Washington, DC: Georgetown University Press.

McNeil, D. (2014). Lax U.S. Guidelines on Ebola Led to Poor Hospital Training, Experts Say, *New York Times*, October 15. Available at: www.nytimes.com/2014/10/16/us/lax-us-guidelines-on-ebola-led-to-poor-hospital-training-experts-say.html (Accessed: May 23, 2018).

Médecins Sans Frontières. (2017). Five Lessons Learned During the Latest Ebola Outbreak in DRC. Report, June 27.

Meltzer, M., Atkins, C., & Santibanez, S. (2014). Estimating the Future Number of Cases in the Ebola Epidemic – Liberia and Sierra Leone, 2014–2015, *Morbidity and Mortality Weekly Report*. doi:10.15620/cdc.24900.

Mexico Ministry of Health. (2009). Outbreak of Swine-Origin Influenza A (H1N1) Virus Infection – Mexico, March–April 2009. *Morbidity and Mortality Weekly Report*, 58(April 30): 1–3.

Mill, J. S. (1974). *A System of Logic: Ratiocinative and Inductive*. Toronto: University of Toronto Press.

Mohan, G., Susma, T., & Hennessy-Fiske, M. (2014). Nurses at Dallas Hospital Describe Poor Safety Measures with Ebola Victim. *Los Angeles Times*, October 14.

Available at: www.latimes.com/nation/la-na-ebola-dallas-20141014-story.html (Accessed: May 23, 2018).

Moon, S., Sridhar, D., Pate, M. et al. (2015). Will Ebola Change the Game? Ten Essential Reforms before the Next Pandemic. The Report of the Harvard-LSHTM Independent Panel on the Global Response to Ebola. *The Lancet*, 386(10009): 2204–2221. doi:10.1016/S0140-6736(15)00946-0.

Moynihan, D. (2009). The Network Governance of Crisis Response: Case Studies of Incident Command Systems. *Journal of Public Administration Research and Theory*, 19(4): 895–915. https://doi.org/10.1093/jopart/mun033.

Moynihan, D. (2012). A Theory of Culture-Switching: Leaderships and Red-Tape during Hurricane Katrina. *Public Administration*, 90(4): 851–868.

NACSPH (National Advisory Committee on SARS and Public Health). (2003). Learning from SARS: Renewal of Public Health in Canada. A report of the National Advisory Committee on SARS and Public Health, October 2003.

Neumann, G., & Kawaoka, Y. (2011). The First Influenza Pandemic of the New Millennium. *Influenza and Other Respiratory Viruses*, 5(3): 157–166. doi:10.1111/j.1750-2659.2011.00231.x.

Nohrstedt, D., & Weible, C. (2010). The Logic of Policy Change after Crisis: Proximity and Subsystem Interaction. *Risk, Hazards & Crisis in Public Policy*, 1(2): 1–32.

Onishi, N. (2015). Empty Ebola Clinics in Liberia Are Seen as Misstep in U.S. Relief Effort. *New York Times*, April 11.

Ontario Nurses Association. (2018). 15 Years Post-SARS: Lessons Learned, Lessons Forgotten. Ontario Nurses Association (April 26, 2018). www.ona.org/news-posts/15-years-post-sars-lessons-learned-lessons-forgotten/ (Accessed: May 25, 2018).

Paquin, L. J. (2007). Was WHO SARS-related Travel Advisory for Toronto Ethical? *Canadian Journal of Public Health / Revue canadienne de sante publique*, 98(3): 209–211. Available at: www.ncbi.nlm.nih.gov/pubmed/17626386 (Accessed: May 9, 2018).

Park B. J., Peck, A., Kuehnert, M. et al. (2004). Lack of SARS Transmission among Healthcare Workers, United States. *Emerging Infectious Diseases*, 10(2): 244–248. doi:10.3201/eid1002.030793.

Plotkin, B. J., Hardiman, M., Gonzalez-Martin, F., & Rodier, G. (2007). Infectious Disease Surveillance and the International Health Regulations, in N. M. M'ikanatha, R. Lynfield, C. A. Van Beneden, & H. de Valk (eds), *Infectious Disease Surveillance*. Malden: Blackwell.

Rittel, H., & Webber, M. (1973). Dilemmas in a General Theory of Planning. *Policy Sciences*, 4: 155–169.

't Hart, P. (2013). After Fukushima: Reflections on Risk and Institutional Learning in an Era of Mega-Crises. *Public Administration*, 91(1): 101–113.

UNDP (United Nations Development Program). (2015). *Human Development Report 2015: Work for Human Development*. New York: United Nations Human Development Program.

UNOG (United Nations Office at Geneva). (2014). Regular Press Briefing by the Information Service: Ebola, April 1.

US GAO (United States Government Accountability Office). (2004). Emerging Infectious Diseases: Asian SARS Challenged International and National Response. GAO Publication No. 04-564 (April): 1–73.

Webby, R. J., & Webster, R. G. (2003). "Are We Ready for Pandemic Influenza?" *Science*, 302: 1519–1522.

WHO (World Health Organization). (2003). Chapter 5: SARS: Lessons from a New Disease, in *The World Health Report 2003: Shaping the Future.*

WHO (World Health Organization). (2013). *International Health Regulations (2005) Summary of States Parties 2013 Report on IHR Core Capacity Implementation Regional Profiles.* Geneva. Available at: www.who.int/about/licensing/copyright_form/en/index.html (Accessed: May 25, 2018).

WHO (World Health Organization). (2014). Ebola Virus Disease, Guinea: Situation as of 27 March 2014. WHO March 2014 Ebola SitReps. Available at: https://reliefweb.int/report/guinea/situation-report-1-ebola-virus-disease-guinea-28-march-2014 (Accessed: May 10, 2018).

WHO (World Health Organization). (2015). One Year into the Ebola Epidemic: A Deadly, Tenacious, and Unforgiving Virus. Report by the World Health Organization (January). Available at: www.who.int/csr/disease/ebola/one-year-report/introduction/en/.

WHO Ebola Interim Assessment Panel. (2015). *Report of the Ebola Interim Assessment Panel.* Available at: www.who.int/csr/resources/publications/ebola/report-by-panel.pdf (Accessed: May 22, 2018).

Wilkinson, A., & Fairhead, J. (2017). Comparison of Social Resistance to Ebola Response in Sierra Leone and Guinea Suggests Explanations Lie in Political Configurations Not Culture. *Critical Public Health,* 27(1): 14–27. doi:10.1080/09581596.2016.1252034.

Wilson, J. Q. (1989). *Bureaucracy: What Government Agencies Do and Why They Do It.* New York, NY: Basic Books.

Wilson, K., Brownstein, J. S., & Fidler, D. P. (2010). Strengthening the International Health Regulations: Lessons from the H1N1 Pandemic. *Health Policy and Planning,* 25(6): 505–509. doi:10.1093/heapol/czq026.

2 The future strikes back

Global public health crises and the rise of preparedness

Loïs Bastide

Introduction

Since the 9/11 attacks, preparedness has become the dominant way of thinking about domestic security in the United States of America (U.S.). This emerging form of "security rationality", caused by a growing sense of a future plagued by unanticipated threats, has resulted in a variety of related activities. In order to foster a "prepared nation", ready to deal with deep uncertainties, laws have been passed, institutions have been created, and preparedness, as a dominant paradigm and as a set of practices, has been organized, promoted and diffused across society. In the process, an increasing range of social activities and "social worlds" (Becker, 1984), such as public health, have been reconfigured in order to incorporate preparedness principles.

This dynamic has been analysed in different ways. Besides rather technical literature mainly concerned with refining preparedness concepts and practices, more critical scholars have located this phenomenon within a broader societal shift, which involves a transforming relationship with the future. Preparedness, it is said, is coincident with a shift in the perception of the future in Western post-industrial democracies, from one of risk, linked to the "insurance" society (Beck, 1992), towards one of uncertainty or even threat. This shift entails important consequences. Indeed, while the idea of risk tends to present the future as a development of current trends, the idea of uncertainty generates a perception of the future as a radical discontinuity (Zylberman, 2013). Whereas in risk thinking the future can still be related to probabilities, uncertainty dissolves this relationship. In this context, an uncertain future (as it is conceived) is only amenable to anticipation through approaches that replace probabilistic thinking, tied to a statistical approach to possible detrimental events, by "possibilistic thinking" (Clarke, 2006), which speculates on scenarios no matter the probability of their occurrence (see: Clarke, 2006; for a critic of this position see: Furedi, 2009). Consequently, in the context of preparedness, only "worst case" possibilities are rationally worth considering, since only they can help prepare for *any kind of threat.*

This approach to the government of future threats is not only infusing the U.S. administrations at all scales of governance. It is also increasingly diffusing internationally, through such a sector as disaster management, culminating in this domain with the release of the 2015 Sendai Framework for Disaster Risk Reduction (UNISDR, 2015). Similarly, it has been capturing ideas and practices in the world of global health emergency management, since the late 1990s. This evolution accelerated significantly after the 2009 A(H1N1) influenza pandemic and the 2014 Ebola outbreak in West Africa, whose international management was widely assessed as succeeding failures. During both episodes, the World Health Organization (WHO) was subject to harsh and widespread criticisms for its perceived inability to uphold its role in leading the international response, as the U.N. organization in charge of public health. These sequences pushed the organization to develop its preparedness organizational models, procedures and techniques.

This chapter intends to shed light on this process of organizational transformation, by assessing the interactions between a consolidating perception of the future as being deeply *uncertain*, the increasing dominance of preparedness as the preferred approach to the management of risks and uncertainties, and real-life crises. It does so by delineating the logic underpinning preparedness, as a form of rationality and a coherent set of practices. It then proceeds to analyse its adoption and diffusion in global health. This process is analysed with a specific focus on the effects of the 2014 Ebola episode in West Africa on the reorganization of the WHO's emergency capabilities.

The logic of preparedness

Several authors have explored the history and properties of preparedness, as a principle for organizing the government of risks (for a comprehensive overview and literature review see: Zylberman, 2013), providing ample elements on the genealogy and ruling mechanisms of this particular approach to planning. Thus, we know that preparedness emerged in the U.S., through an innovative assemblage of concepts drawn from different domains of practice, such as strategic military planning – for scenario planning – disaster management – for the "all hazard" concept (Quarantelli, 1981; Lakoff, 2006; Perrow, 2007, 49) – firefighting – for incident management techniques (Bigley & Roberts, 2001) – or environmental systems studies – for the concept of resilience. This articulation gave rise to an emergent domain of practices, endowed with its own internal rationality and coherence.

At an operational level, preparedness develops a unitary view of disasters, which promotes the expansion of generic capacities, distributed across society. These capacities are meant to be flexibly assembled to respond to *any type* of natural or man-made catastrophes. As such, preparedness shows an intrinsic tendency to extend and "colonize" all domains of practice and dimensions of society – public and private sectors, communities and individuals, to use current bureaucratic language. Conceptually, preparedness is a product of the increasing preoccupation of capitalist societies with the future (Giddens, 2002, 22) and the growing impulse – or pressure – for governments, to *take responsibility for the future*. This has led to the extension of the domain of public action, which now encompasses not only the domain of things present, but also the domain of *things to come* (Ewald, 1986). Historically, this type of governmentality has taken the shape of different regimes of *risk management*, such as insurance, precaution or emergency planning, which all enmesh with specific "techniques of government" (Lascoumes, 2004). What these approaches have in common is their belonging to a "regime of historicity" (Hartog, 2003) – a certain way, related to a given historical configuration, of articulating the past, present and future – where the future is dominantly framed in terms of risks (Beck, 1992).

Likewise, preparedness is co-emergent with a certain way of dealing with time – exploring the future to organize the present. It points towards a transformation of the prevalent regime of historicity, in post-industrial "Western" societies, where the dominant perception of the future comes to be shaped in terms of a radical uncertainty, rather than stochastic risks. Preparedness can thus be viewed as a type of governmentality, aiming at protecting the present by managing future, unpredictable and potentially disastrous events (think of the 9/11 attacks in New York, the 2004 Indian Ocean Tsunami, the Fukushima natural and nuclear catastrophes as timely examples). Under this regime of historicity, preparedness operationalizes an array of techniques aimed at dealing with the present, the past and the future, by articulating risks and uncertainties.

To understand how preparedness shapes the relationships between present, past and future, let us look at a widespread practice, in preparedness processes, called "situational assessments". This type of evaluation reaches into the past and towards the future in order to organize the present. Such iterative evaluations are thus at the core of the temporal processing of preparedness. As they allow delineating current circumstances (according to past events and potential threats), situational assessments are used to define the strategic orientations of preparedness systems, and to keep them up to date and commensurate with identified threats and vulnerabilities. To provide such assessments, two logical paths are available, one backward looking, the other forward oriented.

First, threats and vulnerabilities can be extracted and identified from "real life" lessons imposed by contingent events: in the U.S. administration, the 9/11 attacks or hurricane Katrina acted in this respect as powerful indicators of hitherto "hidden" vulnerabilities. Once identified, these weaknesses are mapped and organized in the form of an "after-action report" and "lessons learned". This first approach remains within the boundaries of probabilistic anticipations, where the past is relied on to forecast *likely* threats. The past is seen as a vehicle to repatriate and animate likely futures, in order to build relevant response capacities.

Second, flaws and loopholes can be identified through scenarios and exercises. This technique opens the way to the careful drafting of "worst case" narratives, which help design simulations of "low probability–high consequences" events, thus putting preparedness systems to a test. Contrary to real-life events, these plots are only loosely dependent on the past (they must remain *plausible*) and can thus be designed to explore the limits of preparedness systems, regardless of their probability of occurrence. Therefore, these two types of situational assessments are used to draw lessons (1) from past events, and (2) from "imaginative enactments" (Lakoff, 2008) conveying "virtual" catastrophes. Through lessons learned, these two strains of events – actual and virtual – are used to improve current preparedness capacities.

To understand this process – learning from the past, anticipating, organizing – it is necessary to underscore a plain and basic fact: that preparedness progresses *in the absence* of its object, considering that, as a domain of practice, it deals with threats located *in the future*, and which are thus, by nature, inaccessible to *praxis* (Bastide, 2017; Anderson, 2010). Hence, this trajectory of organizing relies on ways of "making the future present" in order to fine-tune the ability of preparedness systems to deal with forthcoming events. This "being there of the future" (Anderson, 2010) is realized both through the summoning of past events, and through the careful designing of virtual situations – plausible futures. Thus, it combines a probabilistic stream of thoughts – that which has happened might happen again – with a possibilistic opening – that which has never occurred but must be considered, since its occurring would be so catastrophic as to compromise societal resilience.

The history of planning is replete with examples of the first type of situational assessments, based on classical after-action analyses. To keep with our specific domain of investigation, such practices have been implemented in the U.S., over recent years, following different public health crises. Thus, the large-scale, national response to the 2009 A(H1N1) influenza pandemic was followed, two years later, by the release of the Department of Health and Human Services' (HHS) *An HHS Retrospective on the 2009 H1N1 Influenza Pandemic to Advance All Hazards Preparedness* (Department of Health and Human Services, 2012a). The document is organized along pandemic response domains – surveillance, mitigation, vaccination, communication and education. For each of these topics, past actions are dissected. At the end of each chapter, successes are then identified and "opportunities for improvement" are listed, which are further elaborated in the HHS' *2009 H1N1 Influenza Improvement Plan* (Department of Health and Human Services, 2012b). The newly released *Pandemic Influenza Plan 2017 Update* (U.S. Department of Health and Human Services, 2017) proposes further restructurings of the U.S. public health preparedness system by incorporating lessons from subsequent crises such as the recent Ebola outbreak in West Africa, the 2016 Zika virus outbreak, the Middle East respiratory syndrome (MERS), or ongoing resurgences of the H7N9 influenza strain in East Asia.

However, this type of practice is not specific to preparedness. Thus, let us now turn towards the second, more "exotic" form of anticipation, using scenario planning, which is co-emergent with the shift from risk thinking towards preparedness.

Plausible futures and scenario planning

The rationality of after-action analysis is based on a faith in the possibility to draw useful lessons from the past, in view of managing the present. As such, it is an old practice, which has been systematized in the context of strategic planning. Conversely, scenario planning indicates an erosion of this faith. It is a recognition that this approach, if it should not be discarded, needs to be supplemented, as reality has all too often caught existing emergency management capacities off guard. Therefore, scenario planning is indicative of an important shift in the conceptualization of the future within U.S. preparedness circles.

Historically, scenario planning was first developed as a military tool, in the context of the Cold War, before it spread to other domains of practice, such as corporate planning (Ringland, 1998), the disaster management community (Ericksen, 1975; Alexander, 2000; Tusa, Chin, & Tanikawa-Oglesby, 1996), or public health (Lakoff, 2006). However, this approach gained greater traction following the terrorist threats of the early 2000s. Indeed, the 9/11 attacks created a deep sense of uncertainty in the U.S. administration. The fact that these attacks had been possible at all and that the "unthinkable" had actually occurred was blamed on "a failure of the imagination" (9/11 Commission, p. 304, quoted in De Goede, 2008), pushing scenario planning to the fore of the reorganization process of the U.S. preparedness apparatus. Consistently, the 2002 National Strategy for Homeland Security, a White House document setting the principles of national preparedness, called for a greater emphasis on catastrophic threats entailing "the greatest risk of mass casualties, massive property loss, and immense social disruption" (U.S. Homeland Security Council, 2002, 2).

Subsequently, scenario planning, as a preparedness practice, has been structured and institutionalized, and the responsibility of the drafting and implementation of scenarios, through exercises, has been attributed to the Department of Homeland Security (DHS). This "fictionalization" of strategic planning (Zylberman, 2010), marked by an acute consciousness of being confronted with "fragile futures", was reinforced with the release of the Presidential Policy Directive on National Preparedness (PPD-8) in 2011. While the previous framing of scenarios in the Homeland Security

Presidential Directive (HSPD-8) annex 1 explicitly demanded that national scenarios be focused on the most dangerous *and* the most likely threats, PPD-8 shifted their focus to the incidents identified as posing the greatest threat to the nation's security. Craig Fugate, then administrator of the U.S. Federal Emergency Management Agency (FEMA), referred to these incidences, with a capacity to overwhelm all U.S. countermeasures, as "meta scenarios", to convey the idea of their extraordinary scope (Caudle, 2012). Thus, it was hoped that focusing on events of such scale and implementing the knowledge thus acquired through exercises would stress and, therefore, strengthen preparedness systems surge capacity, the underlying assumption being that once they were calibrated for the worst threats, they would be able to face *any* threat.

Scenarios and exercises have thus become strategic techniques for managing uncertainty, and their organization has grown in complexity. In the latest National Exercise Program (NEP) (U.S. Department of Homeland Security, 2013), which sets the national framework for preparedness exercises, the latter are distributed across every governmental scale (all the way from federal institutions to the individual citizen), across the private and public sectors, and are held iteratively. Following previous experimentations in the early 2000s (for a detailed account see: Zylberman, 2013, 161–164), the first National Level Exercises (NLE) were held in 2009. Such exercises are now implemented on a biennial basis. Likewise, scenarios have grown in scope. Besides narratives aiming at benchmarking specific capabilities, such as the anthrax attack or the influenza pandemic plotted in the 2006 National Planning Scenarios (U.S. Department of Homeland Security, 2006), FEMA has now engaged in long-term scenario planning. In 2010, the agency launched the Strategic Foresight Initiative (SFI), gathering a broad set of actors who worked together to draft scenarios spanning until 2030. The aim is to achieve "(a)n emergency management community prepared for whatever challenges the future holds; and a common sense of direction and urgency to drive action toward meeting our shared future needs – starting today" (U.S. Federal Emergency Management Agency, 2012, V).

In 2013, the SFI released *Toward More Resilient Futures: Putting Foresight into Practice* (U.S. Federal Emergency Management Agency, 2013), the implementation plan following its conceptual statement. As quoted from the document, "This step moves us beyond the analytical world of process and 'theory' toward the real world of practice". The report is divided into three sections. The first section is titled "Sustaining Foresight" and is intended as a move "to spark future thinking" in order to understand "what our future needs will be"; this "requires ... to stretch our imaginations and explore the underlying forces of change – seeking to be more prepared, regardless of how the future unfolds". These statements further document the fact that scenarios have become a critical technique for incorporating the future in the context of U.S. preparedness practices, thus broadening the scope of classical risk analysis.

As we showed, scenarios are means of acting in the present *considering the future*, by constructing *plausible* narratives of forthcoming threats. This said, we agree that scenarios do not aim at forecasting the future, contrary to risk assessments. Indeed, their growing prominence in U.S. preparedness practices is inseparable from the perception that risk thinking is too limited to prepare for a future plagued by growing uncertainties. In a context where the future is increasingly conceived of as unamenable to any form of efficient prospective thinking, specific plots are not selected because they are thought to draw an accurate picture of the future (because they represent *likely* occurrences), but because they offer a broad portfolio of possible threats ("whatever challenges the future holds" … "regardless of how the future unfolds"). These portfolios are designed to stretch preparedness systems to their extreme limits. Thus, preparedness is not achieved by *predicting the future*. Rather, it is achieved through the building of broad and flexible "core capabilities" (U.S. Department of Homeland Security, 2011), which can be combined in discrete configurations to organize a response and face any possible pattern of disaster. What is to be stabilized is not an accurate view of the future, but consistent preparedness capacities.

From capabilities to "whole of society"

PPD-8 set U.S. preparedness on new tracks, as it shifted the focus from wide-ranging scenarios to "worst case" narratives aimed at stressing response capabilities to unprecedented levels (Caudle, 2012). This shift marks a heightened consciousness of the vulnerability of current arrangements and of the possibility of "large-scale disasters" which, as it is understood, could overwhelm all government resources and capabilities. As the "scale and severity of disasters are growing" they will thus "likely pose systemic threats" (U.S. Federal Emergency Management Agency, 2011, 1). In facing such "wicked problems" (Rittel & Webber, 1973) classical capabilities, located in specialized agencies, are deemed insufficient, be they organized according to the all-hazards approach. The only way to face these looming cataclysms is through the mobilization of all components of the national community. Consequently, FEMA launched a national dialogue on a "whole community" approach to emergency in 2010 (U.S. Federal Emergency Management Agency, 2011), seeking to gather inputs from various actors as to the means of organizing relevant response capabilities, in such a fragile environment. This dialogue gave rise to concepts like "whole community", "whole-of-government" or "whole-of-society", which are emerging as a new dominant discourse on preparedness.

This move has two consequences. First, it suggests a shift away from a highly specialized, hierarchized and centralized national preparedness system, which cohered after the 9/11 events, towards a more diffuse form of organization which relies on the ability to mobilize non-specialized resources and actors in times of crisis. This organization leverages resources and capabilities that are presumed to be "latent" in society, in order to foster preparedness and tailor new response processes. As phrased by FEMA, the objective is to "understand community complexity [in order to] recognize community capabilities and needs, empower local action, and leverage and strengthen social infrastructure, networks, and assets".

The second consequence is far reaching. Beyond the notion of the whole community lies the idea of embedding preparedness in the course of ordinary social processes and practices in order to build resilience "within" communities, within the very social fabric. However, the success of this endeavour is premised upon the ability to mobilize individuals within these communities. In order to foster these finely grained social changes and to socialize ordinary social actors to this cultural shift, a number of initiatives have flourished which seek to involve the "whole of society" (government, the private sector, civil society) through participation in exercises or by encouraging individuals to contribute ideas and advice on the future of preparedness. FEMA, for instance, has developed an online crowdsourcing platform to gather inputs and ideas from the public on its preparedness initiatives and reorganizations.[1] In the context of the "whole community" approach, FEMA also seeks to involve individuals through children and youth education programmes on "individual, family and community preparedness", by leveraging social media, or by developing recovery plans "with full participation and partnership within the full fabric of the community". To develop this approach, FEMA has created an Individual and Community Preparedness Division (ICPD),[2] stating that, "Preparedness begins with the individual". In this context,

> FEMA's Individual and Community Preparedness Division (ICPD) serves as the main preparedness link to individuals and families. The Division connects science-based research to communications, education, and tools that empower communities to prepare for, protect against, respond to, and recover from a disaster.

Thus, it seeks to create "citizen responders", able to act before professional agencies can hit the ground.

These techniques of government, as *any* form of government (Foucault, 2004), are thus actively producing *subjects of preparedness* through the exposition and involvement of citizens in/to the preparedness discourse (and hence, to its specific regime of historicity), including in schools, and their enrolment in preparedness practices through disaster scenarios and exercises. These practices participate in framing a particular relationship to the world by diffusing a prevalent, dystopian relation to the future. This subjectivation process – the production of specific subjects of government (Foucault, 1982) – works towards producing citizens amenable and reactive to the preparedness discourse, and responsive to preparedness principles in the context of a catastrophic event.

As we see, there is a logical development between the development of a cultural framing of the future in terms of uncertainty,[3] the rise of scenario planning, and the emergence of the whole community approach in the U.S. preparedness system, thus outlining the constitution of a specific form of rationality. This rationality is currently spreading across governments and international organizations, globally. We now turn to the realm of international public health, as this reading will help us understand its recent developments, in particular during and after the 2009 A(H1N1) pandemic and the 2014 Ebola epidemic in West Africa.

The development of global health preparedness

In the field of public health, preparedness emerged in reaction to the rise of a renewed concern with microbes. Since the late 1980s, virologists and epidemiologists had been increasingly worried about emerging (such as HIV-AIDS) and re-emerging (resistant strains of known bugs) diseases (on this subject see, for instance: Morse, 1990, 1993; Berkelman, 1994; Artsob, 1995; King, 2004). In 1992, the U.S. Institute of Medicine released a report entitled "Emerging Infections: Microbial Threats to Health in the United States" (Lederberg, Shope, & Oaks, 1992). Such mounting preoccupation pushed the CDCs to develop preparedness strategies to address this perceived threat (U.S. Centers for Disease Control and Prevention, 1994, 2002). By the late 1990s, the fear of new pathogens was only growing, as this view seemed to be validated and was sustained by recurrent cases of deadly animal-to-human transmission of the H5N1 strain of influenza virus in East and Southeast Asia, and, later, by the SARS epidemic of 2002. In the U.S., this climate of anxiety was only exacerbated by the fear of possible bioterrorist attacks (Schoch-Spana, 2000, 2004; Keränen, 2011) using weaponized pathogens. Clearly, this blending of concepts, borrowing from distinct "epistemic communities" (Haas, 1992) – virologists/epidemiologists, military planners, emergency management experts – emerged and cohered into dedicated institutions in the U.S., culminating in the structuring of public health as an important branch of the fast expanding national public health preparedness system, in the early 2000s. From the late 1990s, the WHO had followed suit, thereafter contributing to the diffusion of this new domain of practice and new type of organization, merging public health and emergency planning.

The WHO drafted its first influenza pandemic preparedness framework in 1999,[4] setting the stage for international influenza preparedness planning. Influenza was seen as the most likely agent of a potential, deadly pandemic, drawing on memories of the catastrophic 1918 pandemic flu episode (Figuié, 2013) and considering the iterative emergence of new influenza strains in East Asia (Keck, 2010; MacPhail, 2014; Shortridge,

Peiris, & Guan, 2003). This dynamic of institutionalization culminated in 2005: while the U.S. DHS released its National Strategy for pandemic influenza (Kamradt-Scott, 2012), the WHO revised its 1999 plan to take stock of the SARS lessons and to reflect the growing fear of bioterrorism, after the 9/11 attacks. The same year, the revised International Health Regulations (IHR) were signed, which contained provisions for the development and strengthening of public health surveillance systems and capacity building across Member States (Sturtevant, Anema, & Brownstein, 2007). Meanwhile, many countries had started to develop their own pandemic influenza preparedness systems, under the WHO's push. In the domain of public health, the WHO thus acted as a global "clearing house" for preparedness ideas, concepts and practices, contributing to their quick spread at a global level. However, the U.S. model has been altered in the process. Interestingly, this alteration touches upon the most critical foundation of preparedness: its framing of the future. Indeed, as it spreads internationally, public health preparedness, as embodied within the WHO's own organization and objectified in existing instruments promoting the diffusion of preparedness practices, displays distinctive features regarding this specific dimension.

If preparedness is a way of governing the future, or, more accurately perhaps, of governing the present considering plausible futures, then this shift is highly significant. Importantly then, whereas the WHO is now in the process of adopting scenario planning and exercises as routine organizing tools, the organization does not seem to replicate the focus of the U.S. systems on "worst-case scenarios" for the time being. To be sure, the *WHO Simulation Exercise Manual*, released in 2017 (World Health Organization, 2017b), sticks to *likely risks* rather than "black swans" (Taleb, 2007). Likewise, the WHO's approach to preparedness aims at building capacities to deal with: "likely, imminent, emerging, or current emergencies" (World Health Organization, 2015, 20) rather than with low-probability apocalyptic events. Whereas in the U.S. preparedness planning process classical risk thinking is now subjected to the dominant logics of low-probability, high-impact events, the WHO's current frameworks show no such move.[5]

Dealing with international health crises under preparedness models

In 2009, the A(H1N1) flu pandemic put these newly constituted capacities to a test. The handling of the event by national authorities was assessed in rather positive terms in the U.S. and in a few other countries, such as Japan, raising few controversies. In many European countries, it was deemed a semi-failure at best (Flynn, 2010). However, the WHO's role was closely scrutinized and the target of the most violent arguments, being the institution in charge of leading the international response. Its management of pre-established pandemic phases (*Time*, June 10, 2009), the opacity of its decision-making processes during the crisis, its declaration of a Public Health Emergency of International Concern (PHEIC) for a disease which proved, in hindsight, rather mild (*Washington Post*, March 10, 2011), its poor performance in terms of crisis communications (Barrelet et al., 2013), and its putative collusion with "big pharma" (Cohen and Carter, 2010) were all pointed out in harsh terms in the international media. Consequently, the WHO thoroughly revised its preparedness framework. In 2011, it released a revised pandemic plan, the Pandemic Influenza Preparedness (PIP) framework (World Health Organization, 2011) which since then has been (re)evaluated and updated on a regular basis.

International public health preparedness was to reach a new turning point with the 2014 Ebola outbreak in West Africa. The crisis shed light on the risks involved in too narrow a focus on influenza, as the crisis took the WHO and other organizations by surprise. This lack of preparedness shed light on a double "tunnelling effect" (Taleb, 2007):[6] first, an oversized focalization on influenza, as the most likely "coming plague" (Garrett, 1994); second, an entrenched conceptual association between Ebola and Central Africa. Thus, the international community was neither ready to face Ebola as a potential pandemic threat (a status it nearly reached with quickly contained domestic transmission cases occurring in the U.S. and in Spain), nor to deal with it in West Africa, where people were unfamiliar with the disease. Interestingly, our investigations at the WHO headquarters, at the U.S. CDCs, with Switzerland's federal and cantonal authorities, at the Geneva cantonal hospital and at the Swiss branch of Doctors Without Borders, have showed that, during the most heated period of the crisis (March 2014–January 2015), existing emergency systems and procedures were of limited help. Individual initiatives, informal social networks and interactions played a significant role in keeping the response afloat before more permanent structures could be stabilized (see also: Bastide, Chapter 5).

As a whole, the international response to the event and, all the more, the WHO's lead during the episode were abundantly criticized (Moon et al., 2015; Gostin & Friedman, 2014; Gostin, 2015; Clift, 2015), prompting new restructuring of the organization's emergency capacities. In response to the following performance assessments and after-action reports – to date, over forty different assessment reports have been published (Moon et al., 2017), the WHO created the Health Emergency Programme in 2016, along with a large contingency fund[7] to allow the fast projection of response capabilities. Unlike its other programmes, the new department cuts through the three levels of the organization, from its Geneva headquarters to regional and national offices, thus aiming to align practices and create a unified chain of command. These evolutions indicate the broadening scope of public health preparedness within the WHO, while it consolidates as an overarching principle, exceeding pandemic influenza or humanitarian emergencies per se. This move is supported by the release of a series of new preparedness-related frameworks, which import and adapt many organizational elements readily available in the U.S., such as the Incident Management System (U.S. Department of Homeland Security 2008), or preparedness exercises. In 2017, the WHO released *A Strategic Framework for Emergency Preparedness* (World Health Organization, 2017a), which broadens the scope of public health preparedness to any type of emergency with a significant health component. Additionally, the institution is promoting the same type of reorganization on the international stage, through such programmes as the Country Health Emergency Preparedness and International Health Regulations (CPI). Located under the Health Emergency Programme, it supports the development of preparedness capacities in member countries, mainly through technical assistance.[8]

A significant aspect of this circulation and scaling up of preparedness concepts and models is the surfacing, in the WHO's 2017 framework, of the "whole community" approach to emergency planning, which is pervasive in the document. As stated:

> Communities are critical to effective emergency management. Community members are the first responders – and the first victims – of any emergency and, as such, essential members of the preparedness process. They should be represented in all activities around developing and implementing plans for emergency preparedness.
>
> (World Health Organization, 2017a, 3)

Considering this move, it is important to remember that the most significant impediment to the efficient deployment of the international response during the recent Ebola episode rested on the resistance of affected populations to emergency interventions (Niang, 2014; Bastide, 2018; Bastide, Chapter 5). This difficulty made the necessity to involve affected individuals and social groups in the response painfully clear. In the context of such emergency interventions, considering at-risk populations as mere targets of the response had not only proved ethically questionable, but also operationally detrimental (Le Marcis, 2015; Faye, 2015; Calain & Poncin, Chapter 11). Building up the "acceptability" (a term in use among emergency communicators) of such extreme public health measures as confinement, quarantine, triage or safe burials supposes the voluntary and active participation of affected individuals and local social, political and cultural agents.

Similar to the U.S. preparedness system, we can thus analyse the surfacing of the whole community approach as a way of co-opting reluctant populations into the emergency management process. Just like in the U.S., governing disaster situations requires the constitution of "subjects of preparedness", ready to act and re-act according to the requirements and injunctions of preparedness institutions and procedures. Yet, scaled up at the international level, the task appears daunting, if not squarely out of reach. In the U.S. alone, the A(H1N1) pandemic has underscored the need to tailor specific approaches and interventions for minorities and disadvantaged populations (U.S. Department of Health and Human Services, 2012a, 2012b, 31; Uscher-Pines, Maurer, & Harris, 2011). However, international public health preparedness deals, by nature, with considerably more heterogeneous publics. It aims at populations culturally inscribed in highly divergent regimes of historicity – a fact which was made very clear by the recent Ebola response (Bastide, 2018) – which always encompass vernacular ways of shaping the future (Bastide, 2015; Bastide, Chapter 5). If these processes of subjectivation might be thinkable within a single country, where institutions are coincident with national borders and "governed" population, reaching a global scale appears much more problematic.

Conclusion

As a coherent conceptual corpus and set of practices, preparedness is currently reconfiguring international public health emergency planning. If we consider preparedness as inseparable from a specific regime of historicity and as a type of rationality, this scaling process – the diffusion of preparedness from its U.S. cradle to the international stage – still appears incomplete. Indeed, if we accept that the WHO's preparedness models are representative of this internationalization process, it is important to stress that the institution still clings to a stochastic view of anticipation. Considering the difficulties faced while dealing with the A(H1N1) and Ebola episodes, we could thus be tempted to attribute these weak performances to this incomplete adoption of preparedness techniques. Moreover, this argument could be easily reinforced by comparing the WHO's intervention processes to those in place at the U.S. CDCs, where the organization was much quicker to reconfigure and enter into crisis mode. This is fact. However, this would also be a gross underestimation of the specificity of the WHO's position, and of its particular context of intervention. Being the organization in charge of leading the international response to public health crises, it evolves in a highly politicized arena, under unparalleled scrutiny, making its context of actions much more unpredictable and problematic. In these circumstances, there is absolutely no certainty that incorporating the whole preparedness "package" would make the WHO more efficient in the context of future health disasters.

This said, we might be currently witnessing clues that the process of institutionalization of preparedness within the organization is leaning towards a more complete internalization/implementation of its conceptual "economy". In particular, this could be transpiring in the recent emergence, in early 2018, of a discourse on "disease X", which entered the list of pathogens susceptible of triggering a public health emergency.[9] As stated:

Disease X represents the knowledge that a serious international epidemic could be caused by a pathogen currently unknown to cause human disease, and so the R&D Blueprint explicitly seeks to enable cross-cutting R&D preparedness that is also relevant for an unknown "Disease X" as far as possible.

This introduction of uncertainty – disease X – in a list of pathogens whose potential to induce a health crisis is assessed along classical risk assessment lines, was somehow to be expected. Considering that the WHO is currently implementing a whole community approach to preparedness, considering also that this approach intends to turn social actors into active responders in a context of emergency, there is a need to *enrol* people in the preparedness culture – its regime of historicity – to produce *subjects of preparedness.* This process of subjectivation is best facilitated by promoting high-impact uncertainties over known risks. Similar considerations were made by early proponents of scenario planning who argued that creating high-impact narratives – besides its usefulness in terms of capabilities assessment – would also be a way of increasing the awareness and concern for a specific issue, among the public and public authorities alike (see, for instance: Ericksen, 1975). Whether this move will sustain the emergence of more efficient public health crisis management capabilities remains to be seen.

Notes

1 http://fema.ideascale.com/. Accessed May 19, 2018.
2 www.fema.gov/individual-and-community-preparedness-division. Accessed May 19, 2018.
3 On the idea of the future as being a cultural fact, see: Appadurai (2013).
4 Influenza pandemic preparedness plan. The role of WHO and guidelines for national or regional planning. Geneva, Switzerland, April 1999.
5 This might be related, among other things, to the fact that the WHO deploys a logic of action consistent with its commitment to Evidence-Based Medicine (EBM), which promotes more classical risk–benefits analysis.
6 Taleb defines tunnelling as "[a] focus on a few well-defined sources of Black Swans (at the expense of the others that do not easily come to mind)" (Taleb 2007, 83).
7 The fund was set at 100 million U.S. dollars. As of April 2018, it barely reached 60 million U.S. dollars. www.who.int/emergencies/funding/contingency-fund/en/. Accessed May 19, 2018.
8 The promotion of the Revised International Health Regulations is also backed by the Global Health Security Agenda (GHSA), launched at the G7 summit in 2014.
9 www.who.int/blueprint/priority-diseases/en/. Accessed May 15, 2018.

References

Alexander, D. (2000). Scenario Methodology for Teaching Principles of Emergency Management. *Disaster Prevention and Management* 9(2), 89–97.

Anderson, B. (2010). Preemption, Precaution, Preparedness: Anticipatory Action and Future Geographies. *Progress in Human Geography* 34(6), 777–798.

Appadurai, A. (2013). *The Future as Cultural Fact: Essays on the Global Condition.* London and New York: Verso.

Artsob, H. (1995). Emerging Zoonotic Diseases. *The Canadian Journal of Infectious Diseases* 6(4), 208–209.

Barrelet, C., Bourrier, M., Burton-Jeangros, C., & Schindler, M. (2013). Unresolved Issues in Risk Communication Research: The Case of the H1N1 Pandemic (2009–2011). *Influenza and Other Respiratory Viruses* 7, 114–119.

Bastide, L. (2015). Faith and Uncertainty: Migrants' Journeys between Indonesia, Malaysia and Singapore. *Health, Risk & Society* 17(3–4), 226–245. https://doi.org/10.1080/13698575.2015.1071786.

Bastide, L. (2017). Future Now: "Preparedness" and Scenario Planning in the United States. *IRS Working Papers*, University of Geneva. https://archive-ouverte.unige.ch/unige:99430. Accessed May 24, 2018.

Bastide, L. (2018). Crisis Communication during the Ebola Outbreak in West Africa: The Paradoxes of Decontextualized Contextualization. In Bourrier, M., & Bieder C. (eds) *Risk Communication for the Future: Towards Smart Risk Governance and Safety Management*, pp. 95–108, London: Springer.

Beck, U. (1992). *Risk Society towards a New Modernity.* London and Newbury Park, CA: Sage.

Becker, H. S. (1984). *Art Worlds.* Berkeley, CA and London: University of California Press.

Berkelman, R. L. (1994). Emerging Infectious Diseases in the United States, 1993. *Journal of Infectious Disease* 170(2), 272–277.

Bigley, G. A., & Roberts, K. H. (2001). The Incident Command System: High-reliability Organizing for Complex and Volatile Task Environments. *Academy of Management Journal* 44(6), 1281–1299.

Caudle, S. (2012). Homeland Security: Advancing the National Strategic Position. *Homeland Security Affairs* 8(1).

Clarke, L. (2006). *Worst Cases: Terror and Catastrophe in the Popular Imagination.* Chicago, IL: University of Chicago Press.

Clift, C. (2015). *Devil in the Detail for WHO's Ebola Resolution.* London: Chatham House.

Cohen, D., & Carter, P. (2010). WHO and the Pandemic Flu "Conspiracies". *BMJ,* 340, 1274–1279.

De Goede, M. (2008). Beyond Risk: Premediation and the Post-9/11 Security Imagination. *Security Dialogue* 39(2–3), 155–176.

Ericksen, N. J. (1975). *Scenario Methodology in Natural Hazards Research.* Institute of Behavioral Science, University of Colorado, Boulder, CO.

Ewald, F. (1986). *L'Etat providence.* Paris: Grasset.

Faye, S. (2015). L'"exceptionnalité" d'Ebola et les "réticences" populaires en Guinée-Conakry. Réflexions à partir d'une approche d'anthropologie symétrique. *Anthropologie & Santé* [Online] 11. http://journals.openedition.org/anthropologiesante/1796. Accessed May 24, 2018.

Figuié, M. (2013). Global Health Risks and Cosmopolitisation: From Emergence to Interference. *Sociology of Health & Illness* 35(2), 227–240.

Flynn, P. (2010). The Handling of the H1N1 Pandemic: More Transparency Needed. Report of the Social Health and Family Affairs Committee, Parliamentary Assembly, Council of Europe.

Foucault, M. (1982). The Subject and Power. *Critical Inquiry* 8(4), 777–795.

Foucault, M. (2004). *Naissance de la biopolitique.* Paris: Seuil/Gallimard.

Furedi, F. (2009). Precautionary Culture and the Rise of Possibilistic Risk Assessment. *Erasmus Law Review* 2(2), 197–220.

Garrett, L. (1994). *The Coming Plague: Newly Emerging Diseases in a World Out of Balance.* New York, NY: Macmillan.

Giddens, A. (2002). *Runaway World: How Globalisation Is Reshaping Our Lives.* London: Profile Books.

Gostin, L. O. (2015). Critical Choices for the WHO after the Ebola Epidemic. *JAMA* 314(2), 113–114.

Gostin, L. O., & Friedman, E. (2014). Ebola: A Crisis in Global Health Leadership. *The Lancet* 384(9951), 1323–1325.

Haas, P. M. (1992). Introduction: Epistemic Communities and International Policy Coordination. *International Organization* 46(1), 1–35.

Hartog, F. (2003). *Régimes d'historicité: Présentisme et expériences du temps.* Paris: Seuil.

Kamradt-Scott, A. (2012). Evidence-based Medicine and the Governance of Pandemic Influenza. *Global Public Health* 7(sup2): S111–S126.

Keck, F. (2010). Une sentinelle sanitaire aux frontières du vivant. *Terrain* 54, 26–41.

Keränen, L. (2011). Concocting Viral Apocalypse: Catastrophic Risk and the Production of Bio(in)Security, *Western Journal of Communication* 75(5), 451–472.

King, N. B. (2004). The Scale Politics of Emerging Diseases. *Osiris* 19, 62–76.

Lakoff, A. (2006). Techniques of Preparedness. In Monahan, T. (ed.), *Surveillance and Security: Technological Politics and Power in Everyday Life.* New York, NY: Routledge, 265–273.

Lakoff, A. (2008). The Generic Biothreat, or, How We Became Unprepared. *Cultural Anthropology*, 23(3), 399–428. https://doi.org/10.1111/j.1548-1360.2008.00013.x.

Lascoumes, P. (2004). La Gouvernementalité: De la critique de l'État aux technologies du pouvoir. *Le Portique* [Online], 13–14. http://journals.openedition.org/leportique/625. Accessed May 22, 2018.

Le Marcis, F. (2015). "Traiter les corps comme des fagots": Production sociale de l'indifférence en contexte Ebola (Guinée). *Anthropologie & santé. Revue internationale francophone d'anthropologie de la santé*, 11 [Online]. https://journals.openedition.org/anthropologiesante/1907. Accessed May 24, 2018.

Lederberg, J., Shope, R. E., & Oaks, S. J. (1992). *Emerging Infections: Microbial Threats to Health in the United States.* Washington, DC: National Academy Press, Institute of Medicine.

MacPhail, T. (2014). *The Viral Network: A Pathography of the H1N1 Influenza Pandemic.* Ithaca, NY: Cornell University Press.

Moon, S., Sridhar, D., Pate, M. A., Jha, A. K., Clinto, C. et al. (2015). Will Ebola Change the Game? Ten Essential Reforms before the Next Pandemic. The Report of the Harvard-LSHTM Independent Panel on the Global Response to Ebola. *The Lancet* 386(10009), 2204–2221.

Moon, S., Leigh, J., Woskie, L., Checchi, F., Dzau, V. et al. (2017). Post-Ebola Reforms: Ample Analysis, Inadequate Action. *BMJ* 356(j280).

Morse, S. (1990). Regulating Viral Traffic. *Issues in Science and Technology* 7(1), 81–84.

Morse, S. (1993). *Emerging Viruses.* New York, NY and Oxford: Oxford University Press.

Niang, C. I. (2014). Ebola: Une épidémie postcoloniale. *Politique Etrangère* 4, 97–109, [Online] www.cairn.info/revue-politique-etrangere-2014-4-page-97.htm. Accessed May 22, 2018.

Perrow, C. (2007). *The Next Catastrophe: Reducing Our Vulnerabilities to Natural, Industrial, and Terrorist Disasters.* Princeton, NJ: Princeton University Press.

Quarantelli, E. L. (1981). An Agent Specific or an All Disaster Spectrum Approach to Socio-behavioral Aspects of Earthquakes? *University of Delaware Disaster Research Center Preliminary Papers,* 69.

Ringland, G. (1998). *Scenario Planning: Managing for the Future.* Chichester and New York, NY: Wiley.

Rittel, H. W. J., & Webber, M. M. (1973). Dilemmas in a General Theory of Planning. *Policy Sciences* 4(2), 155–169.

Schoch-Spana, M. (2000). Implications of Pandemic Influenza for Bioterrorism Response. *Clinical Infectious Diseases* 31(6), 1409–1413.

Schoch-Spana, M. (2004). Bioterrorism: US Public Health and a Secular Apocalypse. *Anthropology Today* 20(5), 8–13.

Shortridge, K. F., Peiris, J. S. M., & Guan, Y. (2003). The Next Influenza Pandemic: Lessons from Hong Kong. *Journal of Applied Microbiology* 94, 70–79.

Sturtevant, J. L., Anema, A., & Brownstein J. S. (2007). The New International Health Regulations: Considerations for Global Public Health Surveillance. *Disaster Medicine and Public Health Preparedness* 1(02), 117–121.

Taleb, N. N. (2007). *The Black Swan: The Impact of the Highly Improbable.* New York, NY: Random House.

Tusa, W., Chin, P. A., & Tanikawa-Oglesby, S. (1996). Report of the Scenario Planning Group for Medium Climate Change "Apple Fritters". *Annals of the New York Academy of Sciences* 790(1), 183–191.

UNISDR (United Nations International Strategy for Disaster Reduction). (2015). *Sendai Framework for Disaster Risk Reduction 2015–2030.* [Online] www.wcdrr.org/uploads/Sendai_Framework_for_Disaster_Risk_Reduction_2015-2030.pdf. Accessed September 2018.

U.S. Centers for Disease Control and Prevention. (1994). Addressing Infectious Disease Threats: A Prevention Strategy for the United States. *MMWR Recommend,* 43, 1–18.

U.S. Centers for Disease Control and Prevention. (2002). *Protecting Health in an Era of Globalization: CDC's Global Infectious Disease Strategy,* 2002 International Conference on Emerging Infectious Diseases, Atlanta.

U.S. Department of Health and Human Services. (2012a). *An HHS Retrospective on the 2009 H1N1 Influenza Pandemic to Advance All Hazards Preparedness.* Washington, DC: HHS.

U.S. Department of Health and Human Services. (2012b). *2009 H1N1 Influenza Improvement Plan.* Washington, DC: HHS.

U.S. Department of Health and Human Services. (2017). *Pandemic Influenza Plan 2017 Update.* Washington, DC: HHS.

U.S. Department of Homeland Security. (2006). *National Planning Scenarios.* Washington, DC: DHS.

U.S. Department of Homeland Security. (2008). *National Incident Management System.* Washington, DC: DHS.

U.S. Department of Homeland Security. (2011). *National Preparedness Goal.* Washington, DC: DHS. [Online] www.fema.gov/media-library-data/20130726-1828-25045-9470/national_preparedness_goal_2011.pdf.

U.S. Department of Homeland Security. (2013). *National Exercise Program Capstone Exercise 2014: Scenario Ground Truth.* Washington, DC: DHS.

U.S. Federal Agency for Emergency Management. (2011). *A Whole Community Approach to Emergency Management: Principles, Themes, and Pathways for Action.* Washington, DC: FEMA.

U.S. Federal Agency for Emergency Management. (2012). *Strategic Foresight Initiative: Summary Information Packet.* Washington, DC: FEMA.

U.S. Federal Agency for Emergency Management. (2013). *Toward More Resilient Futures: Putting Foresight into Practice.* Washington, DC: FEMA.

U.S. Homeland Security Council. (2002). *National Strategy for Homeland Security.* Washington, DC: White House.

Uscher-Pines, L., Maurer, J., & Harris, K. M. (2011). Racial and Ethnic Disparities in Uptake and Location of Vaccination for 2009-H1N1 and Seasonal Influenza. *American Journal of Public Health* 101(7), 1252–1255.

World Health Organization. (2011). *Pandemic Influenza Preparedness Framework for the Sharing of Influenza Viruses and Access to Vaccines and Other Benefits.* Geneva: WHO.

World Health Organization. (2015). *Framework for a Public Health Emergency Operation Centre.* Geneva: WHO.

World Health Organization. (2017a). *A Strategic Framework for Emergency Preparedness.* Geneva: WHO.

World Health Organization. (2017b). *WHO Simulation Exercise Manual.* Geneva: WHO.

Zylberman, P. (2010). *Neither Certitude nor Peace: How Worst-Case Scenarios Reframed Microbial Threats, 1989–2006.* NCIS Briefing. The Munk Center for International Studies Briefing Series. [Online] http://munkschool.utoronto.ca/wp-content/uploads/2013/05/CPHS_Briefing_07-09.pdf#page=15.

Zylberman, P. (2013). *Tempêtes microbiennes: Essai sur la politique de sécurité sanitaire dans le monde transatlantique.* Paris: Gallimard.

Part II

Lessons learned from the A(H1N1) pandemic and 2014 Ebola virus disease

A multidisciplinary point of view

3 Comparing the 2009 A(H1N1) pandemic and 2014 Ebola virus disease

Of viruses, surprises in outbreak responses and global health work

Mathilde Bourrier

Introduction

The management of the responses to both the A(H1N1) pandemic between 2009 and 2010 and the Ebola virus disease between 2014 and 2016 inspires a certain number of comparative reflections. This chapter seeks to propose a synthesis of the accounts of the actors that we met during the course of our investigation between 2013 and 2016. This summary will also be bolstered by the prolific documentation and the numerous publications that have accompanied the knowledge base of these two epidemics. In the first section, ways in which the narrative of these two epidemics has been influenced by earlier episodes of the flu pandemic and of the Ebola virus epidemics are presented. Anchored conventional wisdoms have unquestionably influenced the cognitive frames that shaped public health responses in both cases. In the second section, a characterization of the surprise effects that molded the response strategies in both crises is offered. Finally, in the last section the challenges faced by key global health actors, during both crises are detailed.

The chapter contends that this comparison makes sense despite the massive differences between the two epidemics. Numerous controversies plagued both responses. Coordination failure, failure of foresight, power plays, group interests, complacency, difficulty in articulating expertise and political decisions, and many more factors played a role in the difficulties that responders faced. However, in retrospect, what could explain the most the magnitude of both crises has more to do with the unrealistic perception of how global health is organized than any of these factors that undoubtedly played their part.

When path dependency matters: on viruses and their conventional wisdoms

The fear of influenza: a common disease with pandemic potential

Despite it already having been around for hundreds of years, the influenza virus A(H1N1) remains somewhat of a mystery for specialists of this disease and for public health professionals. The flu (or influenza) is a disease caused by a virus that attacks the respiratory system and reverberates throughout the body. It normally lasts between three and seven days and can impede a person in his or her daily activities. The virus's composition changes constantly, and it is endemic. This is why we can catch a new flu every year. There exist three types of the influenza virus: A, B and C. Type A is the most dangerous. It has already provoked several deadly pandemics, such as the notorious Spanish flu pandemic of 1918 (Kolata, 1999), which killed more than 50 million people. In 1968, it was the Hong Kong flu's turn to cause a pandemic. The type A virus transforms in very little time, which makes it all the more difficult to combat. In effect, the body has to build up an immune response specific to each new strain of influenza in circulation. The type A virus causes a pandemic about three or four times per century. The type B virus brings about much less serious complications. Its epidemics are localized and are less subjected to modifications than the type A virus. Finally, the type C virus, for which the symptoms present themselves as being similar to the common cold, is also less subject to mutations than the type A virus.

Influenza experts make a distinction between zoonotic, seasonal epidemic and pandemic flu. They have paid critical attention to their most-feared linkages for decades. Influenza attracts mass public health efforts and is the subject of a global surveillance network, the Global Influenza Surveillance and Response System, GISRS. This network has become well established since its inception in 1951, with its stars,[1] its battles and its objectives – a "world in itself" (Kolata, 1999; Dehner, 2012; Caduff, 2014; MacPhail, 2014; Aranzazu, 2013, 2016). The pandemic form of flu has been mobilizing actors around the manufacturing of pandemic plans since the beginning of the 2000s (Zylberman, 2013; Bastide, 2017, Brender & Gilbert, 2018). The WHO, in consultation with the Strategic Advisory Group of Experts on Immunization (SAGE) and the GISRS, with advice from the International Health Regulations (IHR) emergency committee is responsible for decisions concerning the composition of the seasonal flu vaccine twice a year for both hemispheres. The vaccine is not perfect, and, given its hybrid formulation, is more or less effective against the viruses that circulate in a given season. If the seasonal flu can count on the development of two vaccines per year, the pandemic flu, which is by definition unforeseeable, suffers from the catastrophic representation of the Spanish flu pandemic of 1918 and from heightened fears emanating from Asia, where there was a resurgence of avian bird flu H5N1 (type A) in February 2003 in Hong Kong. Avian bird flu is only slightly contagious but has become endemic among domestic poultry in certain countries.[2] It has proven to be quite often (in 60 percent of cases) lethal when humans are infected.

The source of the 2009 virus can be traced to pig farms in the district of Santa Cruz in Mexico and not to poultry farms. In a large majority of cases, the symptoms were hardly distinguishable from an ordinary, benign seasonal flu. Most of the time, those who became ill got better on their own without requiring medical attention. However, in acute cases, some people needed specialized medical attention, such as respiratory assistance or the use of antivirus medication (oseltamivir and zanamivir). But, the virus also infected and killed young people in good health. From the beginning, it attacked segments of the population that were healthy and young and caused higher mortality among children and young adults than the seasonal flu (Brammer et al., 2011). This observation would come to have a persistent influence on the evaluation of risks by global public health authorities (Fraser et al., 2009; Flahault & Zylberman, 2010). Experts were reminded of elements from the Spanish flu epidemic, where it was young adults who paid the heaviest price. In this context, the WHO wasted no time in declaring a Public Health Emergency of International Concern (PHEIC) on April 25, 2009, as was prescribed by the provisions of the IHR, which had been revised in 2005.

In effect, the virus circulated quickly: the United Kingdom and Spain, as traditional entry points of airlines from the American continents, were strongly afflicted. In the span of several weeks, the WHO declared a pandemic on June 6, 2009 (it would come to be declared as over by the WHO on August 10, 2010). This virus implanted itself very rapidly and mutated in an extraordinary manner. The initial strain, called "California", has since become a part of the cocktail used in the manufacturing of the seasonal flu vaccine. The type A viruses are feared by public health experts, particularly in a context where the flu has become endemic. The potential for linkage between the two types of viruses is not impossible. Uncertainties concerning flu virus's circulation, contagiousness, recombination and transmission remain significant despite the number of researchers engaged in research on these flu viruses: "The natural history of influenza is still largely unknown" (Flahault & Zylberman, 2010, 331).

Without a doubt, the 2009 influenza virus A(H1N1) suffered from social misrepresentation from the beginning. The collective reference, for both populations and public health experts alike, came from the Spanish flu, which was also of porcine origin ("Swine flu") and killed between 50 million and 100 million people worldwide, according to some recent calculations (Johnson & Mueller, 2002; Taubenberger & Morens, 2006; Wilson, 2011). Against all expectations, at least in appearance, the 2009 virus turned out to originate from North America, and not from an Asian animal reservoir, which was the expected scenario. In effect, for many years, in lay and expert narratives alike, Asia is depicted as the likely host for all flu viruses (Keck, 2010; MacPhail, 2014, 76).

Ebola: a textbook lethal and African hemorrhagic fever

The Ebola virus was jointly discovered in 1976 by Peter Piot (a Belgian doctor at the Institute of Tropical Medicine in Antwerp) in Yambuku, in the north of Zaire (nowadays called the Democratic Republic of the Congo), and the Congolese researcher Jean-Jacques Muyembe, who was in charge of blood collection. Ebola is the name of the river that flows nearby the small village where the virus was discovered. It was in a hospital of this village where the first case of Ebola hemorrhagic fever was identified, announcing its first epidemic which would then come to infect 318 people and kill 280 of them. Ebola specialists seemed to better understand its *modus operandi* than flu specialists understood the mysteries of the flu virus. It was as if Ebola's simplicity made it an excellent candidate for a first-year student's virology textbook. The Ebola virus, of which several variations exist (the most dangerous is called "Zaire"), appears more stable than the flu virus. It is contagious, but not as contagious as the flu.

Several Ebola epidemics have occurred during the past forty years in the Congo, Sudan, Uganda and Gabon. Each outbreak caused several dozen infections and large numbers of deaths. These Ebola outbreaks remained, up until now, relatively limited and did not kill nearly as massive numbers of individuals as the epidemic of 2014–2016.[3] In the spring of 2014, numerous public health experts understood the situation as follows: this epidemic is a manageable public health emergency, which eventually consumes itself, like a raging fire, and runs its own course, like the dozens of other times it had occurred up until that point. With the term "outbreak", we can imagine a fire breaking out, which we can of course also associate with a forest fire, or a bush fire, what Wald (2008, 7) named "the 'primordial' spaces of African rainforests". As such, the following larger narrative would come to circulate: these flares burn themselves out. And once the virus has been able to attack everything in its path, it retreats and lurks in the forest, among the bats, believed to act as the "guardians" of the virus.[4]

No treatment to fight the disease really exists; the administration of rehydration salts and antipyretics in order to contain the fever comprise the basis of Ebola medical care. At the outset, there is no tested vaccine. Ebola had previously interested virological, epidemiological and ecological research, particularly in the context of the agenda of global health security and the fight against bioterrorism. There was an experimental vaccine, which was stocked in military laboratories, most notably in the United States and in Canada. It had never been tested with humans during an outbreak. In 2014, certain pharmaceutical companies possessed the capacity to produce a potentially effective antiviral. Nevertheless, mass treatment efforts in the first months of 2014 consisted of administering rehydration salts and antipyretics aimed at containing fever.

The Ebola virus epidemic of 2014 was officially confirmed in March 2014 in Guinea by the Institute Pasteur in Lyon (France) and the WHO declared it a PHEIC on August 8, 2014. It is likely that the first epidemic broke out some months beforehand, in December 2013. The index case might be a child who passed away in December 2013 in Meliandou, situated in the Guinean forests in the Guéckédou district. It was thought that the presence of the virus was a result of remote communities who had been living in the forest in close contact with animal hosts of the virus, such as fruit-eating bats: this is the leitmotiv of the traditional narration about Ebola epidemics. This theory is not yet confirmed. After two years of fighting the outbreak, the PHEIC linked to Ebola in West Africa was declared over on March 29, 2016. In total, 28,616 confirmed, likely and suspected cases were reported in Guinea, Liberia and Sierra Leone, and 11,310 people perished (WHO, 2016).

Ebola's symptoms are comparable, in certain cases, to those of cholera or Lassa fever, which makes identifying the disease difficult, particularly among communities and caregivers who are unfamiliar with the disease. This epidemic presented all of the characteristics of an Emerging Infectious Disease (EID). Since the 1990s, due in part to the anthrax attacks in the United States and the growing fear of bioterrorism (Collier & Lakoff, 2008; Boin et al., 2003; Bastide, Chapter 2), viral contagions have been at the heart of collective fears. From this perspective, images circulating about Africa could only reinforce these worries: those who were sick suffered greatly, they died in more than half of the cases, a large majority were women and children, they were not well taken care of, hardship was rampant, the virus took advantage of promiscuous behaviors and was transmitted by direct contact and by bodily fluids.

Deforestation, a growing practice, also likely contributed to the disruption of the ecological balance. As a result, this provided opportunities for the virus to escape from the forest, where it had been confined most of the time. The already historically, socially and politically disadvantaged inhabitants of the Guinean forests would come to find themselves in the center of the most tenacious rumors and as the object of aggravated stigmatization (Epstein, 2014; Faye, 2015).

At the beginning of the intervention, African burial practices and the extent to which they can play a role in contamination appeared to be if not surprising to the public health community (in the corridors of the WHO, CDCs or at Médecins Sans Frontières), who knew about their central role, not culturally handled in an appropriate way. They would end up interfering in the proper handling of the crisis. Funerary practices and the traditional preparations of bodies were quickly blamed by health authorities (national and international) and experts, which created "resistance" and distress without precedent among local populations. This would only further reinforce the image of an Africa struggling with its cultural practices from another era (Kidjo, 2014). Very rapidly, anthropologists mobilized themselves and organized networks in order to counter this simplistic, culturalistic and counterproductive explanation (Fairhead, 2016; Moulin, 2015, Abramowitz, 2017). Anthropologists were called upon as reinforcements everywhere and their knowledge, invoked in numerous arenas, was tried and tested in the field in the three countries (Moulin, 2015; Richards, 2016; Abramowitz, 2017).

However, it is of importance to recall that numerous accounts already existed on how to engage in dialogue with local populations that are struggling with an Ebola epidemic. At the end of the 1990s, Pierre Formenty, the Ebola expert from the Pandemic and Epidemic Diseases department of the WHO, and his colleagues at the time, engaged in collaborations with anthropologists (Barry and Bonnie Hewlett, anthropologists from the University of Washington in Vancouver; Alain Epelboin from the Musée de l'Homme in Paris, notably), which allowed them to write intervention protocols that were informed by local practices. They particularly addressed safe and respectful burial practices, and aimed at increasing knowledge about the modes of transmission of the disease with the objective to communicate them in the most respectful manner possible (Boumandouki et al., 2005; Hewlett et al., 2005; Hewlett & Hewlett, 2008; Brunnquell et al., 2007; Epelboin et al., 2007, 2008). An update followed in 2014 (Formenty, 2014).

The 2014 Ebola virus disease appeared in retrospect as an ultra-dangerous, ultra-contagious virus that was capable of tearing down health systems and shifting entire geopolitical and economic balances. It was a virus that got around: it gained Nigeria by plane in July 2014 and, by autumn 2014, had made its way to Mali, Senegal, Spain, the United States, Great Britain, Ireland and Italy.

The virus also attacked three countries that had already been devastated by civil war and desperately lacked healthcare infrastructures. If the entire world seemed to discover this established fact, this was, without a doubt, not the case for the WHO. Before 2014, the United Nations (UN) institution, through the IHR instrument already pointed out the risks for poor countries and their neighbors of major outbreaks occurring with such weak healthcare infrastructures. On May 28, 2009, during the World Health Assembly, the first female president from an African country, Ellen Johnson Sirleaf (who had been in power in Liberia since 2006), pleaded in front of the delegates:

> I am here to say that people should not simply die because they are poor and because the treatments that are used in the rest of the world are not available … In Liberia, one woman out of 1000 dies during childbirth, 90 percent of Liberians live on less than two dollars per

day. In 1989, Liberia still had 800 doctors. After fourteen years of war, only fifty doctors.

(Quoted in Lempen, 2010, 282)[5]

It would be this very president who would confront the Ebola crisis in her own country.

Both diseases, the flu pandemic and the Ebola virus disease, carried their own histories and powerful conventional wisdoms. These impacted even unconsciously the immediate types of responses that public health officials designed at the outset. In a way, initial cognitive frames left a persistent imprint on organizational collectives of early responders, thus continuing to shape organizational behaviors and outcomes in the long run, even as conditions altered and adjustments were needed. However, as Priscilla Wald eloquently explains: "The outbreak narrative is conventional and formulaic, but it is also evolving. Stories of disease emergence in all their incarnations are so powerful because they are as dynamic as the populations and communities that they affect" (Wald, 2008, 28).

On outbreak responses: coping with surprises

A(H1N1): trapped in initial pandemic plans

From the 2000s onwards, global public health experts, as prompted by the WHO and as a result of lessons learned from the Severe Acute Respiratory Syndrome (SARS), continued to devote efforts to a vast operation to prepare pandemic plans (Brender, 2014, 40–44). This investment in pandemic planning also signaled the move from the WHO to re-appropriate the pandemic influenza issue and regain status in world health leadership (Brender & Gilbert, 2018, 39). The largest preparedness operation in the history of public health was applied at all levels and brought people on board from different professions who during these years learned to get to know one another and to work together (Zylberman, 2013; Keck, 2010; MacPhail, 2014; Lakoff, 2017). Ironically, in April 2009, the WHO had just published its new Pandemic Influenza Preparedness and Response plan.

The informants, particularly in Switzerland, Japan and the United States, that we questioned about this all confirmed that they had been very involved in the drafting of these pandemic plans. All of them remembered the years and the months prior to A(H1N1) and how they had tried to mobilize their respective colleagues in order to successfully prepare themselves the best that they could. All of them remember that these preparations allowed them to forge relationships with other entities (i.e. other sectors) and at various levels (local, regional and national), depending on their initial location within the public health system. They had constituted veritable networks, both formal and informal, made of strong and weak ties. It only seemed "natural" that the pandemic would allow these individuals to activate these networks in order to test out the plans that had been fine-tuned over several long years (Keller et al., 2012). Brender (2014) borrows the term "epistemic communities", forged by Haas (1992), to account for these knowledge and expertise-based networks. To a large extent, these plans proved, at least according to retrospective declarations made by our informants, to be helpful when logistics were involved. They were used as a coordination mechanism but were ultimately set aside because the plans compelled action based on a severe crisis, but the threat would prove to be of a lesser magnitude than anticipated (Keller et al., 2012).

In the case of the pandemic flu, a kind of blindness resulted in not taking into account some of the signals indicating that the flu, albeit very contagious and able to spread very quickly, resulted in only moderate symptoms in most cases. Yes, it was a pandemic; however, as time would tell, it was not a very severe one. It did nonetheless prove to be a lasting one: a "paracrisis", as one of our informants called it. Most experts remained alert and waited for the second wave that, in the historical model of the 1918 influenza outbreak, had been shown to be deadlier. What was particularly worrisome for experts were the possible recombinations and mutations of the virus (Garrett, 2005; Flahault & Zylberman, 2010). Health authorities stuck for the most part to the original outbreak forecasts, which had been strongly influenced by mathematical models of disease transmission (Fraser et al., 2009) and by the associated death scenarios. These models predicted disturbing severity for populations that were young and in good health. By declaring the transition to Phase 6 on June 11, 2009, the WHO was posed to set off the largest order of vaccines and antiretroviral in history: rich economies jumped at their chance and pulled the lever to launch the entirety of their pandemic plans (Abeysinghe, 2013; Pasquini-Descomps et al., Chapter 8). They were bound by their Advance Purchase Agreements and a race against time began. Vaccines were not available for the first wave of the pandemic in the spring of 2009, but experts thought they would be useful when the second wave of the pandemic struck, possibly in the fall season for the northern hemisphere (Saluzzo, 2011).

Each country's over-response should nonetheless be described with greater nuance: the United Sates, for example, adjusted their response, and vaccination campaigns remained targeted towards specific segments of the population such as high-risk populations like first responders and pregnant women. The American campaigns did not attain the same level of scale that was witnessed among the mass campaigns implemented in some European countries – a phenomenon that can be attributed to the vaccine shortage, which did not allow for any other option.[6] In Switzerland or in France, for example, a calculation of two doses per person deemed to be a priority (caregivers; staff serving in sovereign capacities; at-risk populations – pregnant and asthmatic women in particular; and any person wishing to get vaccinated) was proposed.

In Europe, the variance in vaccine coverage between countries was significant (ranging from 4.8 percent to 92 percent, according to the analysis provided by Brien et al., 2012). According to the 2010 VENICE (Vaccine European New Integrated Collaboration Effort) study, of twenty-nine European responding countries, twenty-six organized national pandemic influenza vaccinations. Of the twenty-seven countries with vaccine recommendations, all recommended it for healthcare workers and pregnant women. Twelve countries recommended vaccines for all ages.[7] Most countries identified similar target groups for pandemic vaccine, but substantial variability in vaccination coverage was seen (Mereckiene et al., 2012). In Europe, large centers located in stadiums, military barracks or any kind of large public infrastructures were set up to receive thousands of people to receive their vaccine shots.

However, vaccination campaigns were not always met by population-level adherence, with few exceptions, such as in Sweden (Barrelet et al., 2013). Also in the US, campaigns targeted at pregnant women and healthcare workers have been successful and with lasting effects over the years. Several experts and researchers even hypothesized that in countries where populations have high levels of trust towards their leaders and governmental authorities, vaccination campaigns were met with higher levels of adhesion. By contrast, in countries where trust had been eroded, vaccination measures failed. In Switzerland, for example, not more than 17 percent of the total population was vaccinated (Barrelet et al., 2013). Several researchers have suggested that the failure of this vaccination campaign should not only be interpreted in light of the particular event represented by the 2009 pandemic, and have claimed that the interpretation could go a step further by attributing this failure to a growing mistrust among certain groups of European populations towards vaccination use (Burton-Jeangros et al., 2005; Schindler et al., 2012).

As for Japan, which was used to such strong responses to epidemics and was well equipped for the seasonal flu, its authorities supported and maintained a significant level of engagement, despite critics in the press, due to extra costs in the end incurred by underused vaccines. A total of 17 million doses were supplied by the end of 2009. Large amount of vaccines were imported (GSK and Novartis). Most of them were not used and resulted in significant waste (see Pasquini-Descomps et al., Chapter 8).

Various investment logics were in the works. They concerned the resources that needed to be mobilized, resources that were not only financial in nature, but also organizational, communicational and cognitive. The establishment of pandemic plans along with contingency and business continuity plans within administrations, hospitals, schools, public transportation, the private sector, airports and places with high concentrations of people fell upon the responsibility of hundreds of individuals in order to get ready for the preparedness war front. All the hype about the rolling out of the thought-out plans for one of the most severe pandemics, as well as the difficulty of leaving behind a worst-case-scenario logic, are both strongly engrained in the memories of the actors we met, even five years after the event, which is when we conducted our interviews. Many of them, particularly those who worked in national public health services, attributed this escalation to the strong injunctions provided by the international echelon represented by the WHO.

The WHO responded to critics, who accused its top leaders of a "cry wolf attitude", on June 10, 2010 by referring to the large biomedical uncertainties they faced in handling the flu virus:

> The first human infections with the new H1N1 virus were confirmed in April 2009. Analysis of laboratory samples showed that the new virus had never before circulated in humans. This is a virus of animal origin with a unique mix of genes from swine, bird, and human influenza viruses. The genetic composition of this virus is distinctly different from that of the older H1N1 virus that has been causing seasonal epidemics since 1977.
>
> (WHO, 2010)

To summarize, the response to A(H1N1) was mainly geared towards the production of a vaccine. However, the time it took to produce it, and the difficulties encountered in convincing populations to get vaccinated provoked social controversies, which consistently made the headlines in the press. Interestingly, not being able to provide a vaccine in time was also an issue when the 2014 Ebola epidemic struck.

Ebola: using a classical toolbox for an unfolding disaster

In the spring of 2014, the situation for numerous public health experts was as follows: Ebola was a health emergency that could be controlled and that would eventually run its course on its own, just like all previous outbreaks had done up to that point. So goes the leitmotiv of the traditional narration concerning Ebola epidemics. Our informants attested to this "Ebola normal" scenario that they first thought was unfolding, at WHO headquarters and at the CDCs alike. Lakoff (2017, 158), in his recent book, makes the same observation and calls it a "failure of administrative imagination". The measures that needed to be implemented in order to bring an Ebola epidemic to a close were well known. It generally consisted of the deployment of public health interventions, the operational doctrine of which was as follows: (1) isolation of patients practices and forced quarantines, if necessary; (2) the systematic searching out of those who had come into contact with each patient in order to track down the transmission chain; (3) the implementation of risk communication programs specifically aimed at afflicted communities in order to inform the locals and to avoid the spreading of the disease through risk behaviors; (4) the

implementation of medical care that prioritized rehydration and the provision of painkillers, in the absence of a real cure; and (5) the overseeing
of funerary burial practices. No one suspected that this arsenal of public
health measures might be insufficient.

Yet, populations at the borders of the three countries – Guinea, Liberia
and Sierra Leone – were in fact very mobile (Richards, 2016). For that
matter, before their prohibition, local markets were sometimes held in
one country and sometimes in another, depending on the day of the week.
Contamination, as a consequence, followed the commercial routes and
the paths of the most mobile members of the communities: merchants,
religious leaders, healers, farmers and small-harvest vendors. Hunger, lack
of resources and the disorganization of post-conflict countries brought
these populations to the roads as they sought out better living conditions
and resources for survival. As such, the most active members of these communities navigated non-stop between their villages of origin and the cities
where work opportunities were more abundant.

Two other narrative elements reinforced the initial framing on an
"Ebola normal" outbreak and served to handicap the emergence of a new
representation of the crisis as it continued. The first element was of a logistical nature: the virus would spread into a borderland region where it was
thought that means of communication were lacking and in bad shape due
to war that had raged on for so long. As such, experts projected that the
virus would not spread very easily. However, in reality, the road system was
not as bad as was thought, and, as Richards (2016, 45–48) attests, the roads
were regularly utilized. A second element strengthened the first one: this
time, it was of a meteorological nature. The rainy season might mechanically slow down travelers and hinder both the virus's progression and
further contagion.

The international and national health authorities acted according to
the model of a classic epidemic and rolled out measures designed with this
model in mind. As was customary practice, it was decided that small
contingents of experts from the WHO, the CDC and MSF (Médecins Sans
Frontières), coordinated by the WHO and under the banner of the Global
Outbreak Alert and Response Network (GOARN), would be sent into the
field.[8] These measures had previously proven to be effective elsewhere, as
we were informed in August 2015 by an expert from the CDC who had
been accustomed to these types of deployments.

In April 2014, the number of cases seemed to demonstrate the experts'
capabilities. The curve began to slope downward, leaving the impression
that epidemic hotspots were under control, especially in Guinea. However,
at the end of the spring of 2014, voices were raised to call attention to the
need to reconsider the premises of the first analysis of the situation. These
voices came mainly from actors who were in the center of the action, particularly from MSF. More marginal voices, further from the direct health
response, were raised for example in Geneva-based embassies to the

United Nations of the concerned countries and from anthropologists (Fairhead, 2016).

As the crisis continued, the complexity of relationships between the different levels of the WHO – from the headquarters in Geneva, to the level of the AFRO (Brazzaville) region, down to the level of the afflicted countries – significantly hindered a robust assessment of the situation. The complexity of the WHO's structure was once again called into question (Sridhar et al., 2014; Horton, 2014). Global public health experts again highlighted that the director-general could not act without a mandate from the Member States and that the nomination of WHO regional directors, no more than the nomination of WHO country directors, for that matter, was not within her purview.

Both within the hallways of the WHO as well as outside them, our informants confided to us that declaring a PHEIC does not always suit the governments of the concerned countries. Particularly, this type of announcement inevitably risks having non-negligible collateral effects, in terms of product boycotts, the closure of countries' borders in the region and the slowing down of, or even bringing a complete halt to, business exchanges. Clearly, during these months of this wait-and-see approach, from the point of view of massive assistance, many other considerations were taken into account at the heart of these debates. It is not that nothing happened; only that what happened obeyed other logics, particularly of a global health diplomatic order, so as to not push the governments of the affected countries into a corner.

During the summer of 2014, MSF continued to regularly alert the international public health authorities. For the stakeholders, everyone had a role to fill. The expected course of the outbreak was drifting out of control in the field, but on the global chessboard, the various actors were playing a part that they thought they knew. The WHO occupied the posture of the large UN agency, "prevented" from its duties by its Member States (Lall, 2017) but at the same time as the keeper of the resources that come with diplomatic expertise as well as of capabilities to mobilize resources of supplementary expertise. The figure of "I wish I could, but my hands are tied" was once again over-played by this UN agency, although it would prove nonetheless to be critical, most notably for the speedy coordination of clinical trials, which it would come to achieve (Evans et al., 2016).[9] On the other side of the chessboard, there was MSF, a powerful and rich non-governmental organization with strong reputational capital and advocacy power. As one of our informants told us: "This is normal for MSF to manifest, this is what they do as an organization, and they are in their role". This expected stand might have prevented them from being heard early enough.

Thus, the scenario at the beginning (sporadic outbreaks that could be contained each time, which killed by hundreds and not by thousands, struck at the heart of remote, rural communities) was not reevaluated early enough. As a WHO employed virologist, upon returning from Liberia, confided to us in Tokyo in February 2015:

> The question that we needed to answer was: What do we do once Ebola enters a city? Everything else was essentially secondary. Nobody was able to give an answer to this question. Not on the ground, not in the country, not in the region, not in Geneva. No coordination efforts were working on this fundamental point.

Finally, in the sense that an epidemic with different hotspots leaves room for distinct, separate epidemics, it became vital that the communities themselves take ownership of the struggle against Ebola. On the ground, the public health approach, which was too strictly articulated around biosafety measures and had been used in all of the epidemics before this one, was not working well: numerous anthropologists warned of the risk of not relying on people's expertise in handling contagion (Richards, 2016), which could handicap the measures being implemented in the field (Wilkinson & Leach, 2015; Fairhead, 2016; Anoko et al., 2014; Le Marcis, 2015; Faye, 2015). First responders declared themselves to be floundering and too often incapable of correctly deploying interventions in the field (Médecins Sans Frontières, 2015; CDC, 2015). They particularly cited risk communication operations in relation to the population to be greatly suffering from their overwhelming workload. The deployment of international response teams, which fell into place the best they could, provoked uprisings among the concerned populations, right up until the dramatic Womey episode of September 2014.[10] The hostility and violence towards teams of first-line responders, both local and international teams alike, were, however, not new (Bausch et al., 2007; Fribault, 2015; Calain & Poncin, Chapter 11). Both were particularly well known by our MSF informants.

Global health workers and their responses

In this section, we intend to present three different angles to better apprehend what global health work entails. The first one concerns the flu pandemic responders, the second one deals with the Ebola responders, and the third focuses on international global health workers. Generally speaking, global health workers are medical professionals, drawn from public health, medicine and the life sciences.

Pandemic flu: tailored responses by long-committed experts

The pandemic rapidly mobilized the highest public health and civil security authorities of the Member States, as well as other socio-economic stakeholders possibly impacted by a pandemic. The degree of leadership retained by public health actors differed depending on the country. In France, leadership had to be shared with other pandemic stakeholders (Brender & Gilbert, 2018). Whereas in Switzerland for example, public health officials and experts stayed center stage.

The numerous retrospective feedback reports (international, national and regional) written after the flu pandemic (US Department of Health and Human Services, 2012; ASTHO, 2010; European Commission, 2010; Forster, 2012; Greco et al., 2011; Lister & Redhead, 2009; President's Council of Advisors on Science and Technology, 2009; Delaporte et al., 2010; WHO- Regional Office Europe, 2010; Ernst & Young/OFSP, 2010; WHO, 2011; Door & Blandin, 2010), the numerous academic writings on the subject, as well as our retrospective interviews with actors involved in response efforts, at the WHO, in Switzerland or in Japan, all confirmed that in the case of the influenza A(H1N1), the pandemic plans were activated from the beginning. As our informants told us in their own words: "At the time, we had one concept: the plan". The scenario for the A(H1N1) crisis had a powerful vehicle at its disposal. This vehicle was the framework of action that was "already there", operational and reassuring. Most countries quickly came to focus on two tools: (1) social distancing measures, which consisted of a campaign to raise awareness about safe sneezing practices, frequent handwashing, and limiting one's outings in case of the flu; (2) the development of a vaccine, as quickly as possible, as a response to the most dreaded eventuality, which was the second wave of the epidemic in the autumn of 2009 (with the model of the 1918 influenza waves in mind), which occurred but proved to be even milder.

In accordance with the application of pandemic plans, national and regional public health authorities found themselves in crisis centers which were often coordinated by security actors. This was the case in both France and Switzerland, for example. The paradigm shift in the affairs of surveillance and anticipation of bioterrorism post-9/11 brought about the emergence of new command structures. Such structures placed health authorities in close coordination with security forces aimed at maintaining public order, like in the Canton of Geneva, where the catastrophe plan named OSIRIS was deployed. This plan is coordinated through a crisis center, occupying its own space at the police headquarters, regrouping specific functions under the command of the police chief of staff. Representatives of the Canton of Geneva's Directorate General for Health, the cantonal doctor in charge of infectious diseases, the cantonal pharmacist responsible for "vaccination" records and "stocks of antivirals" (essentially Tamiflu, which is produced by Roche in Switzerland), representatives from public transportation services, flu experts working in infectiology or vaccinology at the cantonal hospital, a representative from the airport, and also a representative from the Fédération des entreprises romandes (the French-Swiss Business Federation) shared a same space. Health experts rapidly gained the upper hand and organized themselves into a sub-crisis "health center". However, their dependence upon federal-level decisions, particularly those of the Federal Office for Public Health (based in Bern), for the dispatching of vaccines and Tamiflu, which frequently resulted in *volte-face* decisions, underscored the OSIRIS's actors (Ernst & Young/ OFSP, 2010). When discussing the proximity between the forces of law and order and health experts, the actors we met offered an ambiguous version of events: with the police or the army, there certainly existed a clear chain of command, but they reported not being able to count on the police forces for any credible expertise in public health. As one key informant, working in the crisis center at the time, explained, "We could not expect everything to come from the OSIRIS apparatus in Geneva".

Certain researchers have already retraced the mixed results that the responders who struggled with these measures were able to take away from the situation (Keller et al., 2012; MacPhail, 2014; Brender & Gilbert, 2018). For certain actors, crisis centers served essentially for them to know on which network of actors they could lean for support: the famous A4 sheet of paper with "all of the telephone numbers on it". For many, the frequent telephone conference calls during the spring, autumn, and winter of 2009 with public health, national, federal and international authorities were an immense waste of time. The cumbersome organizational structuring of the response, stained by the transaction costs for communication charges, revealed itself to be ill-suited to the situation. Pandemic fatigue took place during the fall of 2009.

Yet, the overall picture still needs to be more nuanced. Japan firmly anchored itself in a posture of "super-management" when facing the pandemic. As many experts have pointed out, the Japanese health authorities ("the good student" when handling the seasonal flu, as WHO experts have contented themselves in recounting) habitually employed comprehensive measures in seasonal flu management. The most common measures implemented for the seasonal flu included: keeping social distance from others, mask-wearing behaviors, rapid administration of antiviral medications, school closures, isolation, vaccination and border control. As our informants explained, before 2009, influenza pandemic preparedness focused on early response, through "early medical responses and aggressive measures of containment". Japan had developed since December 2005 a "National Action Plan for Pandemic Influenza", last updated in February 2009. In line with this philosophy, early response to the 2009 pandemic made use of "aggressive border control measures", starting April 28, 2009, including fever screening for all passengers coming from affected countries. Public health authorities also decided to close schools for five days in May 2009 in Hyogo and Osaka Prefectures for example (Kawaguchi et al., 2009). Japanese experts we met in March 2015 at the Ministry of Health, Labor and Welfare recalled that these school closures were successful in containing the virus in the early stage.[11]

Switzerland opted for a strong response (ordering 13 million doses to cover 80 percent of its population) without employing the same systematic measures that characterized the Japanese response. The United States, for its part, adopted a middle-ground approach. In fact, it quickly became apparent that the virus was only slightly virulent. Beginning in January 2010, Janet Napolitano, Secretary of Homeland Security, began to declare that it was no longer the time for a mass uproar but rather the time for a scaling down. Mass vaccination would never have been an option. This was without a doubt more due to the unavailability of the vaccine than due to it being a consequence of a sound political decision. However, at the CDC, as was confirmed to us in the summer of 2015, the Incident Command System, staffed with no less than 300 "Flu guys" at the height of the crisis, compared with sixty people at WHO headquarters, remained active after January 2010.

The variance in pandemic responses is important across European countries, even between countries with a very similar profile. This is one of the puzzles of A(H1N1) research. Despite strong international impetus, resources invested at the country level and similar threats, European countries offered a picture of contrasts. This is especially clear when considering vaccination campaigns (Mereckiene, 2012). Baekkeskov (2016) compared Dutch and Danish 2009 A(H1N1) responses. Tracking the main factors that can explain why such similar countries differed in their vaccination programs (the Netherlands ordered vaccine for all residents while Denmark ordered vaccine for 28 percent of their population), he finally reached the conclusion that what makes the difference is the different pre-formatted norms that national leading experts are using in order to advise their governments: "The Netherlands prepared for an extraordinary deadly influenza solved by general mass vaccination … Danish pandemic flu preparations had focused on the problem as a range of probable, moderately severe influenza, solvable through limited vaccination" (Baekkeskov, 2016, 307–308).

After the crisis, and in line with the observations made in the retrospective feedback reports, the Member States adopted an ambivalent position: one that allowed them to free themselves of the supervision of the WHO in matters of risk evaluation, while at the same time recognizing its central role. Several laws concerning epidemics, which were presented in the years following the pandemic, particularly in Japan and in Switzerland, aimed at reaffirming the necessity of establishing the conditions for independent national risk evaluations. The WHO did not issue a new Pandemic Plan after the 2009 version. It did issue, however, "Pandemic Influenza Risk Management" in May 2017 that updates and replaces the "Pandemic Influenza Risk Management: WHO Interim Guidance" published in 2013. And recently it published a "Checklist for Pandemic Influenza Risk and Impact Management" in January 2018 and a document titled "Essential Steps for Developing or Updating a National Pandemic Influenza Preparedness Plan" in March 2018. These documents are in line with what experts had already pointed out: "European national plans are being up-graded and global leadership is required to ensure that these plans are uniformly applied across regions … Without regional or global leadership in these domains, pandemic preparedness plans could diverge even further across Europe" (Nicoll et al., 2012, 317). One can take note of a change in the vocabulary: checklists and steps are now preferred as plans. Finally, some countries are also moving away from specific pandemic preparedness plans to incorporate a wider range of emergencies, and have built more generic plans, that could be of use in several emergencies and not only health emergencies. The "All-hazards" doctrine is gaining ground.

Ebola: the early commitment of emergency workers pushed to their limit

Prior to the 2014 Ebola virus disease and as the years went by, MSF had become the de facto main medical caregivers during Ebola epidemics. Not surprisingly, during the first months of the management of the Ebola virus crisis, MSF was main actor operating on scene (Casaer, 2015; Hofman & Au, 2017). The Swiss MSF had operated in Guéckédou in Guinea since 2005. They were very familiar with the region, well equipped and set up, and were able to react quickly, not to mention able to cross the Guinean borders by sending a doctor detail when Liberia declared itself to be afflicted by the disease. It is clear that the MSF experts, just like those from the WHO and from the CDC, who were deployed in the first weeks via GOARN, were familiar with Ebola, and they knew it well. The NGO was used to intervening in these situations. It had developed protocols, could count on trained personnel and on powerful logistics.

However, MSF would eventually find itself overwhelmed (MSF, 2015), despite the fact that its teams were composed of the experts on Ebola (Wolz, 2014). The director of MSF international (the umbrella organization of the different MSF sections), Dr. Joanne Liu, for the first time in the history of the organization, on September 2, 2014, made a declaration to the UN in order to request that the Member States mobilize to confront the epidemic that risked decimating African populations. She described the situation as a "global coalition of inaction". And added "The clock is ticking and Ebola is winning … The time for meetings and planning is over. It is now time to act. Every day of inaction means more deaths and the slow collapse of societies" (Liu, September 2, 2014).

Isolation, searching for infected individuals and acceptance of intervening medical teams proved to be recurring challenges in almost all of the afflicted regions and countries. Humanitarian aid workers were regularly met with hostility. This was not the first time that MSF teams met strong reluctance among the populations who were afflicted with the disease. Rumors were rampant and fed off of each other in communities that had not only been profoundly impacted by civil war and where abuses had been committed, but also where tenacious, misguided medical practices had previously been imposed upon African populations by "the white" doctors (Lachenal, 2014; Calain & Sa'Da, 2015; Tilley, 2011). In Liberia, one rumor spread concerning how President Sirleaf herself might have been responsible for unleashing the virus in her country in order to attract the attention of humanitarian aid. Another rumor depicted foreign public health experts as going to and from districts, commissioned by their governments, to bring back biological samples that would later serve in the development of medication and vaccines for their own benefit, without benefiting local populations in Africa. Worse yet was a rumor claiming that certain public health experts were there to traffic organs.

MSF was finally joined at the end of the summer of 2014 by some Cuban doctors, American Christian NGOs, International Medical Corps and the British organization Save the Children. In an open letter to the Swiss French newspaper *Le Temps* on October 31, 2014, Thomas Nierlé, president of the Swiss section of MSF, and Bruno Jochum, the director-general, demanded that roles be respected. They explained that MSF could not be a substitute for international cooperation between countries of the international community. This letter inscribed itself into the same line of thinking as the mixed reviews of MSF's implication in the chronic under-medicalization of the developing world (Péchayre, 2014).

MSF's way of intervening has met with controversies, both internally (Nierlé, 2015) and within the WHO. Two of the many controversies concerned: (1) the choice made early on by MSF to opt for centrally located Ebola treatment centers, whereas other actors within the response – including inside MSF and at WHO headquarters – would rather favor community care centers or home-based care options (for which both organizations had guidelines, e.g. for the WHO's recommendations: see Kerstiëns & Matthys, 1999; Formenty et al., 2003; Roddy et al., 2007; Formenty, 2014; for MSF: see Sterk, 2008); (2) the choice to use "full" personal protective equipment (PPE). Full PPE was an option strongly favored by MSF field managers. They were operating in a very dangerous phase of the response, facing difficulty in recruiting healthcare givers, and overwhelmed by the magnitude of the epidemic despite their early and powerful commitment. One has to recall that by 2015, 815 healthcare givers had been infected with Ebola virus and two-thirds of them had died (MSF, 2015). Proponents of the "sufficient" PPE, however, suggested that it could be more appropriate in settings where basic protection was already difficult to guarantee and resources were scarce. In addition, accounts abound describing the difficulty of actually delivering compassionate care in these outfits, especially to children (Pallister-Wilkins, 2016; Georges, 2015). The "sufficient" PPE option constituted a middle ground that WHO clinicians and some MSF specialists would have favored. It did not propose second-class protection, unduly exposing healthcare workers to fatal risks. It suggested a modulation of the protection depending on the context, allowing for adaptation, when people had only limited resources to protect themselves (only one pair of boots, long plastic bags instead of full PPE), or when circumstances allowed for faces to be uncovered if standing at a distance, over a fence. However, they had to back off when confronted with the opposition mounted by frightened first-line responders (MacIntyre et al., 2014, 2015). In this context and in order to maintain a reasonable flux of new hires, full PPE was recommended (WHO, 2014c).

As our informants would come to tell us, in different points of the global health system, and contrary to what was said at the beginning of the crisis, there was not so much an issue of a lack of money, but rather of trained personnel. This observation was made at MSF where donations were far from lacking. The organization was in fact facing a shortage of qualified staff members, which was also recounted by other organizations in the field, particularly by the Red Cross (Georges, 2015) and the WHO. We turn now to the position of the international global health workers.

International global health workers on all fronts

First, the involvement of the WHO's personnel at headquarters is especially important to follow in both cases. It once again reveals the somewhat paradoxical position in which the WHO's global health workers have been locked for decades (Hein & Kickbusch, 2010). As one of its top representatives in 2014 explains: "WHO is not traditionally involved in direct patients care activities. Our principal mission is to guarantee international health safety" (Jaberg, 2014). Are they expected to provide technical expertise or are they expected to become the general operational coordinator of health emergencies? Many informants we met at the time were not all in accordance on this subject.

Second, the short experience of the United Nations Mission for Ebola Emergency Response (UNMEER) adds yet another example of the complex international governance schemes that vast transboundary crises like the 2014 Ebola epidemic trigger, even if it constitutes a one shot experience.

WHO representatives: as technical experts or operational coordinators?

The WHO's position in the context of both crises reactivated numerous debates and criticisms. In the case of the flu pandemic, the WHO, in the middle of a dense network that had been up-and-running since the 1950s (McPhail, 2014; Keck, 2010) and assisted by Mexican, American, and European health ministers, quickly took the reins in the central coordination of the pandemic in 2009 and would hold on to them over time. Dr. Keiji Fukuda, a former epidemiologist for the Centers for Disease Control and Prevention and flu specialist, served as one of Margaret Chan's assistant directors-general. Undeniably, there were leadership implications on the chessboard of global health politics (Forster, 2012). Criticized for its alarmism, its lack of foresight in the use of pandemic phases, the ambiguous nature of the definition of a pandemic (Doshi, 2011), its dependence upon certain experts with close ties to pharmaceutical industries, the opacity regarding the nomination of members for expert committees whose responsibility was to enlighten the leadership of the UN agency, the WHO faced non-stop controversies (*British Medical Journal*, 2010; Kamradt-Scott & Lee, 2011; Nerlich & Koteyko, 2012) throughout the duration of the pandemic crisis management (particularly the strategy implemented by the Parliamentary Assembly of the Council of Europe, 2010; WHO, 2010).

As a result of the 2010/11 crisis, the UN organization was summoned to reform itself once again (Sridhar & Gostin, 2011) and was subsequently forced to reduce its personnel. Nine hundred positions were cut back and the WHO budget decreased from $4.54 billion in 2010–2011 to $3.96 billion in 2012–2013. WHO headquarters in Geneva lost almost 200 employees in 2011. The Pandemic and Epidemic Diseases department was affected. Its experts became scarce. The link between the epidemic's mega-alert and this personnel reduction was drawn by numerous observers and by members of the organization itself, seeing it as a "punishment". When Ebola emerged, the organization was in the middle of reforming its structures, its resource allocation procedures and its mandates.

In the first months of 2014, in stark contrast, the WHO was only slightly visible on the media front of the Ebola crisis. For several months, there was no veritable leader to represent the fight against the Ebola virus. The difficulties met on the inside of the WHO itself, and the discord surrounding the best ways to approach the problem, were central to the lack of the WHO's ownership of the problem. Following the criticisms the WHO had endured regarding its handling of the flu pandemic in 2009, the organization seemed to be keeping a "low profile".

The WHO's positioning in this regard meant that the organization found itself once again in the middle of heated debates and difficulties in the context of its management of the Ebola crisis. For some of its members and senior staff, the WHO remained a "technical" organization charged with establishing recommendations so as to clarify global health policies as well as the policies of its Member States. In the context of this mandate, the WHO's role was not one that involved deploying its own resources in an operational capacity in the field. For others, in particular those who came from the ranks of emergency response, the organization's responsibilities involved being in the field, where it could deploy its experts to assist health authorities who were closest to the action. Those who shared this line of thinking were team members who had traditionally been involved in interventionist work throughout the world; they had been deployed for natural or industrial disasters, or were experts who had been in charge of large disease eradication programs, such as for polio and malaria. As one of our informants would summarize it: "Two cultures were clashing". On one side, there were the disease specialists who occupied positions concerning a specific *disease focal point* (flu, plague, Ebola). They were experts on the surveillance and the evaluation of the epidemiological risks of these diseases. On the other side, there were experts in force deployment in the field who were used to intervening in mass health efforts and programs.

In this context, an opinion piece published at the beginning of the autumn of 2014 in the *New England Journal of Medicine* from the director of the Pandemic and Epidemic Diseases department allows us to identify some of her colleagues who were working on the fight against the Ebola epidemic (Briand et al., 2014). A little while after this, some of the faces of the highest-ranking officials in charge of the response would come to be better known by the general public.

In the spring of 2014, the provisions of the internal WHO Emergency Response Framework, created in 2013, fell sequentially into place in order to manage the Ebola epidemic. It allows the various levels of the organization to be called upon to pull resources when a crisis exceeds a country's capabilities. Grade 2 of this instrument deployed different forces from the Pandemic and Epidemic Diseases department, but not only. These forces were also able to find support from the GOARN initiatives, which were operating in concert with the various countries and the regional WHO office, AFRO. Then in July 2014, a political and diplomatic path was attempted at the regional level with the proposal of the SEOCC (Sub-regional Ebola Operations and Coordination Centre) solution. It was only in August 2014 that the WHO, in the person of Bruce Aylward, and by implication the WHO director-general and three of her assistant directors-general, drafted up the "Ebola roadmap" (WHO, 2014a). At this date, the WHO Pandemic and Epidemic Diseases department would come to join forces with the Health Emergencies department. This "roadmap" was continually and incessantly revamped and updated in order to accommodate and cover the immense needs that changed on both a daily and weekly basis (WHO, 2014b).

In March 2014, the Global Outbreak and Response Network (GOARN) was beginning to deploy twenty people when the internal organization of the WHO was placed on a Grade 2 emergency. Then, when the warning became "international" – still acting in line with the internal Emergency Response Framework of the WHO – GOARN deployed fifty people. During the second call in June 2014, 100 people were deployed. Grade 3 emergency was attained on July 26, 2014, once the response became regional and implicated all three countries at the same time via the regional coordination structure SEOCC. At this time, GOARN deployed 250 people into the field. In May 2015, 1100 people had been deployed and were active at seventy-three different sites. Since the beginning of the crisis, GOARN had deployed a total of 2000 people.

The "Ebola roadmap" was a work in progress and was rewritten as the news became more and more alarming. The concerned African countries did not really have an emergency public health plan. There were so many other public health emergencies in these countries that Ebola was not, and never had been, a priority. It was thought that GOARN would do the job, like it did in previous Ebola outbreaks. Putting Ebola onto the entire world's agenda turned into an ongoing battle (WHO, 2015a, 2015b). The important actors and the major donors did not tilt in the "right" direction regarding their preoccupations, which came to translate into financial and personnel assistance being granted (or not). The official version of the 2014 situation was as follows: mobilization efforts had experienced organizational difficulties, which could mainly be explained for financial reasons, lack of expert staff and manpower. Other criticisms arose and suggested that it was in the heart of the WHO machine that resources had not been allocated in a timely fashion, nor properly disbursed (Grépin, 2015; UNMEER, 2015).

In December 2014, our informants confided to us, the "work plans" of the different sections, divisions and departments, in charge of a different piece of the international response, had still not been approved officially by higher ranks in the hierarchy. What was missing for the financial backers, accountants and human resources managers in order to approve the work programs of their colleagues and experts, who were responsible, for example, for "clinical management", "clinical training" and "contact tracing"? In the decisive months at the end of 2014, why did the different components of the Ebola response team, orchestrated from WHO headquarters, appear to find it difficult to coordinate and be on the same page?

Political pressures were important as well as uncertainty on the best strategy to choose. Controversies inside the ranks of the WHO, as well as outside, like inside MSF, developed and can be attributed to the great challenges faced by responders. Indecisiveness played a role, as well as the great difficulty in disposing of a safe place to exchange and work on trade-offs. As we came to realize throughout our study, managing outbreaks, no matter their size, scope, complexity or lethality, is plagued with resistances and pre-formatted conventional wisdoms at all levels. There was no rationality at the WHO level, and irrational fears on African soil. There was in fact great difficulty in formulating a blueprint for a "back to basics" strategy that would build something from the situation, bottom-up, and not top-down, superimposing external public health interventions that were known for decades to create resistance in the populations. This does not mean that no help should have been offered. But as many anthropologists and experts have said on numerous occasions, the outbreak response should be designed in accordance with and based on existing knowledge. As Hewlett and Hewlett wrote ten years ago:

> Interventions teams should view local people as allies rather than as enemies in epidemic control efforts ... Although some behaviors need modification, local people are ready and willing to help where

possible. Local people can contribute to disease surveillance … as well assisting health education and social mobilization among family and neighbors.

(Hewlett & Hewlett, 2008, 115)

When UNMEER *intervenes*

In September 2014, in the context of open and political contention regarding the WHO's coordination capacities and facing the fact that the crisis had "become multidimensional with significant political, social, economic, humanitarian, logistical, and security dimensions" – to borrow the terms used by the secretary-general of the United Nations – as well as the impossibility of containing contamination zones, the United Nations sought to coordinate their action and to create a new actor on the global chessboard. This was the first pandemic that gave rise to a Security Council Resolution (Security Council Resolution 2177, September 18, 2014). This is how UNMEER, the first multi-agency mission of the UN (established on September 19, 2014 and closed on July 31, 2015) was created. Based in Accra in Ghana, UNMEER was responsible for coordinating the UN agencies' actions in the battle against Ebola. These were WHO actions, of course, but also those of the World Food Programme, the World Bank, UNICEF, the International Monetary Fund, the UN Development Programme (UNDP), the UN Population Fund, the UN Office for the Coordination of Humanitarian Affairs (OCHA) and the International Organization for Migration. The secretary-general appointed David Nabarro as the special envoy on Ebola, and he named Anthony Banbury as his special representative and head of UNMEER.

Little has been written since then about the role of UNMEER (Garrett, 2015; Benton & Dionne, 2015). Our informants, mainly in the ranks of the WHO and of MSF, painted a contrasting picture of the situation. For many of them, there is no doubt that this institutional creation is the fruit of the WHO having been discredited through its actions in the first months of the crisis. It is the symptom of the non-use of the global health cluster that should have been activated, but which was not, during the Ebola response. The senior experts of the WHO openly criticized this "layer of supplementary bureaucracy", on which the personnel was "entirely" dependent for the information and expertise of the WHO. Other actors, particularly in the embassies in Geneva, provided a different, more forgiving, discourse and indicated the aid offered by UNMEER had been of the utmost importance in order to unify the UN areas of action in these countries.

In the autumn of 2014, a plan for specialization by function, by institution and by country was drawn up. The "Nabarro plan" proposed a division in two phases: a redistribution of the pillars of the response and a territorialization of different operations. Thus, according to the first part of the plan's objectives, the various forces were organized as follows:

(1) UNICEF was entrusted with "community engagement" and "risk communication" in the response; (2) the various Red Cross organizations, aided by the International Red Cross and thanks to a vast knowledge transfer from MSF and WHO teams, were given the responsibility of overseeing safe and dignified burials; (3) the World Food Programme was to take over the dispatching of food supplies, particularly in communities where quarantines had been instituted; (4) the World Bank was to act as the grand financier of programs; (5) the American CDC would coordinate with German laboratories and the European Union in order to look for contacts and to establish 157 laboratories where samples from the sick could quickly be tested; (6) finally, the WHO was to be in charge of the coordination of operations on the ground. This role was so difficult that many in the field recounted an incredible paralysis of WHO deployees on the ground. As one of our informants pointed out, "It's difficult to coordinate so many people who especially do not want to be coordinated". As Nabarro would himself say afterwards: leadership is important as well as "followship" (WHO, 2015c).

However, the partition of these tasks is to be taken with a certain prudence, because, in the details, many organizations have declared in their activity and feedback reports that their interventions were hybrid in nature. On top of the specialization by pillar and by institution, a sharing of geographic zones was put into place. As such, the United Kingdom helped more particularly Sierra Leone, France focused on Guinea, and the United States concentrated on Liberia. The former colonial spheres of influence seem to have reappeared and delegated their action to their armies, hereby espousing the tendency towards the militarization of public health operations, called *global health security*, not to mention the troubling postcolonial influence in all of these schemes.

Abnormal or expected crises of the global health system?

This comparison between both crises leaves open the following questions: are we facing the repeated failures of an international system to fight epidemics, serving as a tangible embodiment of global health, which is insufficiently organized, lacking power, and ill equipped and whose gaps need to be filled (Moon et al., 2017)? Or, rather, are we facing abnormal crises that it would be futile to try to manage, because they are so extraordinary that learning from them, although important will not help us fight the next big crisis, mainly because it will appear very differently? Are we facing a "failure of administrative imagination", in Lakoff's words (2017), and particularly are we all trapped in a fatal illusion to conceive of the possible coordination of global health crises via the intermediary of the WHO (and several large partners) at the center? This analytic error has repeatedly provoked criticism and frustration when facing expectations that are as unrealistic as they are unfounded and which consistently faults medical personnel at local, national and central levels. This is true for the 2009 A(H1N1) pandemic as well as for the 2014 Ebola epidemic. This chapter demonstrates that each crisis has been dealt with using prior knowledge, pre-conception, established yet debated doctrines from all parts. Consequently, reenforcing command and control, leadership and fellowship, providing for better ways to coordinate are certainly important tasks on the agenda. However, in the light of both narratives, establishing a common understanding of ethically acceptable modes of intervention, organizing some mechanisms where distributed knowledge and local expertise are captured efficiently, seems to be more pressing.

Notes

1 On one occasion, invited as an observer to a consultation aiming at determining the composition of the vaccine for the southern hemisphere in September 2014, at the WHO headquarters, we witnessed the tribute paid to one of these stars, Dr. Nancy Cox, Director of the Influenza Division in the National Center for Immunization and Respiratory Diseases (NCIRD), retiring from CDC after more than thirty years of service.
2 According to CDC, six countries are concerned: Bangladesh, China, Egypt, India, Indonesia and Vietnam). www.cdc.gov/flu/avianflu/h5n1-animals.htm.
3 Disagreements over the issue underline that it would not be correct to say that the virus never spread into an urban context. In 1995, the Ebola virus spread to a hospital in Kikwit, a city of the Democratic Republic of Congo with around 400,000 inhabitants.
4 We can ascertain this just as much by looking at the following extract from Preston's 1994 book, *The Hot Zone: The Terrifying True Story of the Origins of the Ebola Virus*, a new edition of which was published in 2014, wherein Preston provided his readers with vivid imagery of the disease for the last twenty years:

> The Ebola in Sudan wiped out several hundred people in central Africa in the same fashion that a fire consumes a pile of straw. When the flames had burned everything up, there remained only a heap of ashes. The virus, in its Sudanese incarnation, had retreated into the heart of the bush, where it continues to live in the present day, circulating indefinitely between unknown hosts, able to modify itself, potentially with the capability of penetrating the human species in a new form.
>
> (Preston, 2014 [1994], 101)

5 My translation from the original text, which was in French.
6 The United States' 1976 experience with swine flu, when 40 million Americans were vaccinated for the new strain, and the pandemic never showed up, may also have played a role in encouraging caution. In addition, at the time dozens of cases of Guillain–Barré syndrome had occurred and prompted lasting distrust in public health decision-making processes (Fineberg & Neustadt, 1978; Saluzzo, 2011).
7 The reported vaccination coverage varied between countries from 0.4 percent to 59 percent for the entire population (22 countries); 3 percent to 68 percent for healthcare workers (13 countries); 0 percent to 58 percent for pregnant women (12 countries); 0.2 percent to 74 percent for children (12 countries).
8 For details on GOARN, see Ansell et al. (2012).

9 In May 2017, when the Democratic Republic of Congo was affected by an Ebola epidemic, a vaccine trial was quickly established. Designed and tested in Guinea in 2015 by MSF (and Epicentre, the Paris-based research team of Doctors Without Borders) and the WHO, the vaccine made by Merck and stored in the United States, has not yet been licensed, and can only be used as part of a clinical trial.

10 The Womey massacre is about a deadly attack on and murder of eight members of a team of healthcare workers, journalists, and government officials who were affiliated with the conflict resolution non-profit Search for Common Ground. In mid-September 2014, they traveled to the Village of Womey in Guinea's southwest region to educate the locate population during the West African Ebola virus epidemic outbreak. The team had come to warn the village about dangers of the Ebola virus disease. The bodies were found in a latrine with evidence of being struck with clubs and machetes, and three were found with their throats slit.

11 In the end, compared to other countries both in the northern and in the southern hemisphere, Japan fared well with a mortality rate, per million population (directly attributable to pandemic influenza A (H1N1) virus infections) of 0.16 compared with 1.32 for Canada, 1.05 for Mexico or 3.3, for the United States (Source: Ministry of Health, Labor and Welfare, Japan).

References

Abeysinghe, S. (2013). When the spread of disease becomes a global event: The classification of pandemics. *Social Studies of Science*, 43*(6)*, 905–926.

Abramowitz, S. (2017). Epidemics (especially Ebola). *Annual Review of Anthropology*, 46, 421–445.

Anoko, J., Epelboin, A., & Formenty, P. (2014). Humanisation de la réponse à la Fièvre Hémorragique Ebola en Guinée: approche anthropologique (Conakry/Guéckédou mars-juillet 2014).

Ansell, C., Sondorp, E., & Stevens, R. H. (2012). The promise and challenge of global network governance: The Global Outbreak Alert and Response Network. *Global Governance: A Review of Multilateralism and International Organizations*, 18*(3)*, 317–337.

Aranzazu, A. (2013). Le réseau mondial de surveillance de la grippe de l'OMS. Modalités de circulation des souches virales, des savoirs et des techniques, 1947–2007. *Sciences sociales et santé*, 31*(4)*, 41–64.

Aranzazu, A. (2016). Surveillance de la grippe d'origine animale à l'OMS. *Revue d'anthropologie des connaissances*, 10*(1)*, 71–93.

ASTHO (Association of State and Territorial Health Officers, US). (2010). www.astho.org/Programs/Infectious-Disease/H1N1/H1N1-Barriers-Project-Report-Final-hi-res/. "NACCHO H1N1 Policy Workshop Report". Minneapolis, MN: NACCHO, 5.05 2010. www.naccho.org/topics/h1n1/upload/naccho-workshop-report-in-template-with-chart.pdf.

Baekkeskov, E. (2016). Same threat, different responses: Experts steering politicians and stakeholders in 2009 H1N1 vaccination policy-making. *Public Administration*, 94*(2)*, 299–315.

Barrelet, C., Bourrier, M., Burton-Jeangros, C., & Schindler, M. (2013). Unresolved issues in risk communication research: The case of the H1N1 pandemic (2009–2011). *Influenza and Other Respiratory Viruses*, 7*(suppl. 2)*, 1–6.

Bastide, L. (2017). Future now: "Preparedness" and scenario planning in the United States. *Institute of Sociological Research, University of Geneva, Working Paper 12.*

Bausch, D. G., Feldmann, H., Geisbert, T. W., Bray, M., Sprecher, A. G., Boumandouki, P., ... & Winnipeg Filovirus Clinical Working Group. (2007). Outbreaks of filovirus hemorrhagic fever: Time to refocus on the patient. *The Journal of Infectious Diseases,* 196*(suppl. 2),* S136–S141.

Benton, A., & Dionne, K. Y. (2015). International Political Economy and the 2014 West African Ebola outbreak. *African Studies Review,* 58*(1),* 223–236.

Boin, A., Lagadec, P., Michel-Kerjan, E., & Overdijk, W. (2003). Critical infrastructures under threat: Learning from the anthrax scare. *Journal of Contingencies and Crisis Management,* 11*(3),* 99–104.

Boumandouki, P., Formenty, P., Epelboin, A., Campbell, P., Atsangandoko, C., Allarangar, Y., ... & Salemo, A. (2005). Prise en charge des malades et des défunts lors de l'épidémie de fièvre hémorragique due au virus Ebola d'octobre à décembre 2003 au Congo. *Bulletin de la Société de Pathologie Exotique,* 98*(3),* 218–223.

Brammer, L., Blanton, L., Epperson, S., Mustaquim, D., Bishop, A., Kniss, K., ... & Finelli, L. (2011). Surveillance for influenza during the 2009 influenza A (H1N1) pandemic: United States, April 2009–March 2010. *Clinical Infectious Diseases,* 52*(suppl. 1),* S27–S35.

Brender, N. (2014). *Global Risk Governance in Health.* Basingstoke: Palgrave Macmillan.

Brender, N., & Gilbert, C. (2018). From emergence to emergences: A focus on pandemic influenza (pp. 35–57), in Morand, S., & Figuié, M. (eds), *Emergence of Infectious Diseases: Risks and Issues for Societies.* Versailles: E-editions Quae.

Briand, S., Bertherat, E., Cox, P., Formenty, P., Kieny, M. P., Myhre, J. K., ... & Dye, C. (2014). The international Ebola emergency. *New England Journal of Medicine,* 371*(13),* 1180–1183.

Brien, S., Kwong, J., & Buckeridge, D. (2012). The determinants of 2009 pandemic A(H1N1) influenza vaccination: A systematic review. *Vaccine,* 30, 1255–1264.

British Medical Journal (2010). Editorial: Conflicts of interest and pandemic flu. 340, c2947.

Brunnquell, F., Epelboin, A., & Formenty, P. (2007). *Ebola: No Laughing matter/ Ebola: Ce n'est pas une maladie pour rire.* DVD, Capa Télévisions.

Burton-Jeangros, C., Golay, M., & Sudre, P. (2005). Adhésion et résistance aux vaccinations infantiles, une étude auprès de mères suisses. *Revue d'épidémiologie et de santé publique,* 53, 341–350.

Caduff, C. (2014). Pandemic prophecy, or how to have faith in reason. *Current Anthropology,* 55(3), 296–315.

Calain, P., & Sa'Da, C. A. (2015). Coincident polio and Ebola crises expose similar fault lines in the current global health regime. *Conflict and Health,* 9*(1),* 1–7.

Casaer, P. (2015). *Film Affliction.* MSF.

CDC. (2015). *The Road to Zero, CDC's Response to the West African Ebola Epidemic, 2014–2015.* US Department of Health and Human Services, July.

Collier, S. J., & Lakoff, A. (2008). Distributed preparedness: The spatial logic of domestic security in the United States. *Environment and Planning. D, Society & Space,* 26*(1),* 7.

Council of Europe. (2010). The handling of the H1N1 pandemic: More transparency needed. Verbatim report of the June 24, 2010, Council of Europe Ordinary Session.

Dehner, G. (2012). *Influenza: A Century of Science and Public Health Response*. Pittsburgh, PA: University of Pittsburgh Press.

Delaporte, E., Iten, A., & Sudre, P. (2010). Bilan épidémiologique de la grippe pandémique (H1N1) 2009 à Genève. Direction Générale de la Santé, Geneva, October.

Door, J.-P., & Blandin, M.-C. (2010). La gestion des pandémies: H1N1, et si c'était à refaire? Compte rendu de l'audition du 14 juin 2010. Rapport de l'Office Parlementaire d'Evaluation des Choix Scientifiques et Technologiques. Paris: Sénat. www.senat.fr/rap/r09-651/r09-6511.pdf.

Doshi, P. (2011). The elusive definition of pandemic influenza. *Bulletin of the World Health Organization, 89(7)*, 532–538.

Epelboin, A., Formenty, P., Anoko, J., & Allarangar, Y. (2007). Humanisation and informed consent for people and populations during responses to VHF in Central Africa (2003–2008). *Humanitarian Borders*, 25–37.

Epelboin, A., Formenty, P., Anoko, J., & Allarangar, Y. (2008). Humanisations et consentements éclairés des personnes et des populations lors des réponses aux épidémies de FHV en Afrique centrale (2003–2008). Mesures de contrôle des infections et droits individuels: Un dilemme éthique pour le personnel médical. *Humanitarian Stakes*, 1, 25–37.

Epstein, H. (2014). Ebola in Liberia: An epidemic of rumors. *New York Review of Books, 61(20)*, 91–94.

Ernst & Young. (2010). Grippe pandémique H1N1 evaluation de l'organisation et des processus de l'OFSP. Office Fédéral Suisse Santé Publique.

European Commission. (2010). Assessment report on the EU-wide response to pandemic (H1N1) 2009 covering the period 24 April–31 August 2009 (excluding vaccine policy issues). http://ec.europa.eu/health/communicable_diseases/docs/assessment_response_en.pdf.

Evans, N. G., Smith, T., & Majumber, M. (2016). *Ebola's Message: Public Health and Medicine in the Twenty-first Century*. Cambridge, MA: MIT Press.

Fairhead, J. (2016). Understanding social resistance to the Ebola response in the forest region of the Republic of Guinea: An anthropological perspective. *African Studies Review, 59(3)*, 7–31.

Faye, S. L. (2015). L'"exceptionnalité" d'Ebola et les "réticences" populaires en Guinée-Conakry. Réflexions à partir d'une approche d'anthropologie symétrique. *Anthropologie & santé. Revue internationale francophone d'anthropologie de la santé*, 11.

Fineberg, H. V., & Neustadt, R. E. (1978). *The Swine Flu Affair: Decision-making on a Slippery Disease*. US Department of Health, Education, and Welfare.

Flahault, A., & Zylberman, P. (2010). Influenza pandemics: Past, present and future challenges. *Public Health Reviews, 32(1)*, 319–340.

Formenty, P. (2014). Stratégie Ebola. Flambées épidémiques de maladie à virus Ebola et Marburg: Préparation, alerte et évaluation. Août 2014. WHO/HSE/PED/CED/2014.05.

Formenty, P., Libama, F., Epelboin, A., Allarangar, Y., Leroy, E., Moudzeo, H., ... & Hewlett, B. (2003). L'épidémie de fièvre hémorragique à virus Ebola en République du Congo, 2003: Une nouvelle stratégie. *Méd trop*, 63, 291–295.

Forster, P. (2012). To pandemic or not? Reconfiguring global responses to influenza. Working Paper 51. Brighton: Steps Center.

Fraser, C., Donnelly, C. A., Cauchemez, S., Hanage, W. P., Van Kerkhove, M. D., Hollingsworth, T. D., & Roth, C. (2009). Pandemic potential of a strain of influenza A (H1N1): Early findings. *Science, 324(5934)*, 1557–1561.

Fribault, M. (2015). Ebola en Guinée: Violences historiques et régimes de doute. *Anthropologie & santé. Revue internationale francophone d'anthropologie de la santé*, 11.

Garrett, L. (2005). *The Next Pandemic?* Council on Foreign Relations.

Garrett, L. (2015). Ebola's lessons: How the WHO mishandled the crisis. *Foreign Affairs*, 94(5), 80–107.

Georges, N. (2015). *Six semaines dans un centre de traitement Ebola: À Macenta, Guinée forestière*. Nantes: Éditions Amalthée.

Greco, D., Stern, E. K., & Marks, G. (2011). Review of ECDC's response to the influenza pandemic 2009–2010. Stockholm: ECDC. www.ecdc.europa.eu/en/aboutus/key%20documents/241111cor_pandemic_response.pdf.

Grépin, K. (2015). Analysis: International donations to the Ebola virus outbreak: Too little, too late? *British Medical Journal*, 350, h376.

Haas, P. (1992). Introduction: Epistemic communities and international policy coordination. *International Organization*, 46(1), 1–35.

Hein, W., & Kickbusch, I. (2010). Global health, aid effectiveness and the changing role of the WHO. *GIGA Focus International Edition English*, 3.

Hewlett, B. S., & Hewlett, B. L. (2008). *Ebola, Culture and Politics: The Anthropology of an Emerging Disease*. Belmont, CA: Cengage Learning.

Hewlett, B. S., Epelboin, A., Hewlett. B. L., & Formenty, P. (2005). Medical anthropology and Ebola in Congo: Cultural models and humanistic care, *Bulletin de la Société de pathologie exotique*, 98, 230–236.

Hofman, M., & Au, S. (eds). (2017). *The Politics of Fear: Médecins Sans Frontières and the West African Ebola Epidemic*. Oxford: Oxford University Press.

Horton, R. (2014). Offline: The case against global health. *The Lancet*, 383, May 17.

Jaberg, S. (2014). Les virus tels qu'Ebola sont le grand défi sanitaire du 21e siècle. SwissInfo.ch, October 17.

Johnson, N. P. A. S., & Mueller, J. (2002). Updating the accounts: Global mortality of the 1918–1920 "Spanish" influenza pandemic. *Bulletin of the History of Medicine*, 76(1), 105–115.

Kamradt-Scott, A. & Lee, K. (2011). The 2011 pandemic influenza preparedness framework: Global health secured or a missed opportunity? *Political Studies*, 59(4), 831–847.

Kawaguchi, R., Miyazono, M., Noda, T., Takayama, Y., Sasai, Y., & Iso, H. (2009). Influenza (H1N1) 2009 outbreak and school closure, Osaka Prefecture, Japan. *Emerging Infectious Diseases*, 15(10), 1685–1685.

Keck, F. (2010). *Un monde grippé*. Paris: Flammarion.

Keller, A. C., Ansell, C. K., Reingold, A. L., Bourrier, M., Hunter, M. D., Burrowes, S., & MacPhail, T. M. (2012). Improving pandemic response: A sensemaking perspective on the spring 2009 H1N1 pandemic. *Risk, Hazards & Crisis in Public Policy*, 3(2), 1–37.

Kerstiëns, B., & Matthys, F. (1999). Interventions to control virus transmission during an outbreak of Ebola hemorrhagic fever: Experience from Kikwit, Democratic Republic of the Congo, 1995. *The Journal of Infectious Diseases*, 179(Suppl. 1), S263–S267.

Kidjo, A. (2014). Don't let Ebola dehumanize Africa. *New York Times*, October 31.

Kolata, G. (1999). *Flu: The Story of the Great Influenza Pandemic of 1918 and the Search for the Virus That Caused It*. New York, NY: Farrar, Straus & Giroux/Macmillan.

Lachenal, G. (2014). *Le médicament qui devait sauver l'Afrique: Un scandale pharmaceutique aux colonies*. Paris: La Découverte.

Lakoff, A. (2017). *Unprepared: Global Health in a Time of Emergency.* Oakland, CA: University of California Press.

Lall, R. (2017). Beyond institutional design: Explaining the performance of international organizations. *International Organization*, 71*(2)*, 245–280.

Le Marcis, F. (2015). Traiter les corps comme des fagots. Production sociale de l'indifférence en contexte Ebola (Guinée). *Anthropologie & santé. Revue internationale francophone d'anthropologie de la santé*, 11.

Lempen, B. (2010). *Genève, laboratoire du XXIe siècle.* Geneva: Georg Editeur.

Lister, S. A., & Redhead, C. S. (2009). The 2009 influenza pandemic: An overview. Congressional Research Service. http://oai.dtic.mil/oai/oai?verb=getRecord& metadataPrefix=html&identifier=ADA510981.

Liu, J. (2014). www.youtube.com/watch?v=niehJb220nY.

MacIntyre, C. R., Chughtai, A. A., Seale, H., Richards, G. A., & Davidson, P. M. (2014). Respiratory protection for healthcare workers treating Ebola virus disease (EVD): Are facemasks sufficient to meet occupational health and safety obligations? *International Journal of Nursing Studies*, 51*(11)*, 1421–1426.

MacIntyre, C. R., Chughtai, A. A., Seale, H., Richards, G. A., & Davidson, P. M. (2015). Uncertainty, risk analysis and change for Ebola personal protective equipment guidelines. *International Journal of Nursing Studies*, 52*(5)*, 899–903.

MacPhail, T. (2014). *The Viral Network: A Pathography of the H1N1 Influenza Pandemic.* Ithaca, NY: Cornell University Press.

Médecins Sans Frontières. (2015). Pushed to the limit and beyond, a year into the largest ever Ebola outbreak. International website of Médecins Sans Frontières. www.msf.org/en/article/ebola-pushed-limit-and-beyond.

Mereckiene, J., Cotter, S., Weber, J. T., Nicoll, A., D'Ancona, F., Lopalco, P. L., ... & Giambi, C. (2012). Influenza A (H1N1) pdm09 vaccination policies and coverage in Europe. *Euro Surveillance*, 17*(4)*.

Moon, S., Leigh, J., Woskie, L., Checchi, F., Dzau, V., Fallah, M., ... & Katz, R. (2017). Post-Ebola reforms: Ample analysis, inadequate action. *BMJ: British Medical Journal* (Online), 356.

Moulin, A.-M. (2015). L'anthropologie au défi de l'Ebola. *Anthropologie & Santé*, 11.

Nerlich, B., & Koteyko, K. (2012). Crying wolf? Biosecurity and metacommunication in the context of the 2009 swine flu pandemic, *Health and Place*, 18, 710–717.

Nicoll, A., Brown, C., Karcher, F., Penttinen, P., Hegermann-Lindencrone, M., Villanueva, S., ... & Nguyen-Van-Tam, J. S. (2012). Developing pandemic preparedness in Europe in the 21st century: Experience, evolution and next steps. *Bulletin of the World Health Organization*, 90*(4)*, 311–317.

Nierlé, T. (2015). Ebola: Un défi à notre identité d'humanitaire – une lettre ouverte au mouvement MSF, written by nine members of the Swiss MSF movement in December 2014, published February 3, 2015 in French newspaper *Libération*. www. liberation.fr/terre/2015/02/03/parfois-le-traitement-symptomatique-a-ete-neglige-voire-oublie_1194960.

Nierle, T., & Jochum, B. (2014). Ebola: MSF n'a pas à remplacer les Etats pour gérer la crise. *Le Temps*, October 31.

Pallister-Wilkins, P. (2016). Personal protective equipment in the humanitarian governance of Ebola: Between individual patient care and global biosecurity. *Third World Quarterly*, 37*(3)*, 507–523.

Péchayre, M. (2014). Impartialité et pratiques de triage en milieu humanitaire. Le cas de Médecins Sans Frontières au Pakistan. *Les Cahiers du Centre Georges Canguilhem*, 125–142.

President's Council of Advisors on Science and Technology. (2009). Report to the President on US preparation for 2009 – H1N1 influenza. President's Council of Advisors on Science and Technology, August 7. www.whitehouse.gov/assets/documents/PCAST_H1N1_Report.pdf.

Preston, R. (1994, 2014). *Ebola, les origines*. Paris: Presses de la cité.

Richards, P. (2016). *Ebola: How a People's Science Helped End an Epidemic*. London: Zed Books.

Roddy, P., Weatherill, D., Jeffs, B., Abaakouk, Z., Dorion, C., Rodriguez-Martinez, J., ... & Borchert, M. (2007). The Medecins Sans Frontieres intervention in the Marburg hemorrhagic fever epidemic, Uige, Angola, 2005. II. Lessons learned in the community. *The Journal of Infectious Diseases*, 196*(Suppl. 2)*, S162–S167.

Saluzzo, J.-F. (2011). *La saga des vaccins, contre les virus*. Paris: Belin.

Schindler, M., Blanchard-Rohner, G., Meier, S., de Tejada, B. M., Siegrist, C. A., & Burton-Jeangros, C. (2012). Vaccination against seasonal flu in Switzerland: The indecision of pregnant women encouraged by healthcare professionals. *Revue d'épidémiologie et de santé publique*, 60*(6)*, 447–453.

Sridhar, D., & Gostin, L. O. (2011). Reforming the world health organization. *Jama*, 305(15), 1585–1586.

Sridhar, D., Frenk, J., Gostin, L., & Moon, S. (2014). Global rules for global health: why we need an independent, impartial WHO. *BMJ*, 348. doi: https://doi.org/10.1136/bmj.g3841.

Sterk, E. (2008). *Filovirus Haemorrhagic Fever Guideline*. Médecins Sans Frontières.

Taubenberger, J. K., & Morens, D. M. (2006). 1918 Influenza: The mother of all pandemics. *Emerging Infectious Diseases*, 12*(1)*, 15–22.

Tilley, H. (2011). *Africa as a "Living Laboratory": Empire, Development and the Problem of Scientific Knowledge, 1870–1950*. Chicago, IL: University of Chicago Press.

UNMEER. (2015). *Report. Global Ebola Response: Making a Difference*. Outlook 2015. January.

US Department of Health and Human Services. (2012). An HHS retrospective on the 2009 H1N1 influenza pandemic to advance all hazards preparedness. US Department of Health and Human Services, June 15, 2012. www.phe.gov/Preparedness/mcm/h1n1-retrospective/Documents/h1n1-retrospective.pdf.

Wald, P. (2008). *Contagious: Cultures, Carriers, and the Outbreak Narrative*. Durham, NC: Duke University Press.

WHO. (2010). The international response to the influenza pandemic: WHO responds to the critics. www.who.int/csr/disease/swineflu/notes/briefing_20100610/en/.

WHO. (2011). Report by the director-general. Implementation of the international health regulation (2005): Report of the review committee on the functioning of the international health regulations (2005) in relation to pandemic (H1N1) 2009. WHO, May 5, 2011. www.srmuniv.ac.in/downloads/ihr_global_public_health_emergency.pdf.

WHO. (2014a). *Ebola Response Roadmap*. August 28.

WHO. (2014b). *Strategic Action Plan for Ebola Outbreak Response*. July–December.

WHO. (2014c). WHO_EVD_Guidance_PPE_14.1_fre.pdf.

WHO. (2015a). *Current Context and Challenges: Stopping the Epidemic; and Preparedness in Non-affected Countries and Regions*. Report by the Secretariat for the Executive

Board, Special Session on Ebola Provisional agenda Item 3, EB 136/26, January 9.

WHO. (2015b). *Response in Severe, Large-scale Emergencies*. Report to the Director-General, 68th World Health Assembly, Provisional agenda Item 15.4, A68/23, May 15.

WHO. (2015c). WHO informal consultation "Anticipating emerging infectious disease epidemics". Meeting Report, December 1–2, 2015, Geneva.

WHO. (2016). Ebola situation report – June 10 2016. http://apps. who. int/iris/ bitstream/10665/208883/1/ebolasitrep_10Jun2016_eng. pdf.

WHO-Regional Office Europe. (2010). Report of the annual WHO European Regional Influenza Surveillance Meeting (Brasov, Romania, September 21–23 2010).

Wilkinson, A., & Leach, M. (2015). Briefing: Ebola–myths, realities, and structural violence. *African Affairs*, 114*(454)*, 136–148.

Wilson, K. (2011). Revisiting influenza deaths estimates: Learning from the H1N1 pandemic. *The European Journal of Public Health*, ckr142.

Wolz, A. (2014). Face to face with Ebola: An emergency care center in Sierra Leone. *New England Journal of Medicine*, 371*(12)*, 1081–1083.

Zylberman, P. (2013). *Tempêtes microbiennes: Essai sur la politique de sécurité sanitaire dans le monde transatlantique*. Paris: Gallimard.

4 Epidemics and risk communication

Why are lessons not learned?

Claudine Burton-Jeangros

Introduction

Addressing another area of controversies associated with global health responses to re-emerging infectious diseases, this chapter is dedicated to the gap existing between risk communication guidelines and actual practices of front-line risk communicators. This component of the response refers to the efforts developed to bridge between the technical response put in place by public health institutions and society at large. The persisting co-existence of diverging views on risks and hence on the proper ways to manage them have modelled risk communication efforts over the last decades. While norms and guidelines of the field have progressively taken into account the large array of social factors affecting communication between different groups of concerned people, this chapter will show how actual practices struggle to take into consideration the knowledge gained in social sciences.

Before moving to the analysis of the risk communication practices developed by front-line risk communicators in the context of the A(H1N1) pandemic and the 2014 Ebola outbreak, recent developments in risk communication should first be situated against the larger background that have shaped responses to epidemics. First, both institutional and public reactions to recent epidemic episodes have been affected by globalization, understood as a process extending far beyond economics (Giddens, 1990). On one hand, global preoccupations towards epidemics reflect a new sense of biological vulnerability, propagated by national and transnational bodies and extended to the whole world through the biosecurity framework (Lakoff & Collier, 2008). Simultaneously, globalization is accompanied by massive developments in communication technologies and the "viral power of communication" (Nerlich & Koteyko, 2012, p. 711) contributes to exacerbate the global awareness of any emerging outbreak. Second, public health action has been progressively guided by alternatives to the risk governance framework, including precautionary and preparedness approaches that not only extend the scope for action but call for early international action on emerging threats (Lakoff, 2017). Third, global health responses are supported by scientific evidence and biomedical measures that typically value individual responsibility towards health while downplaying the importance of social, cultural and economic contexts of risk (Joffe, 1999).

Nowadays, risk communication occupies a central role in the tools put in place to anticipate epidemics. Since major global health agencies had developed risk communication guidelines over the last decades, the A(H1N1) pandemic in 2009–2010 and the 2014 Ebola outbreak both offered concrete opportunities to apply risk communication guidance. This chapter aims at examining how risk communication practices have been challenged by the unfolding events associated with A(H1N1) and the 2014 Ebola outbreak. While agencies had previously strived to develop universal principles and standardized tools to communicate adequately in risk situations, our analyses will show that recurrent difficulties reflect the crucial but underappreciated importance of non-technical matters in responses provided to re-emerging infectious diseases. These matters include, among others, power relationships within and across organizations as well as cultural variations in reactions towards adverse situations.

This contribution, which is part of the project "Unraveling lessons learned from A(H1N1) pandemic to the 2014 Ebola Epidemic", proposes analyses combining social science literature on risk communication, official documents produced by the World Health Organization (WHO) and the US and Swiss national public health agencies as well as data collected through the participation in meetings and interviews with public health professionals engaged in risk communication activities in those settings (see Introduction for more details on the methodology).

The ambitions of risk communication

Risk communication emerged as a specialized field in the 1980s. Building upon the knowledge gained in risk perception research, it is meant to bridge technical risk assessment and social reactions to hazards and crises. While psychologists showed recurrent variations in estimations about the future, along a range of factors affecting the way people perceive risks (Slovic, 2000), social science scholars emphasized that social mechanisms affect the acceptability of risk for different groups (Douglas, 1985; Short, 1984). Taking stock of the idea that technical risk management is insufficient to generate consensus across society, risk communication was thus designed to reconcile contrasted views and integrate the whole society in the process of risk management (Renn, 2008).

Models of risk communication evolved over the last decades, taking into account larger transformations in the relationship between the scientific arena and society (Krimsky, 2007; Leiss, 1996). In its early days, top-down risk communication focused on experts informing the public about the extent of risks and providing messages on how to adopt proper behaviours to mitigate adverse consequences. This first stage relates to a period when access to scientific and technical knowledge was confined to experts, who could decide which information to provide to audiences then considered as passive (Wilkinson, 1999). This narrow view of communication assumes that experts can actually control the public opinion as long as they provide appropriate messages to the media. More recently, as a result of increasing circulation of information through a range of independent channels and along steady public questioning about the value and independence of science, more attention has been given to alternative views about risk, as formulated among different implicated groups. Risk communication has thus been reconsidered and is currently defined as an interactive process of information exchange between a range of concerned stakeholders (Höppner et al., 2012). This deliberative and participatory perspective opens up to the inclusion of contested knowledge, a trend further reinforced by social media developments (Krimsky, 2007). In that new perspective emphasizing two-way communication, audiences are considered active and potential contributors to risk and crisis management.

One could say that these transformations in risk communication thinking reflect the growing contribution of social sciences to risk management. It expanded from a narrow approach focused on "inadequate" risk perceptions towards a broader discussion on the acceptability of decisions taken around a predicted adverse event, emphasizing the political nature of mitigation responses. They can also be seen as a result of the success of anticipatory forms of action, such as precaution and preparedness that attribute a greater importance to non-technical and expert components of risk management (Anderson, 2010). In the regime of precaution, uncertainty implies acting before complete knowledge is available, thus emphasizing the importance of non-technical criteria such as political arguments or value-laden preferences in decision making. In the regime of preparedness, the implication of non-expert stakeholders responds to the need to mobilize all sectors of society so that adequate responses will be put in place when the crisis occurs (cf. Bastide, Chapter 2). Such complexification of anticipatory action clearly favours a more inclusive approach to risk communication.

Risk communication developments have been particularly important in public health. Starting in the 1970s, health education campaigns aimed at informing at-risk individuals on how to modify their unhealthy behaviours (Renn, 2008). Regulatory agencies developed risk communication to the intention of the general public or workers in specific settings to inform them about their exposure to certain environmental, food or drug risks (Glik, 2007). Failures to communicate appropriately in a range of successive public health crises, including the anthrax episode of September 2001 or hurricane Katrina in 2005, prompted the Centers for Disease Control and Prevention (CDC) in the United States to develop dedicated material. The Crisis and Emergency Risk Communication (CERC) manual, first published in 2002, states that "CERC is the attempt by public health professionals to provide information that allows individuals, stakeholders, and entire communities to make the best possible decisions for their well-being during a crisis or emergency" (Centers for Disease Control and Prevention, 2014, p. i). In this continuity, the WHO published outbreak communication guidelines in 2005, establishing a list of best practices (WHO, 2005). These guidelines pursued multiple aims including improved surveillance, promotion of protective behaviours and reduction of confusion. The crucial role attributed to communication has been further emphasized by the revised International Health Regulations (IHR) adopted in 2005. In this document, communication is one of the eight core public health response capacities required for the IHR implementation, which means that capacity in risk communication should be built in each WHO Member State.

Risk communication is considered a "hybrid field" (Glik, 2007) that developed at the intersection of different specialties, including risk perceptions, disaster research, health promotion and communication, and media research. In the current risk governance framework, multiple functions are attributed to risk communication (Höppner et al., 2012). A first goal relates to raising awareness among affected communities and minimizing risk behaviours. A second one, along the now advocated model of two-way communication, aims to reinforce mutual understanding between stakeholders. A third objective is focused on improving coordination and cooperation among actors (within and across institutions) in the mitigation of risks, an issue of crucial relevance in the complex organizational landscape of global health (cf. Bourrier, Chapter 9). Finally, with regard to the importance given to institutional accountability, it is considered that risk communication engages the fiduciary responsibility of regulatory agencies who eventually have to report on the decisions they made to avert crises.

Despite the support of academics and regulatory agencies in this transformation of risk communication, research has documented recurrent controversies in that field (Barrelet et al., 2013). In the context of crises, the media make the risk exist outside of professional circles and thus play a crucial role in the public awareness of risks that are often invisible or remote to most of the population (Roslyng & Eskjær, 2017). At the same time, for institutions striking the right balance between avoiding public complacency in the face of serious threats and creating panic is not easy (Davis et al., 2011). Therefore, experts typically regret what they consider media's inappropriate coverage of crises (Hughes et al., 2006). Against this commonly held grief, studies documented that very large volumes of media content were produced in both A(H1N1) and Ebola contexts, but concluded that media reporting remained mostly factual and neutral (Kilgo et al., 2018; Klemm et al., 2016; Vasterman & Ruigrok, 2013). The assumption commonly held by public health specialists, that media are over-hyping epidemics and could generate panic among the general population, is therefore not supported by evidence. In the case of 2014 Ebola, it has, however, been observed that contents shared through social media, where there is no gatekeeping like in regular media channels, might have exacerbated fears (Kilgo et al., 2018).

Such ambivalent relationships have been characterized in terms of increasingly mutual influences between institutional communicators and journalists (Roslyng & Eskjær, 2017). The media are necessary partners for international and national public health agencies. The former dependency on official agencies has also been observed: in the early stages of the pandemic, media reported the facts provided by the public health institutions (Klemm et al., 2016; Vasterman & Ruigrok, 2013). An analysis of the Dutch media coverage of A(H1N1) even concluded that the concerned tone of some of the coverage was a reflection of the alarmism of official statements (Vasterman & Ruigrok, 2013).

This review of the literature showed that risk communication is considered a cornerstone of public health responses, connecting the views and actions of risk experts with those of the general public. The social amplification model describes this as "the phenomenon by which information processes, institutional structures, social-group behavior, and individual responses shape the social experience of risk, thereby contributing to risk consequences" (Kasperson et al., 1988, p. 181). However, beyond research assessing the volume and content of media reports, empirical research remains limited on risk communication practices as they are shaped and experienced inside public health agencies. Indeed, developed under the lead of a limited number of scholars, the interdisciplinary field of risk communication has been accused of being too intuitive and of lacking an integrative theoretical framework (Dickmann et al., 2015; Gurabardhi et al., 2004; McComas, 2006). This chapter will assess how the operationalization of risk communication objectives and recommendations have actually taken place in the context of two recent epidemics.

Risk communication experiences in the contexts of the A(H1N1) pandemic and the 2014 Ebola outbreak

While the A(H1N1) pandemic and the 2014 Ebola outbreak took place in different contexts and had contrasting impacts, they were both framed as "Public Health Emergencies of International Concern" (PHEIC) and mobilized some of the same risk communication specialists, especially in the WHO and CDC. In the aftermath of both events, a range of commentaries vehemently criticized efforts in that domain as illustrated by the following publication titles: "The price of poor pandemic communication" (Abraham, 2010) or "Ebola crisis: communication chaos we can avoid" (Ratzan & Moritsugu, 2014). This chapter aims at analysing the experience of the front-line risk communicators, in their interactions with the public, the media and professionals engaged in other segments of the response. Interviews were conducted with Swiss and US public health agencies professionals and WHO staff involved in the A(H1N1) pandemic and/or the 2014 Ebola outbreak risk communication. The available empirical data allows comparisons between agencies, countries and epidemics. The triangulation of these data will help to elucidate the gap existing between theoretical models of risk communication and their actual application. After describing the expectations towards risk communication established in the official guidance and documentation, challenges encountered by front-line risk communicators will be analysed around the topics that emerged from the joint analysis of documents and interview transcripts. They include difficulties encountered with actually reaching out to fragmented publics and understanding their needs, struggles with sustainability and coordination of risk communication activities, issues related to professionalization of risk communication, problems met within organizations and frustrations related to reputation management.

Expectations towards risk communication

Over the years, a more and more central role has been attributed to risk communication in responses developed to mitigate re-emerging infectious diseases, as indicated by the development of guidance in that domain by both the CDC and WHO. Next to the role given to risk communication in the revised 2005 International Health Regulations, the 2007 Swiss pandemic plan and the 2006 United States National strategy for pandemic influenza implementation plan developed previous to the 2009 A(H1N1) pandemic included a section or chapter on risk communication. The 2008 WHO Outbreak Communication Planning Guide states that in the early days of an epidemic, when technical solutions (treatments, vaccines, etc.) are not available yet, "effective communication can help limit the spread of a disease" (WHO, 2008, p. 4). The recent WHO Emergency Risk Communication guideline (WHO, 2017) reiterates this: "Risk communication is an integral part of any emergency response" (p. ix).

Front-line professionals confirmed this central role of communication. A Swiss public health professional involved in the A(H1N1) management we interviewed stated that it is "crucial" ("le nerf de la guerre"), a WHO specialist implicated in the Ebola outbreak published a paper in which she claims that communication is "the bedrock of outbreak response" (Odugleh-Kolev, 2014, p. 23). This central role of communication was also emphasized by a range of agencies deployed over the Ebola outbreak, including Médecins Sans Frontières (MSF), the International Federation of Red Cross and Red Crescent Societies (IFRC) and the Overseas Development Institute (Wilkinson, 2016). Official documents updated after the A(H1N1) pandemic further emphasized the importance of risk communication. The 2011 WHO review committee document situates risk communication at the same level as technical skills in the expertise required to tackle a pandemic: "For an influenza pandemic, this expertise would include virology, laboratory assessment, epidemiology, public-health field and leadership experience, veterinary science, risk assessment and risk communication, and methodological expertise in systematic reviews of the scientific literature" (WHO, 2011, p. 18). In the revised Swiss pandemic plan, risk communication moved from chapter 9 in 2007 to chapter 2 in 2018 (Office fédéral de la santé publique, 2018). In the United States, the updated preparedness and response framework for influenza pandemics includes risk communication in the "eight domains used to organize response efforts" (Holloway et al., 2014). And again, in the post-Ebola review of CDC communication a similar idea is formulated: "communication is an essential part of sustainable preparedness and long-term global health security" (Bedrosian et al., 2016, p. 73). In these documents, "effective risk communication" is emphasized not only as way to modify behaviours but also as a strategy to build trust and empathy (WHO, 2012, p. 3) thus underlying the importance of two-way communication: "It [effective risk communication] allows authorities and experts to listen to and address people's concerns and needs so that the advice they provide is relevant, trusted and acceptable" (WHO, 2017, p. 1).

All these guidelines thus set high expectations for risk communication activities. Furthermore, over the years they have not diminished but rather expanded. Against that background, the range of challenges encountered by front-line risk communicators, as they emerged in post-crisis documents and interviews, will now be described.

Communication with the publics and the difficulties of two-way communication

The United States were well prepared in regard to A(H1N1) risk communication – this can be associated with previous crises that triggered anticipation of major public health events, in particular a pandemic flu. The post-A(H1N1) evaluation emphasized the success of the communication strategy: "Communication with the public was one of the more successful aspects of the 2009 H1N1 response" (Department of Health and Human Services, United States, 2012, p. 63). The CERC manual recommendation of two-way communication with a large range of stakeholders including the public, insurance companies, the private sector as well as community and faith-based organizations was actually applied (Centers for Disease Control and Prevention, 2014). Communication was transparent, with uncertainty acknowledged by the CDC director. Interviews with CDC staff confirmed this positive feedback from the inside, they stressed that the flu was well documented and in that domain "risk com[munication] preparedness was mature". Several interviewees attributed the public trust towards CDC to these competencies in communication.

The success was, however, not total since access to minorities was considered insufficient: "Many felt that 2009 H1N1 communication and education efforts did not succeed in reaching minority, disadvantaged, and other hard-to-reach populations, including AI/AN [American Indian/ Alaskan Native], migrant workers, and non-English speakers" (Department of Health and Human Services, United States, 2012, p. 70). However this same report considered that some useful practices had been put in place, such as "building capacity in trusted community and faith-based networks" (p. 70).

In Switzerland, communication to the public was considered clear and coherent at first, but as the epidemic lasted, confusion was generated by contradictory messages (Van-Tam et al., 2010). The post-pandemic review emphasized the need to better plan communication along a range of scenarios, rather than limiting it to the worst-case scenario. In the aftermath of the A(H1N1) pandemic, at the international level, the WHO's reluctance to abandon one-way communication was sharply criticized, with regrets expressed about the persistence of persuasion aiming at convincing the public about the danger of flu and the importance of vaccination (Abraham, 2010).

Indeed, the A(H1N1) pandemic and 2014 Ebola outbreak responses taught risk communicators about the fragmentation of the publics, which seems to have come as a surprise. This was made particularly apparent in the context of the 2014 Ebola outbreak, especially for the Centers for Disease Control and Prevention, who, following their previous international engagements, developed risk communication activities in both the United States and West Africa (Bedrosian et al., 2016). The awareness of public fragmentation came up with the observation that skills necessary to tackle contrasting views and expectations among the public were absent in the communication teams, justifying demands for French speakers and anthropologists. The clash of views between the public health framing of epidemics and locals beliefs was acknowledged by a CDC interviewee who reported feeling helpless in front of cultural aspects, especially when these had concrete adverse consequences such as people dying because of rumours, circulating in West Africa, that salted water could heal Ebola patients. In the post-Ebola lessons learned, the need to integrate local views and to foster community engagement was emphasized by both WHO and CDC staff: "it is communities that control outbreaks and engaging with communities requires a sharing of power which goes far beyond media briefings, press releases, and tweets" (Odugleh-Kolev, 2014, p. 243). As admitted by one interviewee, anthropological knowledge related to Ebola countries actually existed but was not adequately convened. Besides cultural differences, language differences proved challenging in the French-speaking Ebola-affected countries. CDC staff reported difficulties in recruiting deployees who could communicate in French, calling for an ironic statement from one interviewee: "Considering how we miscommunicate in English … imagine in French!"

In the context of Ebola-related communication in West Africa, communication activities were reframed under different terms including "health promotion", "social mobilization" and "community engagement or participation". This shift in terminology reflects the presence on the grounds of different agencies having previously developed their own set of competencies under specific headings. As UNICEF was asked to co-lead the communication component of the response with the WHO, social mobilization and community engagement became prominent (Gillespie et al., 2016). Beyond the terminology, the shift reflected the need felt by communicators to actually understand their audiences before developing communication. As stated by a CDC interviewee, despite their risk communication background, deployees had limited knowledge of the audiences they were addressing: "So we had to get out and seek answers". Such statements directly refer to the two-way communication principle advocated by risk communication theory.

The communication specialists' lack of awareness about the importance of health and illness beliefs was thus made particularly visible in the Ebola context, confirming that culture becomes apparent only when it is obviously different. This would explain why calls for social scientists or anthropologists were much less vocal for A(H1N1) communication occurring in the United States or in Switzerland. Recurrent calls for anthropological knowledge are often associated with a naïve hope that it will act as a cultural broker (McElroy & Jezewski, 2000), and hence provide tools on how to modify local beliefs to make them compatible with the public health framing of the outbreak. Available data indeed shows a persistent focus on the importance of correcting "improper" views, typically associated with social categories situated in a subordinate position. In that vein, the HHS retrospective report highlighted the need to "address the myths and misconceptions about vaccines that may be prevalent within a culture" (Department of Health and Human Services, United States, 2012, p. 58).

These experiences related to the fragmentation of audiences underlie the still too limited awareness of cultural variations in meanings associated with health and risks among risk communication specialists. Oblivious to anthropological knowledge, culture still often appears as an obstacle to global health action. Moving beyond such a position can be possible when two-way communication is actually developed, as a strategy to reduce the social and cultural distance between those who represent public health agencies and targeted publics.

Challenges encountered within risk communication activities

Beyond the difficulties of reaching the publics, professionals who were at the forefront of risk communication activities reported a range of challenges in their daily routines, including resources limitations and coordination issues (see Bastide, Chapter 5).

First, pressures on resources were high. According to a WHO interviewee, the occurrence of the A(H1N1) pandemic actually helped to scale up risk communication activities within the organization. The WHO declaration in April 2009 of a Public Health Emergency of International Concern in relationship to the increasing cases of a new flu generated a very high demand for information. Those involved reported that in the early phase of the pandemic, communication was expected twenty-four hours a day and seven days a week, a rhythm dictated by the 24/7 news channels active at the global scale. According to one of our sources, a hundred press people were actually camping on the WHO front lawn, eager to get any information directly from the WHO. CDC staff also reported feeling completely overloaded by the volume of demands, coming through different formats such as emails, conference calls, meetings, the web etc. (Department of Health and Human Services, United States, 2012). While they strived to respond to this unprecedented demand for information, several interviewees reported feeling overwhelmed and exhausted, with long and recurrent shifts impacting on their private lives. As regards Ebola, demands on risk communication staff were aggravated by the need to deploy professionals to the affected African countries, while taking into account the frequent turnover of those accepting deployment and the necessity to represent a large range of skills necessary to address the wide spectrum of risk communication activities. As stated by one WHO interviewee: "At this point it was clear that we needed nine communication persons per country". Besides this, considerations for the safety of those deployed increased pressure on the head of the team.

Second, intensive communication could not be sustained over time. Indeed, in the WHO, A(H1N1) communication efforts receded at the very moment the organization declared the pandemic in June 2009. In the post-A(H1N1) review, this timing was specifically criticized: "The decision to diminish proactive communication with the media after declaring Phase 6 (for example, by discontinuing routine press conferences focused on the evolving pandemic) was ill-advised" (WHO, 2011, p. 16). While the declaration of Phase 6 revived demands for information, the WHO was not able to respond to these due to the exhaustion of its communication staff over the previous weeks. Similar concerns regarding the difficulty of sustaining communication over time have been reported regarding the Ebola response by one CDC interviewee. In contradiction with the acting early recommendation (WHO, 2005) and the emergency mode of the response, both the A(H1N1) pandemic and the 2014 Ebola outbreak were long epidemics for which early investments had to be sustained over time. Communication thus appeared more complex than first expected, framed as a dynamic process which had to be adjusted to unfolding events and to new evidence gained over time. These difficulties had been foreseen even before the pandemic: "Rather than a single, one-time big event, pandemic influenza is likely to present as a rising tide or prolonged risk incident, with initial uncertainty that decreases (but can re-emerge) as cases accumulate and consensus grows among experts" (Vaughan & Tinker, 2009, p. S326). However, this was not sufficiently anticipated by communication teams. Limitations in resources are further revealed by the fact that the A(H1N1) pandemic response budgets did not contain any indication about the costs of communication (Pasquini-Descomps et al., Chapter 8), suggesting that these activities were considered part of the usual business and not calling for supplementary investments.

Third, numerous problems emerged with regard to the coordination of communication across institutions. Both US and Swiss post-A(H1N1) reviews reported difficulties in the coordination of communication across states and cantons. In Switzerland difficulties in reaching medical doctors, as front-line responders for public preoccupations, were reported. In a survey conducted by the Swiss national public health authority (Office fédéral de la santé publique, 2011), a large majority of medical doctors reported poor communication as the biggest challenge they had to face, considering information had been partial, insufficient and contradictory. The post-A(H1N1) review confirmed that contradictions emerged over time: while messages were consistent and clear at the beginning of the pandemic, the lack of coordination created confusion, leading to a declining credibility of public health authorities (Van-Tam et al., 2010). A CDC interviewee regretted the multiplication of people involved in communication since the lack of strategy and the absence of well-defined lines of authority ended up in unclear responsibilities. This exacerbated coordination difficulties. As described above, global epidemics raise important challenges due to the multiplication of audiences. Concerns about the contradictions in messages provided to the population were raised by others: "As a number of commentators have observed, communication efforts during this time took the form of simplistic, often contradictory, top-down messages telling people what they should or should not do" (Wilkinson, 2016, p. 11).

Fourth, the implementation of risk communication was criticized with regard to the amount of information provided. The CERC motto, printed on the cover of the manual is "be first, be right, be credible". Emphasis on early and intensive communication is associated with the necessity to counter rumours, alternative views and potential panic. Indeed, these social phenomena are considered anomalies in the proper management of outbreaks. Professionals are thus expected to saturate the information channels with "official information". This is explicitly reported in the post-Ebola CDC review on communication activities: "CDC continually addressed these rumors with additional communication products and messages that sought to counter fears of Ebola spreading through handshakes, pets, or mosquitoes, for instance, with facts about transmission" (Bedrosian et al., 2016, p. 72). A CDC interviewee reflected on the fact that this might have been exaggerated: "During the crisis, they went from 14 to 147 web pages on Ebola on the website". Such multiplication of contents and messages put pressure not only on resources, but also on coordination.

Fifth, norms of early and intense communication implies informing the public before evidence can actually be fully established. However, communicating uncertainty is challenging as acknowledged by some interviewees: a CDC staff stated that dealing with the unknown was the biggest challenge for both the A(H1N1) pandemic and the 2014 Ebola outbreak. Others commented that the situation was different in the two epidemics since the flu was much better documented when the pandemic occurred. Nonetheless, in the United States, the capacity of the then acting director of CDC, Richard Besser, to acknowledge uncertainty in the media in the early days of the epidemic was considered crucial (Maher, 2010). In contrast, knowledge was scarce for Ebola: "collectively, the global public health community lacked experience in how to address this epidemic" (Bedrosian et al., 2016, p. 69). In that context, CDC efforts to minimize the uncertainty about the possibility of Ebola transmission inside a US hospital were later criticized (Gilbert & Kerridge, 2015). The norm of transparency, even though it is promoted in the CDC and WHO guidance, is not systematically applied, due to the view held by some communicators that the public is expecting agencies like CDCs "to know everything right now" (CDC interviewee).

The recurrence, in the reviews and interviews, of similar issues across different national scales and outbreaks reveals systematic weaknesses encountered in the application of risk communication guidelines. Furthermore, these difficulties confirm that risk communication is not only about reaching the publics, but is also about streamlining information within implicated institutions and across professional groups.

The professionalization of risk communication

On top of having been prioritized in the Swiss pandemic strategy between 2007 and 2018, the new plan states that "a professional conduct of communication" (Office fédéral de la santé publique, 2018, p. 18) is part of the national public health authority core activities in a crisis situation. The combination of the IHR demand for capacity building, the WHO Pandemic Influenza Preparedness (PIP) Framework and accumulated epidemic outbreaks have exacerbated the need to train communicators at the global scale. The WHO's large efforts in capacity building can be assessed from this quote of a WHO interviewee in November 2014:

> Plus I trained over 200 people in risk communication preparedness over the last 2 weeks. And those are commitments too. So 13 countries … Southeast Asia, 9 countries Europe … 30 countries in Barbados and then all of the Americas countries in Washington DC! So this was in 11 days ah!

Besides such regional meetings, along with the emphasis given to the pre-event phases in communication planning, the WHO established a roster of specialists in 2013. The Emergency Communication Network (ECN) (www.who.int/risk-communication/emergency-response/en/) is composed of professionals from all over the world who receive an intense ten-day training and can then be deployed when needed, based on their availability, for two months per year. Such efforts to recruit and train risk communication specialists provide further confirmation of the importance attributed to communication (see Bastide, Chapter 5). The production of new material (WHO, 2017), the revision of previous documents (Centers for Disease Control and Prevention, 2014) and the development of online training by both the WHO (www.who.int/risk-communication/training/module-a/en/) and CDC (https://emergency.cdc.gov/cerc/training/basic/index.asp) emphasize these important training needs.

Concerning the skills future communicators should acquire, expectations are high: in the ECN video on the WHO website, the head of the team states: "we have to deploy teams that can do everything". One CDC professional also insisted that deployees should be able "to do everything", including media relationships, be knowledgeable in the content area, and be able to conduct behavioural assessment work with communities. However, some interviewees acknowledged that ambitions associated with the job are very high, with most risk communication specialists having limited capacity to actually reach the expectations. For example, one CDC interviewee stated difficulties in mastering the content of the available guidance, such as the CERC manual: "Few people actually master its contents". Indeed, preferences are now set for specialists having prior experience rather than academic training: "Now they favour field experience over diplomas".

Part of training demands relate to the complex landscape of communication nowadays. As already observed in the context of the A(H1N1) pandemic: "expert or official communications about the pandemic had to compete with a plethora of new modes of lay communication" (Nerlich & Koteyko, 2012, p. 711). A(H1N1) communication in the US has been praised for using "a wide array of media venues, including websites (HHS's flu.gov being the primary example), webcasts, podcasts, texting, news briefings, brochures, flyers, and other media outlets" (Department of Health and Human Services, United States, 2012, p. 63). They were widely consulted and could provide updated information. At the global scale, specialists working in the WHO recognized that in the early days of A(H1N1), skills were limited in respect to the communication tools, but over time the staff became proficient in the use of these technologies:

And the things that we … struggled before you know, virtual press conference … things like that are very just second nature now. So we do regular press briefings, virtual press conferences, we tweet information, we … So I think that's much better.

The 2017 WHO guidance actually acknowledges the communication land-scape complexity as a challenge for risk communication (WHO, 2017, p. ix). Overall the professionalization of risk communication is geared towards building capacities to handle the media in their different formats and to reach out to the public. Issues related to the positioning of communication within organizations and to accountability are not part of the training. However, the last two sections will show that their importance should not be underestimated.

Challenges from within organizations

Next to the crucial role attributed to risk communication in the official documents, risk communication specialists acknowledged that their view is not systematically shared within their own professional environment. Their experiences and comments highlighted the persistent power relationships over competence and resources within public health agencies. Several interviewees commented on the changing place of communication, shifting back and forth between a centralized and a decentralized model of communication. For example, in the WHO risk communication was based in departments before the A(H1N1) pandemic; after 2012 a Department of Communication (DCO) was created to bring together all communication activities. These shifts reflect recurrent tensions between subject matter specialists who consider it is their role to communicate and emergency communication specialists. These tensions are likely to have contributed to the coordination difficulties discussed above. According to a professional we interviewed at CDC, the unstable position of communication reflects the fact that its value is not taken for granted: "there is no consensus on the scientific value of communication".

This downgrading reflects traditional hierarchies of public health institutions that value medical, technical and epidemiological know-how over communication skills. Seeing communication as a soft science allows domain specialists to claim their ability to communicate, among a wide range of tasks, instead of delegating it to specifically trained professionals. A clash over temporality was mentioned in that context: developing appropriate communication requires time, even more so if a dialogue has to be established with audiences. However, medical and epidemiology experts consider it too slow to be useful in the response. Such struggles between specialized areas within institutions reflect fights over resources, distributed in different response sectors according to their perceived value: "Several agencies, including MSF and Oxfam, have noted how there was far greater focus on the "hardware" of treatment facilities, beds, specialist burial teams and equipment rather than the 'software' of communication" (Wilkinson, 2016, p. 15). The International Federation of the Red Cross and the Red Crescent reported that communication was not given sufficient attention in Ebola-affected countries, resulting in some of the available budget for mass media communication not even being spent (Wilkinson, 2016, p. 13).

These elements suggest that in public health agencies risk communication is not yet occupying the central place that official documents attribute to it. A communication officer with a long field experience considered that for risk communication to gain more importance, shifts in power relationships are necessary, including a greater political commitment by policy makers and funders (Odugleh-Kolev, 2014). Some sign of a lesson learned following the 2014 Ebola outbreak is the fact that in 2016 half of the WHO Zika budget was dedicated to communication. The need for proper funding is actually one of the recommendations of the 2017 WHO guidance: "ERC requires a defined and sustained budget that should be a part of core budgeting for emergency preparedness and response" (WHO, 2017, p. 23). However, gaining access to sufficient resources will only be possible with a shift in current hierarchies within public health institutions.

Reputation management

Besides disputes over their role within agencies, risk communicators reported having had to face outside reactions to their action, as illustrated by criticisms towards the accountability of institutions in charge of epidemic responses. These criticisms were formulated in the media, in a second stage of the outbreaks, as typically observed in communication about previous emerging infectious diseases, such as SARS and avian flu (Hughes et al., 2006; Nerlich & Koteyko, 2012). When a new and potentially serious danger emerges, the media and the general public at first uncritically endorse official views. When A(H1N1) was declared a pandemic of international concern, journalists were eager to gain information from the WHO and they reported what the agency told them about this new flu. Such unity, however, did not last, as was discovered by WHO risk communicators. As time passed, the flu appeared to be less severe than initially predicted and critical voices started to emerge in both traditional and online media.

This more broadly reflects transformations in the public discourses about risk: in later stages of risk communication, the interest of the outside world shifts towards issues related to accountability (Höppner et al., 2012; Krimsky, 2007). This was confirmed by a WHO interviewee, stating that the low severity of the threat re-oriented the focus of risk communication from behavioural advice to reputation management: "media communication is much more about agencies talking about what they do". This evolution of risk communication over time could have been expected since "questions of accountability and blame often feature prominently in risk reporting" (Hughes et al., 2006, p. 258). Furthermore, the media are eager to report controversy, especially when conflicts arise among stakeholders. In the A(H1N1) context, critics focused on the changing definition of a pandemic and the alleged role of the pharmaceutical industry in the decision to declare A(H1N1) a pandemic that would call for a massive vaccine production. In the case of Ebola, severe criticisms were also addressed to the WHO by the international media, related to the delay in declaring it a Public Health Emergency of International Concern (Kamradt-Scott, 2016). The post-pandemic evaluation report acknowledged that the WHO might have contributed to confusion and suspicion due to inconsistent descriptions of the pandemic and the lack of disclosure (WHO, 2011). On the other hand, accounts from WHO professionals, who had dedicated huge efforts to communication in the spring of 2009 reveal how much they were particularly hit by the accusations of a "fake pandemic" that would have been promoted by the pharmaceutical industry interests. A similar disappointment was reported in the context of Ebola by a WHO staff member who was regretting the media attacks towards the WHO, admitting some difficulties in the response, but expressing discouragement considering her involvement and willingness to do good and the way these efforts were criticized.

For journalists, the media play an important role in regard to accountability, by providing information on how resources were spent and how well undertaken activities responded to actual needs (Wilkinson, 2016). This is actually one of the roles the media should play in modern democracies, i.e. "operating as a watchdog on the performance of corporate and governmental power centres" (Hughes et al., 2006, p. 251). A journalist we interviewed in Switzerland commented on the ambivalence of institutions towards the media: while public health agencies need the media, professionals are at the same time afraid of what journalists could report on their activities. In her experience, WHO staff were not necessary willing to listen to critics after A(H1N1), whereas this is part of their duty to be credible and trusted by the public and their sponsors. The WHO post-A(H1N1) review accepted the criticisms and stated that they should have listened, in an effort to restore the credibility of the organization (WHO, 2011). Such official statements indeed occurred at a time when severe budgetary cuts were imposed on the WHO and a major reform of the organization was initiated (Kamradt-Scott, 2016). These experiences related to reputation management confirm that communication is a complex two-way process, through which a range of stakeholders can formulate their views, including being critical towards the official response.

Conclusion

Risk communication developed as a normative field defining how institutions should reach the whole society when dealing with risks and crises. This chapter unveiled some recurrent challenges around risk communication, in different contexts. In official documents, risk communication is considered a cornerstone of epidemic responses, so norms and guidelines keep being further developed based on the available evidence regarding the impact of communication on different publics and lessons learned from previous crises. The A(H1N1) pandemic and 2014 Ebola outbreak showed, however, once again the difficulty to learn from past mistakes even though they have been widely documented (Ratzan & Moritsugu, 2014).

Difficulties described in this chapter can be related to the progressive shift away from risk management to other forms of addressing future threats, including precautionary approaches and preparedness (Bastide, Chapter 2). These new frames are moving away from the calculability of risks towards the increasing importance of uncertainty. As stated by the CDC director in the context of A(H1N1), "There is an inherent tension between being first and being right" (Maher, 2010, p. 151). Interestingly, next to all the anticipatory discourses and activities, another frame was somehow unexpectedly invoked by Margaret Chan herself when she stated at a media conference after the Emergency Committee meeting:

> Pandemics are unpredictable and prone to deliver surprises. No two pandemics are ever alike. This pandemic has turned out to be much more fortunate than what we feared a little over a year ago. This time around we have been aided by pure good luck.

Chan's words acknowledge that even though no other epidemic had been previously watched so closely, luck still played a part in its unfolding. This stands in strong contradiction with massive references to controllability and manageability of epidemics in both global health and biosecurity frameworks.

Beyond limits in epidemiological predictions, communication also appeared to be a domain difficult to control. Journalists and more broadly members of the public questioned the appropriateness of public health agencies' action. As profusely mentioned in the literature, the impact of communication is intimately related to credibility and trust towards institutions. If in the United States, CDC benefited from its antecedent positive image, the WHO suffered from its unstable position in the new landscape of global health. Like other public health activities, communication is an intervention that can possibly backfire. In the context of Ebola, contrary to the expectations that proper communication could alleviate the number of cases, communication might have been a source of harm for affected communities: "In fact, communication may have contributed to exacerbating the epidemic by – inadvertently – spreading fear, misconceptions and adding to the stigma experienced by those who contracted Ebola" (Wilkinson, 2016, p. 8). This constitutes a warning against the temptation to saturate communication by multiplying content without considering the views and needs of different audiences. Furthermore, the agency of the publics is too often neglected (Davis et al., 2011). Audiences are active: they interpret, compare, challenge official messages and are prone to identify contradictions.

On another front, it has been shown here that the importance of internal communication is underappreciated. Consensus within organizations and across communities of experts is too often taken for granted. Uncertainty associated with early communication generates room for evolving messages and hence for disputes. On the other hand, views from within institutions are not homogenous since competing interpretation frames can cohabit. Even though risk communication is considered to combine both internal and external components (Renn, 2008), experiences documented above suggest that concrete strategies to streamline information inside institutions still need to be reinforced.

As proposed for decades now by the social sciences, risks are embedded in local contexts. It is important to acknowledge the promises of risk communication guidance as a way to reconcile contrasting views about risks, while taking into account the complex array of economic, political, social and cultural factors shaping reactions to adverse events. Only a broader acknowledgement of these mechanisms, calling for a dialogue between concerned parties, can ensure that the norms and ambitions of risk communication will actually be implemented. It is not enough to formulate risk communication recommendations aiming at reconciling global health expectations with locally situated views and experiences of health needs, these expectations now have to actually be put into practice.

References

Abraham, T. (2010). The price of poor pandemic communication. *British Medical Journal, 340*(12 June), 1307–1310.

Anderson, B. (2010). Preemption, precaution, preparedness: Anticipatory action and future geographies. *Progress in Human Geography, 34*(6), 777–798. https://doi.org/10.1177/0309132510362600.

Barrelet, C., Bourrier, M., Burton-Jeangros, C., & Schindler, M. (2013). Unresolved issues in risk communication research: The case of the H1N1 pandemic (2009–2011). *Influenza and Other Respiratory Viruses, 7,* 114–119. https://doi.org/10.1111/irv.12090.

Bedrosian, S. R., Young, C. E., Smith, L. A. et al. (2016). Lessons of risk communication and health promotion: West Africa and United States. *MMWR Morbidity and Mortality Weekly Report, 65*(3), 68–74.

Centers for Disease Control and Prevention. (2014). *Crisis Emergency and Risk Communication.* Atlanta, GA.

Davis, M., Stephenson, N., & Flowers, P. (2011). Compliant, complacent or panicked? Investigating the problematization of the Australian general public in pandemic influenza control. *Social Science & Medicine, 72,* 912–918.

Department of Health and Human Services, United States. (2012). An HHS Retrospective on the 2009 H1N1 Influenza Pandemic to Advance All Hazards Preparedness.

Dickmann, P., McClelland, A., Gamhewage, G. M., Portela de Souza, P., & Apfel, F. (2015). Making sense of communication interventions in public health emergencies: An evaluation framework for risk communication. *Journal of Communication in Healthcare*, *8*(3), 233–240. https://doi.org/10.1080/17538068.2015.1101962.

Douglas, M. (1985). *Risk Acceptability According to the Social Sciences*. London: Routledge & Kegan Paul.

Giddens, A. (1990). *The Consequences of Modernity*. Cambridge: Polity Press.

Gilbert, G. L., & Kerridge, I. (2015). Communication and communicable disease control: Lessons from Ebola virus disease. *The American Journal of Bioethics*, *15*(4), 62–65. https://doi.org/10.1080/15265161.2015.1009564.

Gillespie, A. M., Obregon, R., El Asawi, R., Richey, C., Manoncourt, E., Joshi, K., ... Quereshi, S. (2016). Social mobilization and community engagement central to the Ebola response in West Africa: Lessons for future public health emergencies. *Global Health: Science and Practice*, *4*(4), 626–646. https://doi.org/10.9745/GHSP-D-16-00226.

Glik, D. C. (2007). Risk communication for public health emergencies. *Annual Review of Public Health*, *28*(1), 33–54. https://doi.org/10.1146/annurev.publhealth.28.021406.144123.

Gurabardhi, Z., Gutteling, J. M., & Kuttschreuter, M. (2004). The development of risk communication. *Science Communication*, *25*(4), 323–349.

Holloway, R., Rasmussen, S. A., Zaza, S. et al. (2014). Updated preparedness and response framework for influenza pandemics. *MMWR Morbidity and Mortality Weekly Report*, *63*(6), 1–10.

Höppner, C., Whittle, R., Bründl, M., & Buchecker, M. (2012). Linking social capacities and risk communication in Europe: A gap between theory and practice? *Natural Hazards*, *64*(2), 1753–1778. https://doi.org/10.1007/s11069-012-0356-5.

Hughes, E., Kitzinger, J., & Murdock, G. (2006). The media and risk. In Taylor-Gooby, P., & Zinn, J. (eds), *Risk in Social Science*. Oxford: Oxford University Press, pp. 250–270.

Joffe, H. (1999). *Risk and "the Other"*. Cambridge and New York, NY: Cambridge University Press.

Kamradt-Scott, A. (2016). WHO's to blame? The World Health Organization and the 2014 Ebola outbreak in West Africa. *Third World Quarterly*, *37*(3), 401–418. https://doi.org/10.1080/01436597.2015.1112232.

Kasperson, R. E., Renn, O., Slovic, P. et al. (1988). The social amplification of risk: A conceptual framework. *Risk Analysis*, *8*, 177–197.

Kilgo, D. K., Yoo, J., & Johnson, T. J. (2018). Spreading Ebola panic: Newspaper and social media coverage of the 2014 Ebola health crisis. *Health Communication*, 1–7. https://doi.org/10.1080/10410236.2018.1437524.

Klemm, C., Das, E., & Hartmann, T. (2016). Swine flu and hype: A systematic review of media dramatization of the H1N1 influenza pandemic. *Journal of Risk Research*, *19*(1), 1–20. https://doi.org/10.1080/13669877.2014.923029.

Krimsky, S. (2007). Risk communication in the internet age: The rise of disorganized skepticism. *Environmental Hazards*, *7*(2), 157–164. https://doi.org/10.1016/j.envhaz.2007.05.006.

Lakoff, A. (2017). *Unprepared: Global Health in a Time of Emergency*. Oakland, California: University of California Press.

Lakoff, A., & Collier, S. J. (eds). (2008). *Biosecurity Interventions: Global Health and Security in Question*. New York, NY: Columbia University Press.

Leiss, W. (1996). Three phases in the evolution of risk communication practice. *The Annals of the American Academy of Political and Social Science, 545*, 85–94.

Maher, B. (2010). Swine flu: Crisis communicator. *Nature, 463*(7278), 150–152.

McComas, K. A. (2006). Defining moments in risk communication research: 1996–2005. *Journal of Health Communication, 11*(1), 75–91. https://doi.org/10.1080/10810730500461091.

McElroy, A., & Jezewski, M. A. (2000). Cultural variation in the experience of health and illness. In Albrecht, G. L., Fitzpatrick, R., & Scrimshaw, S. C. (eds), *Handbook of Social Studies in Health and Medicine*. London: Sage, pp. 191–209.

Nerlich, B., & Koteyko, N. (2012). Crying wolf? Biosecurity and metacommunication in the context of the 2009 swine flu pandemic. *Health and Place, 18*, 710–717.

Odugleh-Kolev, Asiya. (2014). What will it take to move risk communication into the twenty-first century? *Journal of Communication in Health Care, 7*(4), 242–245.

Office fédéral de la santé publique (OFSP). (2011). Résultats de l'enquête relative à la gestion de la pandémie A/H1N1 2009, menée auprès des médecins de premier recours. *Bulletin OFSP, 28*, 580–586.

Office fédéral de la santé publique (OFSP). (2018). Plan suisse de pandémie Influenza. Stratégies et mesures pour la préparation à une épidémie d'Influenza (5e édition). Berne: Confédération suisse.

Ratzan, S. C., & Moritsugu, K. P. (2014). Ebola crisis: Communication chaos we can avoid. *Journal of Health Communication, 19*(11), 1213–1215. https://doi.org/10.1080/10810730.2014.977680.

Renn, O. (2008). *Risk Governance Coping with Uncertainty in a Complex World*. London and Sterling, VA: Earthscan. Retrieved from http://public.eblib.com/EBL Public/PublicView.do?ptiID=430168.

Roslyng, M. M., & Eskjær, M. F. (2017). Mediatised risk culture: News coverage of risk technologies. *Health, Risk & Society, 19*(3–4), 112–129. https://doi.org/10.1080/13698575.2017.1286298.

Short, J. F. (1984). The social fabric at risk: Toward the social transformation of risk analysis. *American Sociological Review, 49*(December), 711–725.

Slovic, P. (2000). *The Perception of Risk*. London: Earthscan.

Van-Tam, J., Lambert, P.-H., Carrasco, P. et al. (2010). Evaluation de la stratégie de vaccination H1N1 de la Suisse. Rapport final. Ernst & Young.

Vasterman, P. L., & Ruigrok, N. (2013). Pandemic alarm in the Dutch media: Media coverage of the 2009 influenza A (H1N1) pandemic and the role of the expert sources. *European Journal of Communication, 28*(4), 436–453. https://doi.org/10.1177/0267323113486235.

Vaughan, E., & Tinker, T. (2009). Effective health risk communication about pandemic influenza for vulnerable populations. *American Journal of Public Health, 99*(suppl 2), S324–S332.

Wilkinson, I. (1999). News media discourse and the state of public opinion on risk. *Risk Management, 1*(4), 21–31.

Wilkinson, S. (2016). Using media and communication to respond to public health emergencies: Lessons learned from Ebola. *BBC Media action – practice briefing*.

World Health Organization (WHO). (2005). Outbreak Communication. Best Practices for Communicating with the Public during an Outbreak. Geneva.

World Health Organization (WHO). (2008). World Health Organization Outbreak Communication Planning Guide. Geneva.

World Health Organization (WHO). (2011). Implementation of the International Health Regulations (2005) Report of the review committee on the functioning of the International Health Regulations (2005) in relation to Pandemic (H1N1) 2009. Geneva.

World Health Organization (WHO). (2012). Rapid Risk Assessment of Acute Public Health Events. Geneva.

World Health Organization (WHO). (2017). Communicating risk in public health emergencies. A WHO guideline for Emergency Risk Communication (ERC) policy and practice. Geneva.

5 Emergency capabilities

Deploying the WHO's communication in West Africa during the 2014 Ebola epidemic

Loïs Bastide

Introduction

The 2014 Ebola virus disease (EVD) crisis in West Africa created a very complex work environment for all the actors involved in the response. Fast contagion, propagation to urban, metropolitan contexts, lack of knowledge in all dimensions of the response, state of public health systems in affected countries, scale of the response and variety of involved jurisdictions and agencies (to cite a few factors) contributed to frame a very demanding action setting for professionals deployed in the field. Deployees were compelled to act under circumstances of scarce knowledge, high uncertainty, and in fast-evolving organizational structures. These elements are identified and expected in emergency settings and tackled in contingency plans and public health preparedness systems (Lakoff, 2007; Zylberman, 2013). Nevertheless, they were pushed to a completely new level due to the high fatality rate of the EVD, incomplete clinical and epidemiological information on the disease in this unprecedented setting (West Africa), the regional, transborder scale of the epidemic, and the scarcity of locally available resources to mitigate the impact of the disease.

In this context, experts deployed in West Africa by various organizations faced many obstacles, which kept on derailing the international response, at least until the spring of 2015. As established procedures and action protocols proved ineffective, they had to develop coping strategies to regain agency, in this complex setting. This chapter focuses on this issue, by analyzing first-line responders' activities in the field, in view of identifying:

- the multidimensional challenges that they faced in their work;
- the resources and capacities that they leveraged to develop their actions, in this difficult setting.

The discussion is based on empirical data collected during a joint research project between the Department of Sociology at the University of Geneva and the Department of Communications (DOC) at the World Health Organization (WHO). The project, which took place between March and

June 2015, aimed at gathering and organizing information produced by communication experts deployed in West Africa through the WHO's Emergency Communication Network (ECN), a roster of professionals coming from various organizations, trained in emergency communication by the WHO, and ready to be deployed in public health emergency settings.

In this context, we choose to focus on the ability of the ECN to sustain the agency of its members, thus enabling them to carry on their tasks in this challenging crisis environment. We posit that this "support function" had much to do with the morphological character of the ECN, as a loose, "networked" organization. We show that its properties, as an organizational structure, increased individual experts' agency and ability to work in the field, by providing different types of resources and capacities. To do so, we start by proposing a theory of "situated action" and capability building, by reworking Amartya Sen's concept of *capability*. We stress the fact that, as an organization, the ECN creates collective capabilities, which proved useful in dealing with the many organizational glitches and dysfunctions on the ground. These capabilities, we argue, include specific forms of trust, and the constitution of a "network of networks" which allowed ECN deployees to reach for heterogeneous resources and capacities, according to their needs.[1]

Situated action and capability building in a crisis setting

Contexts of action

The EVD epidemics deeply disrupted response systems and institutions – at local, regional and global levels – and affected societies in West Africa. WHO communicators sent to the field found themselves struggling to make sense of unfolding events and circumstances, and to define appropriate courses of action, despite their training as emergency responders (Bastide, 2018). To shed light on this process of "sensemaking" (Weick, 1995) and of organizing – making sense of the situation and designing efficient actions – it is necessary to assemble a working theory of action that pays attention:

1   to the specificities of the crisis setting, in particular to its high degree of volatility, contingency and indeterminacy;
2   to the origin and to the processes of mobilization of the resources, skills and capacities needed to act in this uncertain environment.

In view of bringing these dimensions under a unified explanatory framework, the chapter develops an analytics of the response in terms of "situated action" (Garfinkel, 1967; Suchman, 1987; Quéré, 1997). Put in plain terms, this approach posits that actions unfold in specific contexts, which contributes to their framing (they are *indexical*). More specifically, it considers that actions and their settings are dynamically connected by feedback loops, meaning:

1   Settings participate in framing actions, considering that they offer specific resources and impose particular constraints upon them. This idea is captured in the notion of "affordances" (Gibson, 1977), which posits that particular contexts facilitate specific practices and make others difficult, or even impossible.
2   The material and symbolic outcomes of past actions re-structure resources and possibilities available to ongoing practices, thus reframing action settings.

Given this understanding, it will be necessary to characterize the EVD as a specific context of action. However, a cautionary methodological note is necessary before we start picturing the setting.

Indeed, if social action (Weber, 1978) is always situated – considering that it should be envisioned as the combined outcome of individual and collective agency and of a given context – it remains that it can be captured and considered at different scales: individual actions can have different reaches (Dodier, 1993; Bastide, 2015, 39–43). For instance, there are long-term, planned and organized actions, aiming at a more or less distant time horizon. In the case of the EVD epidemic in West Africa, such horizon could be the end of transmission, a critical goal of the response (see: WHO, 2015). This aim involved the conception of long-term strategic goals and courses of action, which themselves involved and served as contexts for shorter scale objectives and actions (Grossetti, 2007). Indeed, ending the epidemic required developing a broad range of shorter-term targets – building Ebola treatment centers, designing sensitizing campaigns, developing relevant situational assessments, etc. – in a variety of domains – epidemiology, laboratory analysis, clinical care, logistics, etc. Conversely, broader time frames were also at play. For instance, a relevant temporality concerned the organizational cycle of international epidemic response systems (Zylberman, 2013). It involved the institutional overhauling of existing response capacities. In this particular dimension, stakes were high for the WHO, as its credibility as the main player in public health crisis response was debated and sometimes questioned by Member States, by other international and non-governmental organizations, and by the media. As such, the *organizational crisis* extended well into the post-Ebola period – and is still ongoing at the time of writing (On the post-Ebola reform at the WHO, see for instance: Fleck, 2017; Moon et al., 2017).

We capture the Ebola outbreak, as a specific action setting, by leveraging a rich data set including seventeen semi-structured interviews with ECN deployees and two ECN managers, twenty-nine non-published End of Mission Reports, thirty deployees' Terms of References (Tors) forms and various documents referring to deployments. By triangulating these different types of data and drawing complementary insights from interviews with other professionals at the WHO (fourteen formal, semi-structured interviews and numerous informal interactions) and the CDCs (fifteen semi-structured interviews), we were able to build a consistent picture of the general circumstances in the field. Thus we re-constructed a generic (ideal typical if you wish) characterization of the EVD crisis setting in West Africa. Bearing in mind the nature of our data set, which refers to deployments taking place between March 2014 and February 2015, given also the position of our respondents as first-line emergency responders, we focus the characterization of the context to Liberia, Sierra Leone and Guinea, during this period.

Situated action and capabilities

As mentioned, looking at situated action not only involves characterizing relevant settings, but also identifying the resources and capacities implemented *in situation.* To frame this analysis, we use Amartya Sen's notion of "capabilities" (Sen, 2010).[2] In terms of an analysis of "social action" (Weber, 1978), Sen's approach allows understanding that actual actions are the outcome of:

1   a person's individual resources and abilities (material resources, skills, capacities, know-hows, etc.), obtained by inheritance (i.e. economic capital) or acquired through education, training and experience (Fernagu-Oudet & Batal, 2016) – what he calls functionings;[3]
2   a given social situation, which determines the range of actually achievable/implementable functionings, due to situational constraints and resources (affordances).

Sen thus recognizes that social actors are to be understood as the partial outcomes of their social trajectories. But his approach focuses on the *contextual actualization* of functionings rather than on their acquisition, thus departing from more deterministic approaches to individual trajectories in terms of socialization and dispositions (Bourdieu, 1990; Lahire, 2006). However, we also follow Bénédicte Zimmermann (2006) when she suggests that Sen's situational approach remains somehow underspecified. Hence our re-conceptualization of action settings.

The proposed approach thus posits that a specific skill, in order to be implementable, needs to meet a fitting environment, or it remains latent. This fact is easy to grasp in the case of highly equipped skills, where the availability of appropriate tools is the *sine qua non* condition of a successful activation. For the sake of clarity, it is easy for instance to appreciate that the professional skill set of a computer scientist will be much less useful without an available computer.

Therefore, capabilities should be understood, in this framework, as the set of functionings one is effectively able to reach or implement, under current circumstances. There is thus a need to distinguish between functionings – sets of resources, skills and capacities – and *capabilities*, defined as the capacity to actually implement these functionings, in a particular situation (Fernagu-Oudet & Batal, 2016). This delineation makes it possible to understand why reputedly well-established skills and response systems failed to be activated in the West African EVD setting. It is of upmost importance in the case of crisis management planning since high-stress environments can easily inhibit individual and, possibly, collective ability to act – being paralyzed by fear, or overwhelmed by the extent of uncertainty, for instance. This formalization allows understanding that a high-skill professional's capacities can be deeply impaired in such context. A high-ranking professional at the United States Centers for Disease Control and Prevention (US CDCs), who had been deployed in Sierra Leone, thus explained that he had to "pull out" some people from the field given their emotional distress, due to the "specter of death".[4]

Following Ibrahim (2006), it is necessary to extend the capability approach by considering that capacities are not only individual attributes: building-up work collectives, such as the ECN, is a way to articulate individual resources and capacities to foster *collective capabilities*. Not only through improving coordination mechanisms by means of *sensemaking* practices in an organizational context (Weick and Roberts, 1993; Weick, 1995), but also through more mundane specificities of the ECN, as a *social network*. Collective capabilities work at two levels. On the one hand, the ECN, as a whole, can undertake tasks that no individual actor could possibly tackle. On the other hand, the ECN gathers, pools and *produces* (through training) individual resources and capacities, which support and increase the capabilities of its individual members. The organization thus works both by opening up new fields and possibilities of action, as a collective, and by increasing and improving its members' individual capacity to act by creating, pooling and re-distributing skills and resources, as we will see.

ECN training

To understand the *context* of ECN deployees' interventions in West Africa, it is necessary to offer a glimpse at ECN training, as it participated fully to the structuration of affordances in the field, by providing different types of tools aimed at facilitating action in highly uncertain environments.

Before entering the ECN, experts have to complete successfully an "Emergency Communications Pre-deployment Training" (WHO, 2016), which the research team had the opportunity to observe.[5] This "is a multi-disciplinary, multi-hazard communications training for WHO and external experts". A successful completion of the course leads to the admission to the "Emergency Communications Network" roster, and experts can then be deployed in health emergencies, according to their areas of expertise. The training brings together WHO Communication Officers and experts in communication from other international organizations and international NGOs with the objective of having a group of a variety of practically oriented communication specialists that can be deployed rapidly.

During training, participants go through a week of classroom learning. This first phase is followed by a three-day simulation exercise – the SIMEX, a "serious game" simulating a humanitarian emergency or a disease outbreak. During the exercise, the participants are tested for their ability to work under stress and in a changing environment. Starting with the ECN 2015 training, the participants are accompanied by mentors during the whole session. Those are previous ECN participants, which have already been deployed as ECN members. Each mentor is responsible for a group of ten participants. At the end of training, one to two days are used for a personal and confidential debriefing of each participant with the "faculty" (WHO, 2016). The faculty comprises the director of the Department of Communications, the head of the Capacity Building Unit in the department, the mentor and several other WHO experts as well as experts from external agencies (WHO, 2015, 2016). The objective of the debriefing is to find the best fitting role for the candidate in an emergency, given her/his performance in the SIMEX, and the situation in which she or he can be deployed. By April 2015 the ECN consisted of a pool of 104 communication experts.

Characterizing the EVD setting

When characterizing the working context of interviewed ECN deployees in West Africa, one has to keep in mind that our dataset encompasses the most "turbulent" period of the epidemic, when the very ability of the international response to curb transmission was still at stake.[6] It thus corresponds to a period when the response was disorganized, with few working capacities in place.

Response structure and institutional complexity

In this context, a first challenge related to the institutional complexity of the response context, with local, national and international actors involved. For instance, in Liberia communication was made difficult by the fact that public health issues were dealt with by the Ministry of Health, whereas media resources were concentrated under the Ministry of Information, thus creating a disruption in information flows and coordination. Institutional complexity was also the product of the structures of international agencies. Many deployees found it difficult to understand the organizational workings of the WHO – especially non-WHO deployees.

The even greater complexity of the UN system and the additional intricacy caused by the creation of the UN Mission for Ebola Emergency Response (UNMEER) added to the confusion. This resulted in a general difficulty to identify management patterns. The response structure itself was cumbersome, due in part to the sheer number of involved actors,[7] causing confusion in communication practices.

Another obstacle related to the shifting nature of the response, as the distribution of roles and attributions were fuzzy and continuously renegotiated and adjusted over time, creating uncertainties in terms of action. The demise of existing response systems led to substantial organizational instability, both in terms of the general response structure and within individual organizations, as existing response mechanisms were questioned, sometimes hotly contested, and transformed. This indeterminacy led to the unregulated development of power plays between individual actors, services and organizations involved in the response – a common reality in humanitarian settings (Hilhorst & Jansen, 2010) – which were resented as counterproductive, as they ran counter to the need of increased coordination and cooperation. For instance, tensions emerged within the WHO between different services within the response structure, and between headquarters and the Regional Office for Africa (AFRO), a phenomenon somehow typical of crisis situations at large (Klein, 2007).

This resulted in the absence of a clear emergency response structure, both at the level of the global response and internally, within the WHO. At a global level, the creation of the Sub-Regional Ebola Operations and Coordination Centre (SEOCC – July–September 2014) and its quick demise and substitution by UNMEER (September 2014–July 2015) is a good illustration. At the WHO, the dual location of community engagement competences within two branches of the technical strategy support and standards function of the WHO's Ebola response team structure, as well as the reorganization of deployment procedures during the crisis, are but a few examples. More broadly, the Ebola response team structure at the WHO's headquarters in Geneva, which coordinated the organization's response and was tasked with dispatching responders in West Africa evolved constantly (see Dupras, Chapter 6). In this shifting environment, deployees had a hard time figuring out roles and functions, lines of reporting and authority. It was felt also that successive reorganizations of the response, at all levels, were designed with political agendas in mind rather than according to sound organizational principles aiming at efficiency in the field.

Deployees also stressed the high politicization of Ebola as a public issue, and the difficulties it posed in terms of communication. Political use of Ebola during parliamentary elections in Liberia (*New York Times*, December 4, 2014), Guinea (Aljazeera, October 10, 2015), as in the US during the 2014 mid-term elections (FiveThirtyEight, October 10, 2014; personal interviews at the US CDCs), thus complicated the task of communication officers, by fueling all kinds of controversies – blurring public health messages – and interfered in political decision processes, such as border controls or quarantine. Media were understood as playing an ambiguous role in this respect, by fueling unnecessary controversies and being often too alarmist, thus disrupting the response.

Information management and contextual knowledge

There were also issues with information management and available knowledge to make sense of the situation, on the ground. One of the most important pillars of science-based institutions such as the WHO is a strong commitment to evidence-based actions, informed by state-of-the-art situational assessments to reduce uncertainty and to define clear lines of conduct. However, the early EVD response was plagued by the paucity of reliable information in all dimensions of the crisis (from virology to epidemiology, from cultural patterns to institutional and organizational contexts, and so on) (Garrett, 2014). According to respondents, such basic information as the list of Ebola treatment centers (ETCs) in a country was sometimes impossible to obtain. Therefore, seeking the right information actually became one of the main tasks of many deployees. Importantly, organized information channels were also lacking. In many cases, information was not systematically collected on the ground, and no system was in place to consolidate and dispatch the data coming up from affected localities. Thus, many deployees spent a substantial amount of time trying to identify information bottlenecks and to bridge individuals and institutions in order to create consistent information channels. They ended up engaging in organizational work. This unanticipated part of the job, which concerned the necessity to assemble a work environment supportive of communication activities – to work towards creating more favorable *affordances* – under highly contingent circumstances and in an understructured organizational context, often ended up being a bigger part of deployees' activities than communication per se.

This difficulty with data collection and management, combined with a lack of situational awareness of local social and cultural environments in the field, resulted in difficulties to design locally relevant communication strategies and messages. This situation reflected an organizational weakness in data and knowledge management rather than an information void, since research on the social dimensions of Ebola was in fact readily available, with a substantial share of this corpus having been commissioned by the WHO itself (Bourrier, Chapter 3).

Roles and attributions

At the level of individual ECN deployees, an enduring difficulty had to do with the discrepancy between sketchy terms of reference and pre-departure briefings, and actual circumstances met in the field. Many deployees found the situation on the ground chaotic, with little-functioning structures in place. In this context, many had:

1   to clarify the actual situation on the ground, including relevant part-
    ners, partners' attributions and existing organizational structures;
2   to identify and/or define their own position and attributions within
    this structure and, as a result, to delineate tasks and task contents.

Moreover, too vague expectations about the role of communicators across institutions was also a shared concern. The combination between loose function attributions, inter-agency competition and a lack of under-standing of communication in national governments or in specific agencies resulted in many deployees having to define and carve their own position within the international response structure. This was also caused by a constantly evolving definition of tasks and attributions. For instance, social mobilization tasks diversified and developed into so-called "community engagement" practices (Bastide, 2018). Corresponding tasks, formally located within UNICEF, were progressively taken over by the ECN. A last consequence of this "blurred" environment was that respondents were often required to perform tasks exceeding their formal professional competency sets. For instance, "social mobilizers" were often asked to do interviews with the press, a job some of them did not feel skilled to perform.

The ECN as a social network

Given these circumstances, we now look at how the ECN helped deployees to develop their individual and collective agency in the crisis setting. Our hypothesis is that the ECN's main quality, as a "capacitating organization" (Fernagu-Oudet & Batal, 2016) in the EVD context, was due to its formal structural features as a social network, rather than to the *content* of its training. ECN training creates strong social ties, which facilitate the development of different forms of trust, a critical "moral good" in highly uncertain environments. As we will see, the quality of these social bonds worked towards expanding the resources and skills available to individual deployees *through the network.*

Forms of trust

Observations conducted during the ECN SIMEX 2015 and interviews with ECN members show that training creates lasting social bonds among the participants. This is particularly true for those being part of the same team during the drill, since they spend three very intense, emotionally charged days together, collaborating tightly around the same tasks. In the process, they get familiar with their respective working styles. Off-duty time, during meals or in shared bedrooms, provides further opportunities for personal interactions beyond these small groups. This intimacy and a common exposure to extraordinary circumstances seem to create a strong *esprit de corps* among participants, a significant identification to the ECN and a lasting commitment to the collective entity.

Many deployees thus stressed the particular relations that they have with their colleagues from the ECN. ECN deployees mentioned that the training created a feeling of closeness and belonging among the participants: "The community value is there". They "have that connection because [coming] from ECN, you have that sense of belonging. You can count on one another. You immediately hand in support and seek support".

These ties are defined in terms of friendship or even a family-like relationship. Thus, being part of the ECN is described as "being part of a network or family". Closeness among the participants is also mirrored and reinforced by their connection through dedicated Facebook groups, for every batch of alumni. Through these groups they can stay in contact and link up with each other at any time, including during deployments.

In addition to the density of social relations within the network, social bonds among ECN participants seem to be characterized by a high degree of trust. If trust is an ambiguous notion (Marzano, 2010), it certainly remains a critical functioning in situations of high uncertainty as it allows the quick development of cooperation and facilitates collective action. As phrased by one interviewee: "finding good people quickly, that you trust on. It's absolutely crucial to do your job".

Thus:

> It's nicer [to work with ECN members]. It's nicer yeah. It's faster too. You can just hit the ground running already. You know what they know, you know their level of skills because you've seen them working together, you've worked with them together as well. And that trust we were talking about is already there.

Complicity trust

As an organizational feature, the kind of trust relations developed in the ECN have different components and can take different forms.

A first form of trust is tied to intimate interpersonal knowledge developed during training, as part of the network, and reinforced during shared deployments. It often involves strong intersubjective ties, including affective bonds. To this extent, this type of trust appears to be unevenly distributed within the ECN, as it supposes shared personal experiences. Bonds of trust based on positive affects (friendship) and intimate interpersonal knowledge are likely to be stronger between people of a given group formed for the purpose of the SIMEX, among members of the same promotion, or between people who are in regular contact (be it because they work in the same organization, because they are deployed on the same operations, or through sustained relations through communication technologies):

INTERVIEWER: So it's one of the values of the ECN? Making links, strong links between people?
INTERVIEWEE: Yes, definitely. And especially if you have shared the same training with them. So ... If you have been in the same training with them, you feel that you are one. You feel closer to them. Before ECN I used to work with so many people in here. And we ... We did not ... We were just colleagues. But now, after ECN ... Especially because we were trained together, we feel that we are from the same batch and we are like friends now.

We call this type of trust *complicity trust* to stress the anchoring of this type of social bond in shared, face-to-face situations, involving substantial inter-subjective and affective engagements. These bonds are thus strictly limited in demographic terms. However, regarding this latter point, it is important to stress that the recent introduction of mentoring during ECN training is a way of widening "trust chains" (Roulleau-Berger, 2011, p. 155) among members, by promoting inter-promotion bonds.

> [The ECN] continues to expand, which is really nice. So being here as a mentor is wonderful because I get to meet this new batch of people. ... So the first year I was a participant, the second year I was a role player just in the simulation exercise, I wasn't there for this part. And then you meet people there and then two months later you're working with them in the field in an emergency. It's pretty ... It's pretty amazing.

The relationship with mentors, who have been through the same training before and are experienced concerning deployments, may help develop and broaden similar forms of trust. Such trust relations are integral to this function, since mentors will be involved in supervising the trainees and giving advice and backup, including after the training, during deployment.

Recognition trust

More broadly, many respondents recognize that the sole fact of being part of the ECN creates a sense of immediate connection between individuals. Another type of trust is thus based on the sheer knowledge of a shared background as ECN graduates, and of shared frames of reference, as well as a shared body of technical skills and professional attitudes related to emergency response. It can thus extend beyond direct relations, if involved individuals have been through the training. ECN members share a basic level of skills, a common language and common tools in terms of risk communication. "Although some of them have more experience, you have a common background ... and you have the same information on how to phase those situations how to phase difficult situations".

Being "part of the same community", having "the same goal together" and knowing it is implicit in the relationship was thus pointed out as an important element. These shared ways of framing situations, a shared language and shared toolboxes are instrumental in facilitating work relations, as they provide a common ground, thus reducing greatly the need to negotiate a common framework of work and action. As far as time is concerned, as is the case of course in an emergency, this is a valuable asset.

Beyond its formal role as an emergency deployment organization, the ECN thus has a more "latent" efficacy in terms of crisis management. On the one hand, it is similar to the Global Outbreak Alert and Response Network (GOARN), a well-known "networked" organization operating in the domain of public health emergencies (Ansell, Sondorp & Stevens, 2012), as it allows the quick identification, mobilization and deployment of trained responders from various organizations. However, it also provides additional capacities in terms of interpersonal and collective coordination. The ECN aligns goals and values among communication professionals with various backgrounds, focuses and streamlines practical norms and methodologies, and provides cognitive routines in the unstable environment of an emergency.

Therefore, by certifying the existence of a common base of knowledge, values and norms, the ECN acts as a "trust device" (Karpik, 2010) and ascribes a set of known attributes to all of its members. As a result, it formats and stabilizes mutual expectations. This "labeling" greatly facilitates working relations in the field since individuals know what can be expected from each other, even in the absence of existing personal relationships and/or when formal role attributions lack, making the ECN a particularly "loosely coupled" organization (Weick, 1995). We call this second type of trust *recognition trust*. The importance of this latter form is made obvious when it is lacking:

> If there is no such team [ECN team], if the team relationship is not working properly, then you have to build your own network, and to build trust takes a lot of time. And by the time you have built strong ties, then you have to go back.

While complicity trust is based on "thick" relationships and substantial interpersonal and intersubjective knowledge, recognition trust is thinner and pertains to the labeling power of the ECN. Bonds related to the first type of trust are multidimensional and involve people emotionally, while bonds related to the second type are more focused, professional in kind (Table 5.1). Complicity bonds are related to a certain degree of intimacy

Table 5.1 Complicity trust and recognition trust

	Complicity trust	Recognition trust
Type of bonds	Personal	Impersonal
Interpersonal commitment	Strong	Weaker
Scope	Focused	Extensive

between individuals, while recognition bonds relate to a formalized body of practices, knowledge, norms and values. The former are more restrictive in scope, as they encompass fewer individuals, but commend deeper interpersonal commitment, while the latter extend further, as they are less demanding to create. Complicity trust is more local and idiosyncratic, while recognition trust is more mobile and more easily transferred, connective.

Pooling social capital

As a property of social relations, these forms of trust hint towards another characteristic of the ECN: as a social network, it greatly enhanced the ability of its members to reach out for different kinds of scarce goods and resources – functionings – in a highly strained environment. This ability to broaden individual and collective capabilities through social ties fits with the concept of "social capital", as it allows understanding how these relations affect positively or negatively the ability to implement or develop one's other bodies of resources and capacities (Bourdieu, 1980), under given circumstances.

To understand this aspect, it is useful to draw on Daniel Aldrich's (2017) definition of social capital. For him, social capital can be delineated according to three different forms – different types of links – namely *bonding*, *bridging* and *linking*. The first form of social capital is constituted by links between people whose association is based on a tendency to link up with persons with similar social properties (according to a logic of *homophily*). Conversely, *bridging* allows connecting people with heterogeneous social characteristics. Eventually, *linking* allows reaching for "power brokers, authority figures and decision makers". Importantly, each of these channels provides different types of resources. Our hypothesis is that the ECN combines these three dimensions.

Bonding

Complicity trust can be associated most closely with *bonding social capital*, as it combines objective commonality (being an ECN member) and subjective ties (including affects). However, whereas Aldrich applies this type to characterize social relations between "family, kin and close friends", we extend it to characterize the social bonds created between given ECN members. To do so, we posit that there is a more fundamental underlying principle than homophily underpinning *bonding*, as a relational type: it is based on a *subjective sense of belonging* (Brubaker and Cooper, 2000), commanding specific forms of reciprocal obligations and loyalty. This sense of belonging and commonality is salient between ECN members and underpins specific forms of solidarity:

> [T]he ECN operates like I know he [generic ECN colleague] knows what I'm going through, and he was like: "Okay, whatever you need, you call me": And then I also, you know, I was calling him because I knew he was away when the thing … happened. So, you know, we're kind of supporting each other. And then I did have [several] members of my ECN team that weren't in the area, that weren't in the Ebola response kind of helping me from outside, like sending me materials, you know, checking "how are you doing?"

Bonding social capital thus shapes the ECN as a close-knit collective with multiple connections between its members. ECN management has leveraged this property by creating the figure of the *mentor*, a way of improving the *clustering coefficient*[8] of the network by fostering inter-promotion relations. In contrast with Aldrich's approach, we thus accept that this sense of belonging can develop *across* social differences (as such, it does not concern only relations ruled by homophily). ECN training is conducive to the development of such bonds, as it gathers professionals with diverse backgrounds and helps developing strong social bonds between them as they are put into intense, shared social experiences. The ECN *generates* bonding social capital by creating and broadening commonality between its members.

These bonds – feeling of belonging and communality – were also produced and/or deepened by the shared experience of field deployment during the EVD outbreak. This high-risk, emotionally draining environment fostered mutual recognition and strong mutual commitment between ECN responders. These relations facilitated the expression of and collective dealing with difficult and potentially impairing affects, such as fear. These social dynamics sustained the development of caring practices within the network, which helped deployees deal with the specificities of the EVD crisis – as a perceived high-risk environment.

Bridging and linking

The ECN also contributes to develop and pool a great volume of the *bridging* and *linking* types of social capital. The network draws members from various organizations with different professional backgrounds and with diverse roles and positions within organizational hierarchies. In the 2015 training, participants originated from all WHO regional bureaus, from the WHO HQ, the International Federation of Red Cross (IFRC), the US CDCs, and Qatar's Ministry of Health. It also included independent communication specialists, sometimes with a journalism background, some with substantial experience working for international NGOs such as Médecins Sans Frontières (MSF).[9] The high turnover of workers in international organizations and NGOs, with individual careers typically bringing professionals to work for different organization, only reinforces this variety. As a result, individuals in these professional worlds are often well connected. This variety creates efficient "bridges" to reach out across various organizations and to mobilize power brokers. Importantly, it allows doing so by using direct interpersonal relations rather than through institutionalized communication channels and processes:

> Heads of office continue to get communications training, … they work closely with communications officers even outside of emergencies so they get to know us. Not just understand the role, but actually know us individually and trust us individually. Because it's … Actually if you think about, if I put myself in the shoes of the man I was working with in [country], he's never met me before. I'm some [foreign] girl from headquarters who's not even WHO staff, I'm a consultant. How does he know if I'm trustworthy, if I'm sending secret messages to my friend at *The New York Times*? He doesn't trust me because he doesn't know me. Even though you can be very … You can be as good as you can be in his presence, he doesn't have that long-term relationship with you. So that's why it's good to be able to build it up, to have these trainings, so that let's say you arrive in the country office, you trained with one of the country office people and they can tell their boss: "Yes she's good" or "he's good". So these networks are very important.

Mixing people from different backgrounds thus offers the possibility to tap into their respective networks. In this respect, the ECN functions much like a "network of networks", more than most other agencies where interactions are essentially contained within the organization. As a result, complicity trust and recognition trust developed within the ECN can extend considerably through these secondary relational systems, by building "trust chains" (Roulleau-Berger, 2011, p. 155) across ECN members' personal social networks.

Conclusion

During the 2013–2016 EVD outbreak in West Africa, the ECN displayed specific qualities, as an organization. Importantly, it combined efficiently different types of social capital, helping to cut across institutions and reaching out for help and assistance in a radically resources-deprived environment. In particular, it helped circulate information. In a context of high uncertainty, with few channels of communication in place among involved actors in the response system, information proved a highly critical good for deployees, especially at the onset of the response, when organization was still very much lacking: "That was a great thing with the ECN, because through that you had other persons that you could rely on and ask for advice. So, in the beginning I was totally relying on that".

Information was vital for actors to be able to qualify (or *assess*) situations, and to take informed decisions on appropriate courses of action. Whatever capacities one possesses, lack of information has a debilitating effect on the possibility to implement them.

To keep with our analytical vocabulary, the ECN, as a professional network, thus increased responders' capabilities in the West African setting. The network itself emerged as a "capacitating organization", thus becoming a significant element of the emergency setting, a defining dimension of the context for its deployees. It contributed to shape flexible affordances – such as trust, information channels, but also, for instance, forms of mutual caring – thus partly offsetting resource deprivation in the field. Its combination of flexible and strong social bonds and low level of proceduralization (or high level of personal autonomy) proved efficient at gathering, articulating and implementing specific resources and capacities, given unfolding events and circumstances.

Notes

1 The interviews are covered by a clause of strict confidentiality. As a consequence, we are not allowed to provide any personal identifier when quoting interviewees, including deployments locations.
2 This is undoubtedly a restrictive use of the author's approach, as it detaches his core conceptualization from its broader theoretical context, as a constitutive element of a theory of justice. The theoretical discussion proposes an adaptation of Sen's propositions in the context of a theory of action.
3 Functionings are states of "being and doing". Being in good health is an instance, or being able to achieve a certain type of specialized action.
4 Interview at the US CDCs headquarters, Atlanta, GA, August 13, 2015.
5 Two interns in the research team were embedded in the 2015 ECN training, as participant observers, namely Beatrice Nass and Kayla Jenni. The analysis of the training relies heavily on their accounts.
6 Personal interview, US CDCs.
7 UNMEER, WHO, MSF, the United Nations Development Program (UNDP), the United Nations International Children's Emergency Fund (UNICEF), the World Food Programme (WFP), the United Sates Centers for Disease Control and Prevention (US CDCs), the International and National Red Crosses, the International Organization for Migrations (IOM), to mention a few.
8 In graph theory, the clustering coefficient indicates a high density of ties within a social group. A high clustering coefficient means that each individual within a group is directly connected to most of its other members.

9 Statuses differed during deployment according to individual professional situations: some communication specialists were deployed as consultants, some as WHO personnel. The WHO was responsible for medical evacuation under deployment contracts.

References

Aldrich, D. P. (2017). The importance of social capital in building community resilience, in Braun, B. (ed.) *Rethinking Resilience, Adaptation and Transformation in a Time of Change.* Philadelphia, PA: Taylor & Francis, 357–364.

Ansell, C., Sondorp, E., & Stevens, R. H. (2012). The promise and challenge of global network governance: The global outbreak alert and response network. *Global Governance: A Review of Multilateralism and International Organizations,* 18(3), 317–337.

Bastide, L. (2015). *Habiter le transnational: Espace, travail et migration entre Java, Kuala Lumpur et Singapour.* Lyon: ENS Editions.

Bastide, L. (2018). Crisis communication during the Ebola outbreak in West Africa: The paradoxes of decontextualized contextualization, in Bourrier, M., & Bieder, C. (eds) *Risk Communication for the Future: Towards Smart Risk Governance and Safety Management.* Cham: Springer.

Bourdieu, P. (1980). Le capital social. *Actes de la recherche en sciences sociales,* 31(1), 2–3.

Brubaker, R., & Cooper, F. (2000). Beyond "identity"'. *Theory and Society,* 29(1), 1–47.

Dodier, N. (1993). Les appuis conventionnels de l'action. Eléments de pragmatique sociologique. *Réseaux,* 11(62), 63–85.

Fernagu-Oudet, S., & Batal, C. (2016). *(R)évolution du management des ressources humaines: Des compétences aux capabilités.* Villeneuve d'Ascq: Presses Universitaires du Septentrion.

Fleck, F. (2017). WHO's new emergencies programme bridges two worlds. *Bulletin of the World Health Organization,* 95(1), 8–9.

Garfinkel, H. (1967). *Studies in Ethnomethodology.* Englewood Cliffs, NJ: Prentice-Hall.

Garrett, L. (2014). Opinion: Why Ebola epidemic is spinning out of control. CNN. com. Available at: http://edition.cnn.com/2014/07/24/opinion/garrett-ebola/ (Accessed December 16, 2014).

Gibson, J. J. (1977). The theory of affordances, in Shaw, R. E., & Bransford, J. D. (eds) *Perceiving, Acting, and Knowing: Toward an Ecological Psychology.* Hillsdale, NJ: Lawrence Erlbaum Associates, 56–60.

Grossetti, M. (2007). Trois échelles d'action et d'analyse. *L'Année sociologique,* 56(2), 285–307.

Hilhorst, D., & Jansen, B. J. (2010). Humanitarian space as arena: A perspective on the everyday politics of aid. *Development and Change,* 41(6), 1117–1139.

Ibrahim, S. S. (2006). From individual to collective capabilities: The capability approach as a conceptual framework for self-help. *Journal of Human Development,* 7(3), 397–416.

Karpik, L. (2010). *Valuing the Unique: The Economics of Singularities.* Princeton, NJ: Princeton University Press.

Klein, N. (2007). *The Shock Doctrine: The Rise of Disaster Capitalism.* London: Penguin.

Lahire, B. (2006). *L'homme pluriel: Les ressorts de l'action.* Paris: Hachette Littératures.

Lakoff, A. (2007). Preparing for the next emergency. *Public Culture,* 19(2), 247–271.

Marzano, M. (2010). Qu'est-ce que la confiance? *Études,* 412(1), 53–63.

Moon, S., Leigh, J., Woskie, L. et al. (2017). Post-Ebola reforms: Ample analysis, inadequate action. *British Medical Journal,* 356(j280).

Quéré, L. (1997). La situation toujours négligée? *Réseaux,* 15(85), 163–192.

Roulleau-Berger, L. (2011). *Désoccidentaliser la sociologie: l'Europe au miroir de la Chine.* Paris: Editions de l'Aube.

Sen, A. (2010). *The Idea of Justice.* London, New York, NY, Toronto: Penguin.

Suchman, L. A. (1987). *Plans and Situated Actions: The Problem of Human–Machine Communication.* Cambridge and New York, NY: Cambridge University Press.

Weber, M. (1978). *Economy and Society: An Outline of Interpretive Sociology.* Berkeley and Los Angeles, CA and London: University of California Press.

Weick, K. E. (1995). *Sensemaking in Organizations.* Thousand Oaks, CA: Sage.

Weick, K. E., & Robert, K. H. (1993). Collective mind in organizations: Heedful interrelating on flight decks. *Administrative Science Quarterly,* 38(8), 357–381.

WHO. (2015). *WHO Strategic Response Plan: West Africa Ebola Outbreak.* Geneva: World Health Organization.

WHO. (2016). 'A pre-deployment training for the Emergency Communication Network: Course brochure'. World Health Organization, Department of Communications.

Zimmermann, B. (2006). Pragmatism and the capability approach challenges in social theory and empirical research. *European Journal of Social Theory,* 9(4), 467–484.

Zylberman, P. (2013). *Tempêtes microbiennes: Essai sur la politique de sécurité sanitaire dans le monde transatlantique.* Paris: Gallimard.

6 The use of matrix structure in epidemic management

Alexandrine Dupras

Introduction

Each time a disease outbreak or a public health emergency occurs, the World Health Organization (WHO) is thrown under the spotlight and scrutinised by its Member States and the media who do not hesitate to criticise publicly its response, as was the case for the 2014–2016 Ebola outbreak (Kamradt-Scott, 2016). And this was not the first time this international organisation received such reviews (Godlee, 1994a; Godlee, 1994b; Godlee, 1994c; Liden, 2014). Yet, the UN agency's work is not limited to outbreak response but ranges from maternal and child health to microbial resistance, from health systems and ethics to mental health. As a reminder, the UN agency has the mandate to handle any health issue and to support all Member States to prepare and respond to "any hazard of public health consequences" (WHO, 2013, 29).

The WHO is also a public organisation which depends upon the funding and decisions of its Member States. Unlike private entities, public organisations seek to "address complex social functions, providing goods and services that cannot be easily packaged for exchange in economic markets" (Pandey & Wright, 2006, 513). They rely on public resources and have the mandate to meet public needs, which makes them "heavily influenced by their external environment" (Pakarinen & Virtanen, 2016, 232). The complex nature of these organisations' work requires an internal management of labour that goes beyond a strict division of labour and standardised work processes. Matrix management is often perceived as a solution "to manage public organisations as complex systems" (Pakarinen & Virtanen, 2016, 232) and some studies have shown that a matrix structure can enhance organisational performance over traditional functional management (Gobeli & Larson, 1986; Kuprenas, 2003). In the past, matrix management was also adopted within the WHO on a smaller scale. Considering its large-scale mandate, it is interesting to look more closely at the structuring of the organisation to tackle such massive crises. This chapter will analyse to what extent matrix management has been applied within the WHO and its impact on the efficiency of the organisation to respond to a health emergency, using the 2014 Ebola response as an example.

Matrix management

Developed as an alternative to rigid silo work in order to bring flexibility over production (Kuprenas, 2003), matrix management can be traced back to the 1960s (Lawson, 1986). A matrix structure is supposed to "combine the efficiency of functional design with the flexibility and responsiveness of a multi-divisional organisation" (Pakarinen & Virtanen, 2016, 232). It is composed of two elements: the functional units and the project units. Functional units (e.g. departments) are, most of the time, discipline-oriented and mobilise "organisational resources around specialities" (Lawson, 1986, 64). In other words, they have the expertise and resources needed for a project or a programme. On the other hand, project units gather the expertise from diverse functional departments in order to achieve objectives in a multidisciplinary perspective. As Baber et al. (1990, 236) explain, a matrix structure "has a dual authority structure, with task oriented work groups drawing members from various functional departments". Workers are asked to think "out of the box" and to bring their expertise to achieve a specific project, as opposed to a traditional (functional) management where objectives are "established by upper management" and "elements of the project are then assigned to relevant functional areas" (Gobeli & Larson, 1986, 72). Functional management provides "stability, maintenance of core values, and long-term development" while, on the other side, "projects are believed to be more appropriate for change, flexibility, and action orientation" (Arvidsson, 2009, 99).

Based on the literature, matrix management can bring complexity of work in organisations. Indeed, matrix management, with its two command lines, might create confusion over roles and responsibilities, obstruct clear decision-making, add additional layers of bureaucracy and cause conflicts between functional and project managers to obtain control over funds for their interests (Davis & Lawrence, 1978; Stuckenbruck, 1997; Laslo & Goldberg, 2008). In order to overcome these challenges, specialists suggest a drastic change in the organisation's culture is needed to enhance worker's autonomy and team spirit (Hall, 2013).

Methodology

From February to October 2015, I embarked on an internship (financed by the University of Geneva and associated with the larger Swiss national science project co-led by Bourrier, Brender and Burton-Jeangros) at the WHO and was asked to produce a literature review on matrix management. At that moment, the WHO was criticised for its handling of the

Ebola outbreak and some organisational restructuring was debated internally. Managers and staff were thus reflecting upon better working and structural approaches to respond to an emergency in a more efficient manner. Seeking suitable solutions to tackle hurdles, the concept of matrix management offered at the time an option worth investigating. The literature review I was then asked to produce turned into an internal report using the Ebola response team as a case study. The data collected for the report on matrix management serves as a background for this chapter, developed three years after the fact. The organisation has changed since then and this chapter reflects only debates that occurred at the time.

This chapter is organised as follow: the first section analyses the WHO in relation with its environment and its funding system, with the help of secondary literature. The second section deals with the different steps taken by the WHO to develop its response to the 2014 Ebola outbreak. Having a closer look at the concept of matrix management, the third section will seek to analyse the extent to which it is suitable for emergency responses.

The WHO in a changing landscape

In order to assess to what extent matrix management has been applied within the WHO and its impact on the efficiency of the organisation's response, it is important to look more closely at the organisation itself. Not only matrix management represents a challenge in itself, but attempting to implement it within the WHO, like within any large and complex organisation, might create specific difficulties.

Founded in 1948, the WHO's mission is to foster "the attainment by all peoples of the highest possible level of health" (Article 1, WHO Constitution). Although the WHO's mandate is large and all-encompassing, unlike other organisations, many other agencies are working on handling health problems. Indeed, the period between the late 1990s and the early 2000s is characterised by a booming number of NGOs and public–private partnerships working on health issues (Liden, 2014), symbolic of the increasing interest in this field around the world which led the WHO to evolve within a more competitive environment. It is widely acknowledged that the proliferation of numerous global health organisations has weakened the WHO's authority (Brown et al., 2006; Prah Ruger & Yach, 2008/2009; Chorev, 2013; Chorev et al., 2011; Liden, 2014). In the midst of new international players who are financially powerful – such as the Global Fund, the Gates Foundation, pharmaceutical companies and the G8 – the WHO's authority on health governance is often seen as being threatened.

Moreover, its international influence and reputation largely depend upon how its management of global epidemics is perceived. For instance, Liden (2014) stresses that the "SARS epidemic in 2003 re-established the

WHO as a global authority and coordinator on disease outbreaks" whereas "WHO's widely criticised reaction to the avian influenza outbreak [sic] in 2009 weakened the organisation's authority" (Liden, 2014, 145). Nonetheless, the WHO remains a central player in the global health system. The WHO's actions and declarations have a huge impact on global perceptions of health threats, remaining an important normative agency, as stressed by Abeysinghe (2015), who showed that the WHO's narratives on epidemic developments highly influence proceeding responses. Also, the revision of the International Health Regulations (IHR) in 2005 has reinforced public health surveillance systems (Calain et al., 2009, 24), giving more legitimacy to the WHO in asking for greater cooperation from Member States with regard to disease control, due to the need to control potential global health threats (Baker & Fidler, 2006, 1058).

The WHO is a decentralised organisation, comprising the headquarters in Geneva, six regional offices and 147 country offices (Lee, 2009, 27). This structure highly impacts the organisation's functioning. Indeed, it is well acknowledged that the autonomy given to each institutional level causes recurrent tensions, as each of the organisation's levels seeks the legitimacy to make decisions (Lee, 2009, 45). Internal tensions arise at the headquarters level as well. Back in 2015, the WHO comprised twenty-six departments that were collectively in charge of fulfilling the organisation's broad mission. In order to understand the organisation's internal dynamics and the implementation of the matrix structure, it is important to further grasp links between the organisation's funding mechanisms and its compartmentalised structure.

Initially, the WHO's activities were mainly funded by "assessed contributions" from its Member States, but the constitution always allowed for the collection of extra-budgetary funds from non-state actors (Lee, 2009, 38). These extra-budgetary funds (also called voluntary or earmarked donations) imply that the donor attributes the grant directly to a specific project. Over time, this extra-budgetary source of income grew and became more important. As a result, the organisation currently relies heavily on extra-budgetary donations that increased from 20 per cent in the 1970s to 60 per cent of its total income in the 1990s (Chorev, 2013, 640). In 2014, 78 percent of the WHO's income stemmed from voluntary contributions (WHO, 2015, 3). In addition to this, an austerity policy of "zero nominal growth" to Member States' contributions was adopted in 1993, reducing the WHO's budget in subsequent years (Lee, 2009, 39; Chorev, 2013, 640). Having only a fifth of its budget guaranteed through the assessed contributions, the WHO is constantly in a fundraising mind-set.

The WHO is governed by Member States that gather once a year during the World Health Assembly (WHA) in order to decide the overall direction of the organisation and to vote on the annual budget (Lee, 2009, 25–26). During the 68th WHA, I observed how this annual meeting provided a good opportunity for departments to advertise their programmes and projects and to seek funding. I saw how this dynamic is engrained into the staff's routine work. In front of meeting rooms, stands were set up and staff members were encouraged to come and talk to country delegates. Informative leaflets, colourful stands and attractive videos completed the visibility strategy. One team had even deployed a tent to expose their latest versions of personal protective equipment (PPE).

The WHO acknowledged that "some donor-based investments are time-limited, particularly when the specific results are achieved or donors' priorities or circumstances change" and is thus actively seeking to increase the proportion of assessed donations (WHO, 2016b, 4). Other than allowing "a small number of rich countries to bypass the World Health Assembly" (Chorev, 2013, 640), the WHO's funding system also influenced internal functioning. Since the donations were granted to specific programmes or projects, it was incumbent upon each of the twenty-six departments of the headquarters to manage the funds that were given for a specific programme or project.

Since the 1990s, the WHO has been evolving in the midst of growing private health organisations which increased the competition with regard to its status of influence in this field. Linked with its funding system, the WHO's independence from external actors was lacking (Moon et al., 2017, 3). Its funding system divided up by departments imported a logic of marketing and rivalry into programmes and within the organisation. Several studies were able to show the impact the environment has on an organisation's strategy and structure (Kolodny, 1979, 544–545). On this topic, Kolodny (1979) stated that "each stage an organisation moves through in evolving toward a matrix organisation should be commensurate with the demands of the environment at that particular stage" (Kolodny, 1979, 545). The WHO was embedded within a specific environment and, in the case of the Ebola outbreak, the pressure from external actors was considerable.

Responding to Ebola

On March 23, 2014, the WHO African Regional Office reported an outbreak of Ebola virus disease in Guinea (WHO, 2016a). This outbreak emerged mainly in three countries in West Africa (Guinea, Liberia and Sierra Leone), affecting more than 28,000 people and causing 11,310 deaths (June 2016) (WHO, 2016a). The Ebola crisis was unique for many reasons. First, this disease crossed two borders in a very short period of time in countries where Ebola had never been encountered before. Second, health care systems of affected countries were not prepared to respond to this outbreak and international support was much needed. Third, unlike previous Ebola outbreaks, the disease was transmitted mostly in big cities (WHO, 2016a).

Internally, the management of this outbreak went through different stages. At first, on 25 March, 2014, the WHO declared the outbreak a

Grade 2 emergency according to its 2013 Emergency Response Framework (ERF), which implied that the outbreak was to be managed by the regional office. The experts were applying the "standard" approach to an EVD outbreak (isolation of cases, treatment of cases, contact tracing and safe burial) (MSF, 2013; Global Ebola Response, 2015, 8) and a decreasing number of cases in Guinea in April and May 2014 (Global Ebola Response, 2015, 11) suggested the outbreak was under control. At the end of June, Médecins Sans Frontières (MSF) declared the outbreak "out of control" and urged the international community to mobilise more resources and to intervene quickly as the number of affected cases was increasing rapidly (MSF, 2014). The WHO established the Sub-Regional Ebola Operations and Coordination Centre (SEOCC) in July 2014 with the aim to better coordinate the response through the three most affected countries and declared the outbreak Grade 3 on 26 July. According to the ERF, Grade 3 is supposed to increase the organisation's capacities (WHO, 2013). One interviewee explained that this mechanism "is an institutional means to mobilise resources from the entire organisation". On 8 August, the WHO International Health Regulations Emergency Committee regarding Ebola convened and declared the outbreak a Public Health Emergency of International Concern (PHEIC).

When any outbreak is declared, the WHO HQ would normally gather professionals from different units or departments in order to create a "task force" – a matrix-type structure – to provide the required support to relevant country's authorities or the WHO's regional or country offices. In the case of the Ebola outbreak, the WHO first activated the same system, but soon realised that it was insufficient. Between March and the beginning of August 2014, at the HQ level, support was provided by two departments, concerned with epidemic diseases and response capacities, with the support of one additional department that deals with risk communication. These departments at WHO headquarters are usually involved in any other major outbreak. A technical officer explains:

> At the beginning of the outbreak, two departments were mainly involved. Technical support by other departments was still informal at that time, so their support was limited by their daily work; they were not deployed to the Ebola response team yet.

The declaration of Grade 3 and PHEIC significantly impacted the WHO's headquarters' Ebola outbreak management. This classification triggered the implementation of new internal procedures. The responsibility of the response was retrieved from the hands of two initial departments and given to a completely new team, composed of staff from different departments according to an enlarged matrix structure. From this point, many other departments got involved and new staff and consultants – with sometimes limited experience on outbreak response – were hired to work exclusively in this structure that constituted the Ebola response team.

A few months in, I was requested to give a presentation on matrix management, as a way to shed some light on the implications of working in such an environment. Some staff members had indeed limited experience of this type of managerial structure. Yet smaller matrix teams were common practice across the organisation (such as for the vaccine team and Pandemic Influenza Preparedness (PIP) Framework team). The matrix structure of the Ebola response team was staffed with people from six different programmes and the office of the director-general, and then split into five thematic sub-teams or project units, led by project managers: (1) Enabling Functions; (2) Epidemiology and Information Management; (3) Planning; (4) Technical Strategy, Support and Standards; (5) Partner Coordination and Logistics. A disease outbreak of this scale required a large deployment of resources and direct operational intervention. As a way to address this issue and according to the WHO's Emergency Response Framework, this cross-cutting structure had been put into place in order to gather and coordinate all essential resources. Staff from each of the departments were assigned to work on this outbreak sometimes full-time, sometimes part-time. At the height of the crisis, more than a hundred employees were dispatched in this matrix structure, full or mainly part-time.

Matrix structure challenges

When responding to an outbreak, the WHO normally brings expertise from different departments together according to a matrix structure. In the case of the Ebola response team, recurrent problems arose from the way the Ebola response team was functioning in such a volatile environment: lack of decision-making, unclear definition of roles and responsibilities and overwhelming workload were some of the typical challenges of a matrix structure identified in the literature (Hall, 2013).

It is possible that the prevalence of the conventional structure over the newly implemented matrix team prevented project units from gaining complete authority from functional departments at the WHO. Indeed, the traditional structure of the international organisation was well entrenched in employees' minds and was hard to overcome. As an example, certain employees would not agree to receive direction from staff in a lower relative position in the conventional hierarchical structure. At the employee level, the dual management line could lead to a loyalty conflict or confusion over reporting (Davis & Lawrence, 1978). People used to reporting to an established manager on their daily work can find it very challenging to report to someone else. It is acknowledged that functional managers often keep their initial authority because they are seen as the natural boss and their departments are perceived as the "home base" (Stuckenbruck, 1997, 217).

During the Ebola crisis, two organisational cultures (Hofstede, 1997) were at play: the scientific technical dimension and the operational humanitarian dimension. One employee summarised this observation:

Before the WHO was a technical agency that was hiring mostly highly technical employees. It changed when Member States required the WHO to be more operational. It led to the hiring of many humanitarian employees who have more a voluntary mind-set for which working in limited conditions is okay.

The scientific technical approach considered that the WHO's fundamental role lay in monitoring data, producing knowledge and making its expertise available to Member States while the operational humanitarian view point implied the WHO was to act as a deployable agency able to provide direct assistance in case of emergency. From the understanding that the WHO was composed of two distinct cultures arose the debate over the main mandate of the organisation. Internal debates questioned the possibility of the WHO responding to emergencies and recalled that the WHO's mandate was mainly technical, not operational.

Notwithstanding this important distinction, the role of the UN agency was a source of debate within the organisation, and of course outside. Indeed, research on public organisations has shown that ambiguity (by no means extraordinary) over an agency's goal can lead to ambiguity over personnel roles, which has a direct impact over work perspective (Pandey & Wright, 2006). Barnett and Finnemore's (1999) analysis of "pathologies" of international organisations sheds some light on the deficiency to which different organisational cultures can lead:

> Different segments of the organization may develop different ways of making sense of the world, experience different local environments, and receive different stimuli from outside; they may also be populated by different mixes of professions or shaped by different historical experiences. All of these would contribute to the development of different local cultures within the organization and different ways of perceiving the environment and the organization's overall mission ... Consequently, different constituencies representing different normative views will suggest different tasks and goals for the organization, resulting in a clash of competing perspectives that generates pathological tendencies.
>
> (Barnett & Finnemore, 1999, 724–725)

On one hand, the scientific technical field of work wanted evidence-based decisions and relied strongly on data, which takes time to establish. On the other hand, the operational humanitarian field of work intended to be ready for anything and plans in advance with the aim to respond quickly. These complementary mind-sets were brought into the Ebola response team. Pakarinen and Virtanen (2016, 247) have shown in their study that a major impediment to a successful implementation of a matrix structure is adhesion to the organisational culture in people's minds.

For project units to obtain authority over decision-making in matrix management, it is important that functional managers delegate power to project managers (Gobeli & Larson, 1986). A concrete manifestation of the delegation of decision-making is the delegation of funds. It is generally acknowledged in the literature that direct access to funding presents a difficulty when working in a matrix structure. Horizontal or transversal projects have a hard time getting funded because they fall under the responsibility of several managers and several budgets.

Conflicts over resource allocation are a typical challenge of matrix structures (Laslo & Goldberg, 2008). In their research, Laslo and Goldberg (2008) observed conflicts between functional and project managers to obtain control over funds for their interests. The interest of project managers is mainly to meet project deadlines, while that of functional managers is to reach long-term effectiveness. These conflicting goals impact the performance of matrix management by preventing the organisation from acting as a cohesive entity.

As the departments were the gatekeepers of the voluntary contributions – which constitute three-quarters of the WHO's budget – the devolution of funding, thus of power, represented a major obstacle to implementing decisions. Ultimately, the matrix team encountered some difficulty in making decisions over the regular functional structure. At all levels of the organisation, it was agreed that the matrix management implemented at the WHO represented a challenge. In the midst of such a massive response, it took time for employees to feel comfortable. Besides this, the outbreak response had been overwhelming for involved staff; most of them had to work overtime for a long period of time.

Overall, it seems that the implementation of this matrix structure ran into classic pitfalls identified in the literature. Besides, this enlarged task force was also taking place in an unstable workplace. The uncertainty of employment also affects the work. The staff turnover made it difficult to make long-term plans. Lots of people worked on short-term contracts. This situation led to uncertainty on a daily basis and may have had other consequences such as losing the sense of ownership of their work. At the WHO, and in the UN system at large, it is common practice to be employed on temporary contracts for many years. Department restructurings had happened in the recent past and could happen again.

Discussion: matrix structure and managing epidemics

At the time the 2014–2016 Ebola outbreak struck, the WHO was used to implementing small matrix structures in the form of a task force to respond to an outbreak involving traditional technical departments leading the response. In 2014, for the first time, employees from more than ten departments related to six different bigger programmes were working under the same roof, gathering more than a hundred employees at the height of the crisis. In light of the above, matrix management was taking place in a specific and complex organisation and this way of working faced common issues identified in the literature.

This thus raises the question: was matrix management the best way to respond to an outbreak? One manager commented: "For emergencies, a clear line of command with vertical decision-making power is needed. We need to create an incident management focus system". More than a simple emergency, an epidemic relies on scientific knowledge. Ansell and Keller (2014) reported on the US Centers for Disease Control and Prevention (USCDC) and underlined the fact that an outbreak response differs from any other humanitarian interventions. It demands rapid scientific mobilisation and knowledge-based deployment (Ansell & Keller, 2014, 25). Technical scientific knowledge is at the core of an outbreak response and this requires time. The USCDC chose to elaborate a specific outbreak response mechanism that "maintains a cadre of specially trained experts – epidemic intelligence service officers – who can be dispatched as needed for outbreak investigations" (Ansell & Keller, 2014, 12). This mechanism follows the principles of the Incident Command System (ICS) approach – initially developed by firefighters in the 1970s – which implies the "rapid establishment of a single chain of command" (Ansell & Keller, 2014, 9). USCDC adapted the concept in the context of public health by, for instance, integrating outside expert panels to mobilise "rapid authoritative knowledge" (Ansell & Keller, 2014, 22) and to make decisions. However, what may work for USCDC, a bilateral organisation, may not work for the WHO, a multilateral organisation.

Conclusion

Over the last thirty years, the WHO has been struggling to position itself in the global health system. Since the review of the IHR (WHO, 2005), the implementation of the Emergency Response Framework (WHO, 2013), the WHO had been appointed a larger role than its initial knowledge-based mandate. Therefore, at the time of the 2014–2016 Ebola outbreak, it still needed to develop internal managerial ways to meet the expectations of being a leader in emergency responses. The WHO had dealt with many emergencies in the past, yet its response to the 2014–2016 Ebola epidemic was perceived as lacking strength and authoritativeness.

Some would argue that matrix management is not suitable for an organisation such as the WHO when it comes to tackling outbreaks. The organisation experienced some resistance from its staff to work on transversal projects because different organisational cultures co-exist within this large agency. More importantly, the WHO's funding system leads to competitive behaviour among departments that are seeking to support their own projects and programmes. As a result, there is a strong attachment to the department and its culture, which challenges the work of a cross-cutting team. In that sense, a direct command line may seem more applicable.

On the other hand, one could also argue that the WHO was previously used to matrix management, although not at this scale. Gathering expertise from different sectors and departments, a matrix structure thoughtfully implemented could be appropriate to tackle an epidemic as it requires a multidisciplinary response.

But is there any form of internal organisation and management that would be fully suitable to manage public health emergencies? Following the Ebola epidemic, it seems that the WHO opted for the establishment of an incident command control structure. The headquarters went through another set of reforms and decided to put into place a new structure dedicated to emergencies called the "WHO Health Emergencies Programme" which seeks to be "one workforce, one budget, one set of rules and processes and one clear line of authority" (WHO, 2017). This time a contingency fund for emergencies was specifically attributed to manage public health emergencies which could potentially solve some internal issues of access to financial resources. It will be interesting to see in the future if this programme will bring more efficiency in terms of response to emergencies.

References

Abeysinghe, S. (2015). *Pandemics, Science and Policy: H1N1 and the World Health Organisation*. New York, NY: Palgrave Macmillan.

Ansell, C. & A. Keller (2014). *Adapting the Incident Command Model for Knowledge-Based Crises: The Case of the Centers for Disease Control and Prevention*. IBM Center for the Business of Government.

Arvidsson, N (2009). Exploring Tensions in Projectified Matrix Organizations. *Scandinavian Journal of Management* 25, 97–107.

Baber, W. F., R. V. Bartlett & C. Dennis (1990). Matrix Organisation Theory and Environmental Impact Assessment. *The Social Science Journal* 27(3), 235–252.

Baker, M. G. & D. P. Fidler (2006). Global Public Health Surveillance under New International Health Regulations. *Emerging Infectious Diseases* 12(7), 1058–1065.

Barnett, M. N. & M. Finnemore (1999). The Politics, Power, and Pathologies of International Organizations. *International Organizations* 53(4), 699–732.

Brown, T. M., M. Cueto & E. Fee (2006). The World Health Organization and the Transition from "International" to "Global" Public Health. *American Journal of Public Health* 96(1), 62–72.

Calain, P., N. Fiore, M. Poncin & S. A. Hurst (2009). Research Ethics and International Epidemic Response: The Case of Ebola and Marburg Hemorrhagic Fevers. *Public Health Ethics* 2(1), 7–29.

Chorev, N. (2013). Restructuring Neoliberalism at the World Health Organization. *Review of International Political Economy* 20(4), 627–666.

Chorev, N., T. A. Rey & D. Ciplet (2011). The State of States in International Organisations: From the WHO to the Global Fund. *Review Research Foundation of State University of New York* 34(3), 285–310.

Davis, S. & P. Lawrence (1978). Problems of Matrix Organisations. *Harvard Business Review*, 131–142.

Global Ebola Response (2015). *Making a Difference*. Progress report 2015. Retrieved on 16 June 2015 from https://ebolaresponse.un.org/progress-2015.

Gobeli, D. H. & E. W. Larson (1986). Matrix Management: More Than a Fad. *Engineering Management International* 4, 71–76.

Godlee, F. (1994a). The Regions: Too Much Power, Too Little Effect. *British Medical Journal* 309, 1566–1570.

Godlee, F. (1994b). WHO in Crisis. *British Medical Journal* 309, 1424–1428.

Godlee, F. (1994c). WHO in Retreat: Is It Losing Its Influence? *British Medical Journal* 309, 1491–1495.

Hall, K. (2013). "Making the Matrix Work". Executive Summary. Retrieved on 9 July 2015 from www.global-integration.com/articles/executive-summary-making-matrix-work/.

Hofstede, G. (1997). *Cultures and Organizations: Software of the Mind*. London, McGraw-Hill.

Kamradt-Scott, A. (2016). WHO's to Blame? The World Health Organisation and the 2014 Ebola Outbreak in West Africa. *Third World Quarterly* 37(3), 401–418.

Kolodny, H. F. (1979). Evolution to a Matrix Organisation. *The Academy of Management Review* 4, 543–553.

Kuprenas, J. A. (2003). Implementation and Performance of a Matrix Organisation Structure. *International Journal of Project Management* 21, 51–62.

Laslo, Z. & A. I. Goldberg (2008). Resource Allocation under Uncertainty in a Multi-Project Matrix Environment: Is Organisational Conflict Inevitable? *International Journal of Project Management* 26, 773–788.

Lawson, J. W. (1986). A Quick Look at Matrix Organisation from the Perspective of the Practicing Manager. *Engineering Management International* 4, 61–70.

Lee, K. (2009). *The World Health Organisation (WHO)*. New York, NY: Routledge.

Liden, J. (2014). The World Health Organisation and Global Health Governance: Post-1990. *Public Health* 128, 141–147.

Médecins Sans Frontières (MSF) (2013). *Clinical Guidelines: Diagnosis and Treatment Manual*.

Médecins Sans Frontières (MSF) (2014). "Ebola en Afrique de l'ouest: Mobilisation exceptionnelle requise". Retrieved on 1 May 2016 from www.msf.ch/news/communiques-de-presse/detail/ebola-en-afrique-de-louest-mobilisation-exceptionnelle-requise/.

Moon, S., Checchi, F., Fitzgerald, G. et al. (2017). Post-Ebola Reforms: Ample Analysis, Inadequate Action. *British Medical Journal* 356, 1–8.

Pakarinen, M. & P. Virtanen (2016). Solving Organisational Conflicts in Public Matrix Organisations. *Qualitative Research in Organizations and Management: An International Journal* 11(4), 232–252.

Pandey, S. K. & B. E. Wright (2006). Connecting the Dots in Public Management: Political Environment, Organizational Goal Ambiguity, and the Public Manager's Role Ambiguity. *Journal of Public Administration Research and Theory* 16, 511–532.

Prah Ruger, J. & D. Yach (2008/2009). The Global Role of the World Health Organisation. *Global Health Governance* 2(2), 1–10.

Stuckenbruck, L. C. (1997). Integration: The Essential Function of Project Management. In D. I. Cleland & W. R. King (eds) *Project Management Handbook*, second edition. Hoboken, NJ: John Wiley & Sons: 56–82.

World Health Organization (WHO) (1946). *Constitution of the World Health Organization*. Retrieved on 14 June 2016 from www.who.int/governance/eb/who_constitution_en.pdf.

World Health Organization (WHO) (2005). *International Health Regulations 2005*, second edition. Geneva: World Health Organization.

World Health Organization (WHO) (2013). *Emergency Response Framework*. Geneva: World Health Organization.

World Health Organization (WHO) (2015). *Financial Report and Audited Financial Statements for the Year Ended 31 December 2014*. Retrieved on 1 April 2016 from www.who.int/about/resources_planning/A68_38-en.pdf?ua=1.

World Health Organization (WHO) (2016a). *Ebola Outbreak 2014–2015*. Retrieved on 30 October 2016 from www.who.int/csr/disease/ebola/en/.

World Health Organization (WHO) (2016b). *WHO's Financing Dialogue 2016: A Proposal for Increasing the Assessed Contribution, Ensuring Sustainable Financing for WHO*. Retrieved on 18 February 2018 from www.who.int/about/finances-accountability/funding/financing-dialogue/assessed-contribution.pdf.

World Health Organization (WHO) (2017). *WHO Health Emergencies Programme*. Retrieved on 23 April 2017 from www.who.int/about/who_reform/emergency-capacities/emergency-programme/en/.

7   Shaping A(H1N1) pandemic response

Money will follow

Nathalie Brender, David Maradan and Hélène Pasquini-Descomps

Introduction

The A(H1N1) pandemic revealed an estimated case fatality ratio of 0.02 percent[1] (Van Kerkhove et al., 2013), at least ten times lower compared to the influenza pandemics of 1918–1920 and 1957–1959 (Potter, 2001; Viboud et al., 2016). Past studies on cost-effectiveness were pointing towards vaccination and antiviral stockpiling as successful strategies, rejecting others, such as school closures and air traffic restrictions. But these interventions were launched based on cost-effectiveness under more severe conditions and without re-considering the mildness of the pandemic. This resulted in perceived overreaction by the authorities, which led to questioning the actions of governments (Barrelet et al., 2013) and the WHO, particularly in Europe. Reinforced by the financial crisis, the cost of the measures taken to control the pandemic was subject to harsh controversies: the money spent on the A(H1N1) pandemic response was considered a waste of public funds to the detriment of other public health missions.

The perception of the benefits and costs constitutes a central dimension of risk assessment (Renn, 2008). In the context of re-emerging infectious diseases, investing in mitigation actions is expected to limit the overall costs during and after a pandemic. Cost–benefit analysis is usually part of risk governance and, more specifically, of risk assessment activities (ISO, 2018; ISO, 2009). A risk assessment process entails a cost analysis: the costs to be incurred in the present time should lead to the avoidance of other present and future costs (i.e., benefits), since these measures would reduce either the impact or the likelihood of occurrence – or both – of uncertain feared events such as pandemics. Similarly, if different options are available, the most cost-effective one should be chosen, if all options provide the same positive effects in terms of risk reduction. However, if comparing costs and benefits is usual for investing in corporate projects, it is rarely used for managing public programs. Power games between political players as well as the level of uncertainty, the availability of data and the time pressure may render this analysis challenging for global pandemic risks (Murray et al., 2000) and even unethical when human lives are at stake. This is particularly well illustrated in the assessment of the 2009 A(H1N1) influenza pandemic.

While the debate on A(H1N1) pandemic costs was largely relayed in the media in Europe, the issue of pandemic costs and their role in decision making has remained understudied in the academic field. It raises, however, several questions about the role and perception of costs in the political and administrative decision-making process. Is evidence available on the cost of the A(H1N1) pandemic? Was someone in charge of forecasting the costs of implementing the measures and/or tracking them down during the crisis? Were costs reported to policy makers when approving and implementing the measures? Did the costs constitute a decision factor in managing the influenza pandemic risk? This chapter aims at answering these questions by exploring how costs and benefits are taken into account when selecting and implementing mitigation strategies against the A(H1N1) influenza pandemic.

In order to address these issues, we studied official documentation, collected key financial data and conducted semi-structured interviews with policy makers, public officers and experts at the WHO, in Switzerland, Japan, and the United States. We consider them "decision makers" at their own levels of responsibility.

We analyzed costs at three different levels. First, we investigated how the cost dimensions were integrated in pandemic planning, mostly how cost estimates were integrated – or not – in pandemic plans, and how planning has evolved since the A(H1N1) pandemic. Second, we examined whether costs were an element of discussion in formulating the pandemic mitigation strategy. Finally, through the interviews, we analyzed whether and how costs played a role in the implementation of the mitigation measures.

The first two sections present our findings from the official documentation and literature review. Over 2000 documents were collected for the whole project (see Introduction for more details about the methodology) out of which 275 were specifically economic related. We studied these documents that mainly cover approaches to estimate pandemic costs (macroeconomic cost and cost–benefit analysis) and cost consideration in pandemic plans (how pandemic costs are addressed in pandemic plans). Budget extractions have not been included in this documents' inventory because they were mostly presented on an ad hoc basis, sometimes included in reports or other documentation. The subsequent sections explain how costs are taken into account in pandemic risk analysis "ex ante", "in" and "ex post" and discuss the insights gained from the interviews combined with literature analysis.

The research team performed informal and semi-directed interviews with decision makers, public health officers and civil servants involved during the A(H1N1) crisis, both at national and regional levels, as well as public health officers and health economists at the WHO. We established an interview guide and a standard protocol specific to costs that were essentially organized around three main axes: (1) cost information that was available to take decisions regarding the 2009 A(H1N1) pandemic, (2) cost forecasting, monitoring, and reporting, (3) the role of costs in decision making.

Interviewees were selected by reviewing the people in charge of the pandemic activities at the health ministry in the three countries (for instance, the officers cited in post-pandemic reports), and at the WHO through the officers in charge of pandemic preparedness. In addition, the authors performed twenty cost-focused interviews with the respondents identified as having a specific knowledge of the economic dimension of pandemic management. Further inquiries about the relevant people to contact were performed during the interviews.

During our research, the Ebola outbreak occurred. However, we did not include in our analysis the Ebola outbreak since the countries under study (the United States, Japan and Switzerland) were not primarily affected by this epidemic. We only used data to check and contrast our analysis on the A(H1N1) pandemic when it was available and relevant. For example, we discuss how costs were considered when managing the hospitalization and treatment of the Ebola Cuban patient admitted at the Geneva University Hospitals.

We analyzed the twenty cost-specific interviews that we performed with interviewees having economic knowledge and/or a health economics background, using a pre-defined analysis grid. We developed a grid of analysis in order to analyze systematically the content of our interview transcripts for the three countries as well as the WHO and identify trends and patterns in answers. Our grid of analysis allowed us to report the discussions around economic themes across forty-eight items organized around the following main themes: characteristics of measures; cost of measures and their use in decision making; cost of inaction; types and content of cost data and expectations in terms of cost estimates for the management of future pandemics.

We also analyzed the other interview transcripts that were not cost-specific. This allows us to investigate if costs constitute a key issue or a minor issue (more than a hundred interviews were completed for the whole project covering the three pillars of organization, communication, and costing, see Introduction). We searched whether the "costing" and "costs" theme was mentioned in the interviews, as well as in the studied documentation. We were thus able to examine if interviewees were spontaneously mentioning costs, investigate how they were referring to costs, and capture relevant quotes that could support or contrast the twenty cost-specific interviews.

Ex ante pandemic costs

Pandemic cost estimates

The literature mainly presents two types of pandemic cost estimates: (1) the macroeconomic literature provides estimates of the impact of a pandemic on the overall economic system; and (2) cost–benefit analysis provides evidence on the cost of specific measures while trying to determine the most cost-effective options for risk mitigation.

Macroeconomic costs of pandemics

Different studies have assessed the impact of infectious disease risks on economies (McKibbin & Sidorenko 2006 and 2007; Rossi & Walker 2005; Burns et al., 2006; Asian Development Bank, 2003) based on the estimates of the statistic value of life and/or of production losses. These economic and social disruption costs are mainly expressed in terms of the proportion of GDP and/or total estimated costs. Models mostly present different scenarios that postulate various durations, transmission rates, and mortality rates of the pandemics as well as the efforts of agencies to limit the spread of the disease. For example, Brahmbhatt (2005) estimated the cost of a human pandemic at US$800 billion if the pandemic lasts one year, which corresponds to a 2 percent loss in the worldwide GDP. A "small" influenza outbreak that infects 0.5–1.0 percent of the population (compared to 2–3 percent for SARS and around 25 percent for the 1918–1919 Spanish Influenza), resulting in up to 65 million people infected and lasting around two to three years, would generate economic losses of US$1 to 2 trillion dollars per annum based on 2005 GDP data (Asian GDP loss of US$150–200 billion) (Rossi & Walker, 2005). The global impact of an influenza pandemic would range from US$200 billion (Rossi & Walker, 2005) to US$4.4 trillion (McKibbin & Sidorenko, 2006) depending on the duration of the pandemic, its transmission rate, and the mortality. For example, according to various studies, Switzerland plans for a loss of 0–6 percent of its GDP (FOPH, 2018, 106). World Bank experts (Burns et al., 2006) have estimated that the economic cost of an influenza pandemic could range from 0.7 to 4.8 percent of GDP, which was finally estimated to less than 0.5 percent of GDP for the A(H1N1) pandemic (Jonas, 2013). A study estimates that a pandemic influenza outbreak could result in GDP losses of US$45.3 billion without vaccination and US$34.4 billion with vaccination in the United States (Prager et al., 2017), taking into consideration the severity, the economic impacts from changes in medical expenditures and workforce participation, and different types of avoidance behavior and resilience actions not previously fully studied, and shows that vaccination reduces the cost of a pandemic.

Ex ante cost projections, mostly estimated in terms of expected losses of GDP, have been used to justify and calibrate pandemic mitigation measures. They have usually been mentioned in order to support the setting of strategies (pandemic plans) by the international community and at the country level. The argument in favor of investments in pandemic preparedness has largely relied on the expected losses that an influenza pandemic could generate and is still used in pandemic planning (FOPH, 2018; WHO, 2017; US HHS, 2017). If these losses, or in other words, the expected costs to be incurred to implement pandemic mitigation measures are less important than the expected GDP loss, then it is worth adopting these measures for public authorities.

Cost–benefit analysis of mitigation measures

The public health cost–benefit literature addresses the implementation costs of specific mitigation measures, such as vaccination or social distancing, with respect to the expected benefits of such measures. In such a framework, the proposed mitigation measures represent costly actions to be undertaken upfront to deal with the risk if it materializes. These upfront measures are expected to avoid costlier future actions that would have to be taken in an emergency without prior preparation. Possible costs can, therefore, be associated with a probability of occurrence, while benefits or losses (the consequences) should be discounted over time, as they will happen in the future. This cost-saving relationship depends on the probability of the occurrence of the risk and on the discount rate used to evaluate the future costs (Renn, 2008, 18). This cost-saving relationship can be expressed in monetary or non-monetary terms, such as human lives saved.

Information on costs and benefits is seldom available during the management of the crisis; thus, it seems relevant to analyze the existing information for the A(H1N1) pandemic to draw lessons for future crises. Cost–benefit analysis remains, however, difficult to apply in this context for the following reasons. First, for global risks such as pandemics, the level of uncertainty remains high, the availability of data is low, and the time pressure is challenging. Such an approach indeed requires a large amount of data and is time-consuming, and the integration of context-specific social concerns in the calculation of cost-effectiveness is difficult to communicate (Murray et al., 2000). For example, in the case of H5N1, human life losses have been estimated as possibly ranging from 2 million to 1 billion by different experts, with an initial estimate published by the WHO from 2 to 7 million and a revised estimate from 2 to 50 million (with 7 million as best-case scenario) (WHO, Epidemic and Pandemic Alert and Response, 2004). These estimations have, however, been widely debated by experts (Brender, 2014, 131–133). Similarly, the estimation of the quantity of drugs and vaccine needed is based on hypotheses. This estimate could be effective (matching the needs) or ineffective (excess stockpiling or lack of drugs); both would generate costs to be compared to the initial estimates, for which we usually have no indication (Brender, 2014).

Cost–benefit analysis, then, can be a complement to informed decision making regarding risk. However, this analysis can take different forms along different risk fields, as acknowledged by the European Union in its impact assessment guidelines (European Commission, 2009). Cost–benefit analyses of specific health measures cannot systematically be performed since cost considerations may be prohibited by law (Stern et al., 1996), e.g., by safety regulations, or it may be considered unethical or politically incorrect when dealing with risks where human lives are at stake (Renn, 2008). Concerns have also been raised with respect to the fact that cost–benefit analysis could dominate the debate and the decision-making process to the detriment of exchanges about conflicting values regarding the risk (Stern et al., 1996). Therefore, cost–benefit analysis is often replaced by cost-effectiveness analysis (Hutubessy et al., 2003; Murray et al., 2000), which compares the relative costs and effects of two or more measures.

Finally, existing cost–benefit analyses are often made on an ad hoc basis, fragmented by the type of countermeasures and/or areas, and they are not integrated within the risk analysis itself (Brender, 2014, 4). Decision makers access a range of potentially contradictory information about cost-effectiveness of influenza pandemic measures based on different valuation approaches and model assumptions. In the case of A(H1N1), various analyses have focused on specific measures taken at national or regional levels (Lugnér & Postma, 2009). Yarmand et al. (2010) examined vaccination and isolation, the two most common measures to control a pandemic such as A(H1N1), and identified which one is more effective. Their search grid allows the determination of a "near optimal" policy: while at low levels of intervention,[2] vaccination is more effective than self-isolation in improving the performance measures, self-isolation is more effective in relatively high levels of intervention. Yarmand et al. (2010) thus suggest adopting vaccination at the beginning of an outbreak, and after a while, if the outbreak is not contained and the disease continues to spread, self-isolation should be implemented.

Most studies pertain to the cost-effectiveness of vaccination (Wang et al., 2012; Durbin et al., 2011; Sander et al., 2010; Yarmand et al., 2010; Brouwers et al., 2009; Khazeni et al., 2009; Medlock and Galvani, 2009), followed by antivirals (Lavelle et al., 2012; Gonzáles-Canudas et al., 2011; Prosper et al., 2011; Lee et al., 2011; Lee et al., 2010; Perlroth et al., 2010; Nagase et al., 2009), and school closure (Brown et al., 2011; Halder et al., 2010; Prosper et al., 2011; Perlroth et al., 2010). Durbin et al. (2011) also examined the mass vaccination strategy implemented to mitigate the effects of the 2009 pandemic influenza A in Ontario (Canada) and concluded that the vaccine is cost effective from a societal viewpoint. Similar findings on vaccines have been established by Prosser et al. (2011), Sander et al. (2010) and Khazeni et al. (2009). Brown et al. (2011) examine social distancing measures focusing on the cost-effectiveness of school closures. Their results suggest that school closures during the 2009 A(H1N1) epidemic could have generated substantial costs to society, as the potential costs of lost productivity and childcare could have far outweighed the cost savings in preventing influenza cases. Halder et al. (2010) compare several measures showing that the most cost-effective strategies involved treatment and household prophylaxis using antiviral drugs combined with limited-duration school closures, with costs ranging from US$632 to US$777 per case prevented. Dan et al. (2009) studied the cost-effectiveness of different hospital responses targeting infected patients in Singapore by simulating outbreaks of SARS, the 2009 A(H1N1) pandemic, and the 1918 Spanish influenza. The results indicate that the protection measures on the susceptible patients only yielded the lowest incremental cost per death averted for the A(H1N1) pandemic, or said differently, greater cost-effectiveness.

While these studies account for cost-effectiveness analyses in various countries, no specific results are available for Switzerland and Japan. In fact, the review of Switzerland's A(H1N1) immunization strategy (Ernst & Young, 2010) does not consider the cost-effectiveness of the vaccine strategy. At the country level, the United States report highlights that US$4.17 billion were spent out of the budget of US$6.15 billion that was made available for the A(H1N1) pandemic response but without assessing the cost-effectiveness of the measures taken (US GAO, 2011).

The 2009 A(H1N1) lessons-learned document stipulates the need for a cost estimation of the pandemic response during the risk assessment phase and calls for further studies in this area. Additional cost-effectiveness studies on the pandemic interventions, including school closure were published after the pandemic. The review of these studies (Pasquini-Descomps et al., 2017) indicates that hospital quarantine, vaccination, and usage of the antiviral stockpile are highly cost-effective, even for mild pandemics, while school closures, antiviral treatments, and social distancing may not qualify as efficient measures, for a virus like 2009's A(H1N1) considering a willingness-to-pay threshold of US$45,000 per disability-adjusted life-year. The severity of the pandemic constitutes one of the main determinants of the relative efficiency of pandemic interventions. Indeed, school closures, antiviral treatments, and social distancing may become cost-effective for severe crises. Pasquini-Descomps et al. (2017) shed light on the cost-utility of various interventions and provide a standard for cost-utility comparisons, which may support decision making, among other criteria, for future pandemics.

Costs in pandemic plans

Whether and how pandemic plans address the costing issue provides interesting information about the *ex ante* consideration of pandemic costs by public authorities and health institutions. In particular, it gives insights on how costs were – or were not – included in preparedness activities, and whether or not they could constitute a formal element that was analyzed and presented in pandemic planning. In the spring of 2009, just before the A(H1N1) influenza pandemic started, the WHO had issued the Influenza Pandemic Plan meant to serve as a reference on a worldwide basis for government officials to develop their own plans. While each country's authorities are prepared, informed, and guided by the WHO, they will ultimately have to decide on the extent of their response and implement their own set of measures at the onset of the pandemic. Therefore, an important role of the WHO is to make sure that each country has implemented a pandemic preparedness plan, and that this plan will be revised and tested regularly to incorporate local determinants and experience from past crises. In 2009, at the time of the A(H1N1) outbreak, 74 percent of the 194 WHO Member States had a pandemic preparedness plan (Fineberg, 2014). The WHO estimated that 68 percent of the 119 revised national plans were based on the WHO plan, but only 8 percent had been tested (WHO, 2011, 66).

The 2009 WHO Influenza Pandemic Plan was the output of several consultations with a broad constituency from November 2007 to April 2009 and included guidelines for tracking risk and its possible sources, as well as for determining the causal chain of a pandemic risk and proposed actions in affected and unaffected countries (Brender, 2014, 182). This plan comprised six phases: Phases 1 to 4 addressed virus transmissibility and the possibility of rapid containment while Phases 5 and 6 addressed sustainable human-to-human transmission (WHO, 2009). The difference between Phases 5 and 6 (Phase 6 being the pandemic in progress phase) mainly relates to the grading of the geographical spread of the disease. At least two countries in one WHO region set Phase 5 and an additional country in another region set Phase 6.

The criteria for the pandemic declaration had been met for a few weeks already when the WHO Director-General declared Phase 6 on June 11, 2009. As a result, pandemic measures were deployed as prescribed in most national plans. Such phasing triggered public expenses and generated post-pandemic criticism about their deployment despite the moderate severity and fatality of the disease. However, at the beginning of a pandemic, its severity assessment remains difficult mainly due to the unavailability and unreliability of data about the cases (Van Kerkhove & Ferguson, 2012), viral characteristics, and reproduction rate. In addition, an influenza pandemic requires significant upfront measures such as vaccine orders and antivirals purchases (WHO, 2011), based on the anticipation of the disease's clinical pattern at the time of decision. This uncertainty was not reflected in the interpretation of most pandemic plans, including the WHO's, therefore leaving aside any possibility to adjust the measures during the course of the pandemic. The response mechanism based on automatic implementation of the WHO plan and national plans was criticized, mostly given the fact that the pandemic turned out to be mild and the pandemic response costs incurred were thus perceived as too high (Brender & Gilbert, 2018).

Pandemic costs depend on the development of the pandemic mitigation strategy. They follow from the objectives of a pandemic plan, its organizational provisions and the state's legal framework. Therefore, we review below the pandemic plans of Switzerland, Japan, and the United States at the time of the A(H1N1) pandemic and the adjustments or lessons learned since 2009 until December 31, 2017. The 2009 A(H1N1) pandemic was the first pandemic to be managed under the revised International Health Regulations (IHR) framework. It triggered a large-scale lesson-learning exercise and initiated the revision of the plan at the WHO and in many countries. In Table 7.1, we show the plans in place in 2009, and the post-A(H1N1) updates or lesson-learned documents, at their corresponding dates of issuance for the WHO, the United States, Switzerland, and Japan. We also indicate the legislative changes that occurred in regard to pandemic influenza, since the revision of the pandemic plans might have motivated a reform of the pre-existent legal framework in order for the national authorities to enforce the actions listed in the new preparedness plan. Finally, we also include additional documents that the governments publish together with preparedness plans on the same public internet website as these general documents may provide additional information on how the governments intend to handle a pandemic.

In the 2009 Swiss pandemic plan, the objectives are to detect a new stream of influenza as early as possible, limit its spread, and when it cannot be contained anymore, reduce the population's morbidity and mortality (OFSP, 2009, 8). In comparison, the 2013 Swiss pandemic plan objectives are to reduce the consequences of a pandemic for the people and society (FOPH, 2013), and the 2018 plan is "designed to protect the life and health of the population" (FOPH, 2018, 7). Both pre- and post-A(H1N1) pandemic plans are addressed to the federal and regional authorities, rather than the public, to help them prepare the health system for handling a pandemic. The 2018 plan integrates the IHR, WHO guidelines and is based on the Epidemics Act of 2013. It defines the division of labor between the Confederation and the cantons to allow for consistent planning of measures throughout Switzerland (FOPH, 2018, 7). In the 2013 plan, a summary of the medical and statistical assumptions and of the characteristics of the disease has been moved from the first part to the end of the document, but is not associated with the costs of measures. In the 2018 plan, this section has also been integrated towards the end and provides a table of expected values that are also not associated with the costs of measures (FOPH, 2018, 105). The plan also aims to clarify the role of the federal versus the regional authorities and suggests that regional pandemic plans should be made using this federal plan as a guideline. In

Table 7.1 Pandemic preparedness plans at the WHO and at the federal level in the United States, Switzerland, and Japan

WHO	United States	Switzerland	Japan
Availability of plans			
WHO website www.who.int/ influenza/preparednewss/ pandemic/en/	Flu website www.flu.gov/ planning-preparedness/federal	Federal office of Public Health www.bag.admin.ch/influenza/	Ministry of Health, Labor and Welfare www.mhlw.go.jp/ english/topics/influenza/
New plan(s) and lessons learned			
• Pandemic Influenza Risk Management WHO Interim Guidance (June 2013) • Pandemic Influenza Risk Management – A WHO guide to inform and harmonize national and international pandemic preparedness and response (2017)	• 2009 H1N1 Influenza Improvement Plan (May 2012) • HHS Retrospective on the 2009 H1N1 Influenza Pandemic (May 2012)	• Swiss Influenza Pandemic Plan (Oct. 2013, Jan. 2018) • Review of Switzerland's H1N1 immunization strategy (April 2010)	• Report of the Review Meeting on Measures against Pandemic Influenza (A/H1N1) (June 2010)
Pandemic plans during the 2009 A(H1N1) pandemic			
• Pandemic Influenza Preparedness and Response: A WHO Guidance Document (Apr. 2009)	• HHS Pandemic Influenza Plan (Nov. 2005) • National Strategy for Pandemic Influenza (Nov. 2005) • National Response Framework (Mar. 2008)	• Swiss Influenza Pandemic Plan (Jan. 2009)	• Pandemic Influenza Preparedness Action Plan of the Japanese Government (Oct. 2007)
Legislative framework revisions			
• International Health Regulations IHR 2005 (2007)	• Pandemic and All-hazards Preparedness Re-authorization Act (Mar. 2013) • Pandemic and All-hazards Preparedness Act (Dec. 2006) *Amendment to the Public Health Service Act.*	• Adoption of the revised Epidemics Act (Sep. 2013)	• Amendment to the Infectious Disease Act and other laws (May 2008) *In order to control pandemic influenza, provides recommendation of hospitalization and border control measures such as detention*

both the new and old plans, the federal government has to provide information, ensure coordination and issue recommendations on the course of action, while the regional authorities (cantons) are in charge of executing the actions and organizing the health network accordingly (FOPH, 2013, 7). The articulation of this chain of command was not without issues during the A(H1N1) as Bourrier explains it in Chapter 9 of this volume. With the 2013 Epidemics Act, the Confederation takes on a stronger role in management, target-setting, oversight, and coordination, while the cantons retain the responsibility for enforcement (FOPH, 2018, 8). Besides this, Swiss authorities also secured access to vaccine purchases, via specific arrangements with Novartis, and planned for an urgent procedure to obtain supplementary credit (FOPH, 2018, 68).

The automatic implementation of national plans following the WHO's pandemic declaration in 2009 was not always considered adapted to the situation, which resulted in some authorities willing to distance themselves from the WHO guidelines and recommendations. For example, the 2018 Swiss influenza pandemic plan provides for the right to deviate from WHO guidelines by explicitly mentioning that guidelines are "primarily of global significance and are thus not automatic triggers for measures in Switzerland" (FOPH, 2018, 11). Similarly, the Swiss Epidemic Act allows the Confederation to decide specific measures in particular and extraordinary situations (without delay in the latter). However, a Public Health Emergency of International Concern (PHEIC) declared by the WHO is classified as a particular situation the Swiss authorities will examine before enacting measures, in order to understand if it constitutes a threat to public health or not (FOPH, 2018, 11).

Switzerland was the first of the three countries under analysis to come out with a new pandemic preparedness plan in 2013, updated in 2018, which follows these revised phases and simplifies the pandemic plan. Switzerland kept the flexibility to declare its own phases asynchronously with the WHO phases. It is indeed an important move for government authorities to maintain flexibility and sovereignty in terms of risk assessment and adaptation of the pandemic mitigation measures to the progression of the disease within their country. This need for flexibility at the country level has been a major reflection on the lessons learned from past pandemics together with the requirement to prepare for the next pandemic. In terms of costs, the 2009 plan indicates that preparedness costs remain minor in comparison to the direct costs estimated at CHF400 million while the 2018 plan indicates a total cost (individuals, environment, economy, and society costs) in the low tens of billions according to the Federal Office of Civil Protection analysis (FOPH, 2018, 106). While mentioning that indirect costs are higher than direct costs, mainly due to absenteeism, the latest plan provides neither an estimate of indirect costs nor a split between indirect and direct costs.

The Japanese pandemic plan's stated objectives are slightly different. Its goal is to avoid socio-economic collapse by delaying the onset of pandemic influenza as much as possible through the proposed measures. This vision, that contagion can be limited by using appropriate measures, is very resurgent through the whole plan. The plan's goal is to state the mitigation measures that need to be taken in each pandemic phase, with the necessary materials that must be distributed to the relevant parties so that they can start buying or preparing the supplies (JMHW, Inter-ministerial Avian Influenza Committee, 2007, 9). Up until December 31, 2017, Japan had not issued a new pandemic plan, and we can therefore assume that the provisions of the 2005 plan (JMHW, Inter-ministerial Avian Influenza Committee, 2007) are still valid and should be considered in conjunction with the recommendations of the Report of the Review Meeting on Measures against Pandemic Influenza A(H1N1) (JMHW, 2010). The Japanese pandemic plan does not mention pandemic costs, but the lessons-learned report highlights the fact that decision-making processes should be clarified with the cost of vaccinations (including the prices of the vaccines) and procurement of overseas vaccines (JMHW, 2010, 13).

The US plan's goal is to reduce the impact of a catastrophe and limit social and economic disruption. It was a manifest from the United States Department of Health and Human Services about the activities it will handle before and during an influenza pandemic that was initially published in 2005 (US HHS, 2005, 4). This plan works in conjunction with the incident management framework (National Response plan) that handles the mobilization of assets from the public (federal, state, and local) and private sectors. The national strategy plan for pandemic influenza explains the strategy of Homeland Security for engaging the public, private sector, and citizen in preparedness and response. In addition to these plans, the CDC published its updated framework "Updated Preparedness and Response Framework for Influenza Pandemics" in 2014, which should serve as a set of guidelines and recommendations for risk assessment, decision making, and action in the United States. The pandemic plan was updated in 2006, 2009, and 2017. The 2017 pandemic plan presents the accomplishments since the 2005 plan and sets objectives in seven key areas (against four for the 2005 plan): (1) surveillance, epidemiology, and lab activities, (2) community mitigation measures, (3) medical countermeasures (diagnostic tests, vaccines, treatments, and respiratory devices), (4) healthcare system preparedness and response, (5) communications and public outreach, (6) scientific infrastructure and preparedness, and (7) domestic and international response policy, incident response, and global partnerships.

Although the United States' 2017 plan does not focus on costs, it addresses the question of resources planning in its Appendix A "Planning Scenarios". It provides the estimate of US$181 billion for the direct and indirect health costs alone (not including disruptions in trade and other costs to business and industry) for a moderate pandemic (similar to those in 1957 and 1968) with no interventions (US HHS, 2017, 42), and presents the pandemic's features in a table according to the pandemic's severity (moderate to very severe) and estimates of illness (transmissibility, illness cases, types of care and deaths). Cost data are not included in this table.

Overall, a detailed examination of pandemic plans in place in 2009 in the United States, Japan, and Switzerland shows a lack of cost assessment during the risk assessment and response phases. It suggests that costs do not play a role at the stage where the pandemic mitigation strategy is developed. We did not find any other administrative documents or reports devoted to the estimates of costs of the planned measures.

The lessons learned at the WHO highlighted the need to have pandemic plans taking into account the cost–benefit analysis during the pandemic risk assessment phase (WHO, 2011). The 2017 WHO guidance does not, however, provide guidelines about cost analysis but mentions its relevance in the newly prescribed context assessment, which should be part of each national risk assessment (WHO, 2017, 29). The WHO proposes to consider the following elements in the cost assessment: direct and indirect financial costs including loss of household income, hospitalization costs, impacts on tourism and trade, and impact on the continuity of essential services. The latest Swiss influenza pandemic plan of 2018 presents a section that is dedicated to economic consequences of an influenza pandemic, in terms of direct costs and impact on GDP. It also assigns costs of measures to the Confederation or other institutions, clarifying the roles and responsibilities of federal, cantonal, and local authorities. However, it does not provide monetary estimates for the described measures. The same is true for the United States' 2017 pandemic plan update, which does not provide cost estimates, and the Japanese influenza preparedness plan, which has not been updated since the A(H1N1) pandemic.

Various explanations for the lack of consideration about costs in the pandemic plans might be given. First, estimates of the costs of measures are not considered reliable because they are related to the pandemic severity and will thus vary from one pandemic to another, or during a single pandemic (Pasquini-Descomps et al., 2017). Furthermore, indicating the potential costs of the measures might strengthen the debates and complicate the adoption of the plan. A third explanation refers to the professional background of the audience, or the users of the pandemic plan, mainly hospital clinicians. They are more concerned by medical-effectiveness or by the minimization of the risk for medical workers rather than by the costs.

Cost in decision making

This section examines whether costs were an important decision-making driver during the A(H1N1) pandemic either for building the strategy or for managing the interventions. One difficulty in pandemic management is that decisions need to be made at an early stage when the parameters of a pandemic, i.e., its severity, remain unknown or highly uncertain.

Overall, we found out that cost was not a driver in decisions in handling the A(H1N1) pandemic at the WHO, in the United States, Japan, and Switzerland. Such results do not contrast with the previous findings on pandemic plans. While decision makers declare that they are aware of the medical-effectiveness of measures, they often ignore their actual costs as well as their distribution among the public and the private sectors. One exception is vaccination, which has been largely studied, both from a medical-effectiveness and cost-effectiveness point of view (indeed, per unit vaccination costs have been cited during the interviews). Decisions seem to be largely based on other drivers such as the number of human cases that the pandemic mitigations measure will avoid, the usefulness and effectiveness of prevention or medical means, as well as the availability of health infrastructures and capabilities. A declaration of a United States CDC officer we interviewed on August 24, 2015 illustrates this point: "For deciders in public health, they have a budget and their mission is to prevent illness. Costs do not come into line".

Facing major uncertainty about the degree of severity of the virus, the strategy was based on a "no regret" or "precautionary" strategy favoring early actions in order to avoid the potentially high damages (evaluated in percentage of GDP loss or potential number of deaths) that could happen if the severity of the virus finally appears to be high. As stated before, a "costs should not count" principle is followed by the representatives of the WHO and national health authorities according to our interviews. In other words, their quasi-option value (i.e. the welfare gain associated with delaying a decision when there is uncertainty about the payoffs of alternative choices) was too small to justify delaying actions. Two justifications are given. First, delaying actions for avoiding unnecessary expenses would be ethically problematic when human lives are at stake. Second, delaying actions could drastically reduce the effectiveness of the measure.

However, such justifications deserve further attention since the unnecessary expenses linked to a misleading anticipation of the pandemic's severity have an opportunity cost and are not available for alternative projects, leading to welfare losses (and also potentially to a loss of human lives). Furthermore, potential measures for fighting a pandemic face different timeframes for being effective. In the case of the A(H1N1) pandemic, the effectiveness of vaccination might be lower if the deadline for producing vaccines is considered in conjunction with the available knowledge about the severity of the pandemic. Decision makers indeed state that costs should not be part of the picture when the crisis is declared. This could delay actions and potentially degrade the whole intervention mechanism. Furthermore, when a pandemic occurs, actions are expected by the population even if they appear to be very costly or face a high risk of not being useful at the end of the day. Risk communication strategies have a crucial role to play in such context. It is indeed easier to reassure the population when strong actions can be announced.

A first explanation for the fact that costs might not be a relevant para-meter when the crisis happens is related to their timescale. Planning and preparedness costs are incurred at the very beginning of the pandemic, even without the outbreak of a crisis. For example, organizational activ-ities, stockpiling medical treatments and material, development of the sur-veillance system, training, as well as maintenance of health infrastructures (e.g., separation of buildings to ensure a quarantine) are undertaken even if no crisis is upcoming. Furthermore, the decision to develop and produce vaccines has to be taken when information about the pandemic remains scarce. As a consequence, refusing some additional measures, such as distributing vaccines, due to their costs at the time of a potential crisis, would render these preliminary expenses meaningless. If the pan-demic appears to be mild, it is difficult for policy makers to stop the meas-ures that have generated high sunk costs, even if such decision is justified. One might oppose the previous argument stating that part of the prelimi-nary measures, such as maintenance of infrastructures or further develop-ment of the surveillance system, would remain available for the future and be useful to strengthen health systems for the next crisis.

A second explanation for the low importance of costs lies in the capa-city to pay. Public officers in charge of the implementation of the pan-demic mitigation measures declared themselves to be unconcerned with cost as long as they have the available budget line at their disposal. They are thus mainly concerned with the legality of the expenses (i.e., authori-zation to spend). Generally, budget lines include exceptional or unplanned situations making it easy to draw on them when necessary. Otherwise, additional specific budgets can also be voted for, as was the case in the United States, Japan, and Switzerland for the A(H1N1) pan-demic. Furthermore, as indicated later in this chapter and in detail by Pasquini-Descomps et al. (Chapter 8), pandemic costs are low compared to the overall health budget. Note that the indirect costs generated by the measures (cost of time for getting vaccinated, for example), which will mainly be supported by the private sector, are, however, not considered.

Costs reach more significance when it comes to the settlement and the final allocation of costs to be incurred by the different collectivities involved in the management of the pandemic. Decisions made about measures to be taken to respond to a pandemic imply orders, deliveries, invoices, and cash settlements that can occur weeks or months after the order, depending on the products purchased. Once commitments have been made to purchase the material or medicine and conduct the neces-sary medical acts such as vaccination, front-line institutions such as hos-pitals engage costs and have to advance the payments. Cost comes into play when the front-line institutions do not have the cash to pay for the actions in advance. One Swiss interviewee, an officer of the Canton of Geneva, summarizes the situation: "There is a federal plan, but the one who orders is the one who pays". This could be critical in the case of cash shortage at an institution because settlement discussions, especially in federal countries, occur once the pandemic is over and are subject to further negotiations about final cost allocations between the federal state, regional authorities, and insurers. In such situations, the officer requires the authorization to spend from his/her hierarchy and the level of costs is discussed and monitored.

Note also that while the envelope has been established, there can be a time lapse and an amount gap between the funds pledged and the funds really paid. Also, in order to protect populations and receive the vaccines on time, government authorities have to proceed to the orders before securing the funds. Similarly, hospitals must provide patients with adequate treatment, care measures, and equipped facilities, involving expenses that must be paid up front. To our question "Can one proceed without having the funds?" a departmental head at the Geneva University Hospitals explained on January 9, 2015 "Yes. Exactly, in the end, I proceed before having the funds". The capacity to pay, rather than the amount of expenses, therefore constitutes an important factor for implementing decisions. During the A(H1N1) crisis, the budget covered the expenses even though budget lines were neither estimated *ex ante* nor monitored in detail during the implementation phase. By contrast, actions taken for fighting the Ebola outbreak in Africa have faced budgetary constraints, as they mainly concerned developing economies where the necessary public resources were not available. Indeed, Grépin (2015) shows that the financial needs during the Ebola outbreak were covered by international donors. The lack of resources among the countries directly influenced the management of the crisis, as donor support reached the affected countries more than six months after the WHO was alerted to the outbreak. "These delays in disbursements of funding may have contributed to spread of the virus and could have increased the financial needs" (Grépin, 2015).

Overall costs are not a decision factor. They are neglected, unless the capacity to spend is missing, either for legal reasons or a lack of cash. In such situations, pandemic policies are subject to the failures of the public budget and bureaucracy process (Wildavsky & Caiden, 1997). These failures include dissociating the decision to act from the knowledge of the cost of actions, dissociating the decision to spend from the availability of funds, or favoring action instead of non-action and putting pressure on the use of the available budget.

Cost as ex post fact

At the time the measures are taken, their cost, as well as their distribution among stakeholders, are poorly documented. Accountability appears as a major driver for ex post cost analysis. In fact, cost analysis is mostly performed once the health crisis is over, to justify the use of budget and to identify opportunities for cost saving in the future. In the United States, it is part of a standard procedure of the United States Government Accountability Office. In Switzerland, the Confederation gave a mandate to a private audit firm to perform an analysis of the pandemic response, in particular the vaccination campaign in response to politicians' questions in parliament (Ernst & Young, 2010). An inventory of the costs was made by the Canton of Geneva, to break down which costs were covered by the federal government, the insurance companies, the Canton and the Geneva University Hospitals. During our interviews, we discovered that the costs of pandemic measures were often not known at the time the measures were engaged, but instead analyzed ex post to justify the use of public funds, as a unit head at the Geneva University Hospitals, interviewed on January 19, 2015, underlined it: "I will have to compute if one really wants to know".

The WHO was strongly criticized, not only for its inadequate A(H1N1) pandemic response, but also for the poor and insufficient quality of its risk communication and the high costs of the selected measures, especially the mass vaccination program, relative to the mild disease severity. It was also accused of squandering resources (Council of Europe, 2010), particularly in Europe. Debate about the necessity of the WHO's expenses and the national public expenses devoted to the A(H1N1) pandemic remains, however, somewhat superficial. None of the factors that led to such a situation seem to have been identified by the public officers: they repeat that they had no other legitimate and ethical alternative at the time they had to decide. However, the interlinkages between the known characteristics of the pandemics (severity, stringency, reproduction rate), the timing of actions taken (measures that need long preparation such as vaccination versus measures that could be implemented overnight like school closure), and the potential overspending on the measures have been neither assessed nor documented ex post. During the interviews, public officers and politicians recognized that the selected measures appear to be rather costly according to the severity of the pandemic. However, they are not questioning ex post the reasons why the information they used to select the measure (the potential human impacts, the cost-effectiveness analysis) might in the end have been misleading and how the strategy could better integrate the uncertainty about the stringency of the pandemic when measures have to be taken.

Controversies must be balanced against the relative importance of costs. According to our research and as explained by Pasquini-Descomps et al. (Chapter 8), pandemic budgets did not represent a major disruption to the public finances: an average extra budget of 0.24 percent during the fiscal year 2009 between the United States, Japan, and Switzerland, with a maximum of 0.44 percent for Japan, 0.14 percent in the United States, and 0.15 percent in Switzerland was spent. The A(H1N1) response burden (analyzed in detail in Pasquini-Descomps et al. in Chapter 8) accounted for 4.2 percent of the Swiss Federal Office of Public Health (FOPH) budget, respectively 6.3 percent of the United States Department of Health and Human Services (HHS) budget and 1.6 percent of the Japanese Ministry of Health, Labor and Welfare (MHLW) budget.

The WHO's lessons learned emphasized the fact that cost evaluation should be made during risk assessment and response phases: "A methodology for measuring the economic costs of interventions and the overall pandemic should be taken into account during pandemic preparedness" (WHO, 2011, 1). The Swiss pandemic plan of 2013 mentions an evaluation of direct costs of CHF400 million compared to CHF300 million for the seasonal flu. In its latest version of 2018, the estimation rises to several billion Swiss francs based on macroeconomic studies of the costs of pandemics. However, a methodology to allow decision makers to assess the costs of measures and their benefits, and reassess them during the pandemic, is still missing. Thus, the capacity to forecast and monitor the cost of pandemics will remain poorly developed, leading to potentially substantial waste in the future.

The questions of responsibility and accountability have not been solved yet. Which bodies should ultimately be in charge of the cost assessment and bear the cost of the response is not clearly established. Arbitrage about the final allocation of costs between the different institutions involved in the management of the crisis is often decided afterwards. In Switzerland, the Communicable Disease Legislation Epidemics Act (EpidA), voted for in September 2013 and put into force on January 1, 2016, clarifies the activities of the Confederation and the cantons, setting up a coordinating body, and aiming to enable timely detection, monitoring, prevention, and control of crisis events. For example, this law prescribes that costs of the measures affecting individuals are borne by the authority ordering them, unless the costs are otherwise covered, for example by social insurance (Art. 71 let. a and Art. 74 para. 2 EpidA). It also lists which measures are the Confederation's responsibility and for which it should assume the cost.

Finally, there are blurred responsibilities in financing the influenza pandemic response. On one side, decision makers manage yearly budgets that face cost reduction pressure and on the other side, emergency funds can be drawn upon quickly, with little upfront discussion, few limits, and almost no control over the nature and extent of expenses. Supplementary budgets were voted for in the United States, Japan, and Switzerland without difficulties. Once the A(H1N1) pandemic was over, cost analysis was performed, trying to reconstitute the total costs paid and associating them with specific measures, including the use of infrastructures, the purchase of material, and the costs of medical acts.

Vignette

Ebola: the Cuban patient in Geneva University Hospitals

A WHO healthcare worker was infected by Ebola in fall 2014. The Geneva University Hospitals in Switzerland reorganized their emergency service to provide care for this patient (see Parfaite, Chapter 10, for a detailed description of the Cuban patient case). This type of situation usually triggers a change in the chain of command, and the usual cost-efficiency settings and cost parameters are left aside in such emergency context. Safety of the medical staff must be as high as possible, whatever its cost. We had access to the cost breakdown of the Geneva University Hospitals and estimated the total cost of this operation at around CHF600,000–700,000. The WHO announced that the organization would cover the costs. However, only direct costs (around 30 percent) were to be paid by the WHO. Such information was barely relayed by the media, indicating that the cost (Who pays? What amount?) was not important. Indeed, the priority given to safety over costs has not been questioned as it would not be ethical to expose the medical workers to higher risk in order to save costs. However, one question remains open: the money that could have been saved here could have been saving more lives in Sierra Leone, for example. We could restate the question differently: is it ethical to give higher importance to the safety (and lives) of the staff taking care of the Ebola patient than to that of doctors or nurses occupied by other communicable diseases? The ethical perspective might thus not be relevant in justifying not to consider the costs.

The ethical perspective is indeed presented frequently as an argument to ignore costs. Costs may be left aside because their evaluation and discussion upfront is considered taboo. Cost–benefit analysis would also clearly show upfront how much is spent on specific cases and would provide information about the perception of one emergency compared to others. The amount of money spent on one case compared to usual cases of infection would then be transparent and generate questions, or even result in stepping back.

For these reasons, we argue that costs should be included in the decision-making process and not be investigated (and sometimes debated) only ex post. The forecasting and accounting of costs would show how much is needed and spent for a specific crisis and provide information about the perception of one emergency compared to others.

Conclusions

We explored how costs and benefits are taken into account when selecting mitigation strategies against the A(H1N1) influenza pandemic. We studied official documentation, collected key financial data and conducted semi-structured interviews of decision makers and experts, at the WHO, in Switzerland, Japan, and the United States. We developed a grid of analysis to systematically compare the interview transcripts and the documentation, and analyzed their content to explain how pandemic costs are addressed in pandemic planning and the setting of pandemic plans, and in the design of the pandemic mitigation strategy as well as in the decisions to implement the selected mitigation measures.

First, to the question "Is evidence available on the cost of the A(H1N1) pandemic?" our results show that only a little evidence is available. Available evidence concerns largely general macroeconomic studies (comparing investments for fighting pandemics and the expected loss of GDP that the pandemics might cause), or specific cost-effectiveness results justifying the implementation of one measure instead of another.

Second, to the questions "Was someone in charge of forecasting the costs of implementing the measures and/or tracking them down during the crisis?" and "Were costs reported to policy makers when approving and implementing the measures?", we answer that neither was the case. Furthermore, decision makers rarely ask for and consider evidence of the costs. As a result, public expenditure analysis is mostly performed ex post to justify and evaluate the relevant and proportionate use of public funds, in response to a political inquiry or a debate in the public arena, leaving the questions of transparency and accountability in pandemic management unresolved. Our findings thus question the ability of decision makers to reassess the true efficiency of all possible interventions during a longer and/or more severe pandemic and to allocate resources effectively among health issues.

Finally, to the question "Did the costs constitute a decision factor in managing the influenza pandemic risk?" we conclude that, in high-income countries, information on the cost of measures played only a minor role in shaping the A(H1N1) response, from pandemic preparedness to its management, and did not constitute a constraint for decision makers. Indeed, the total amount of expected expenses remains marginal in comparison to the public health budgets of the United States, Japan, and Switzerland. Besides this, public authorities assume that current budget lines (and their allowable extensions in case of emergencies) will absorb overspending. Furthermore, financial commitments are not an issue as long as front-line institutions have the cash available to purchase materials and hire the required personnel.

A lack of systematic cost evaluation during a health crisis causes several issues in the long term, such as depleting the financial resources left to handle other risks or health issues, lowering the confidence of citizens in their institutions to evaluate a situation accurately. Our findings show that costs were mainly computed ex post in the case of the A(H1N1) pandemic. However, this cost evidence is seldom used to question why the information and methods that decision makers use to define the strategy have not prevented an overreaction.

The question of costs in pandemics is not an easy one to tackle. We found that in Japan, the United States, and Switzerland costs do not seem important in managing an influenza pandemic, which raises some issues in terms of responsibility of the ultimate payer and ethics. The fact that costs may be considered important and taken into account in making decisions may not guarantee that the authorities would select the most cost-effective and most ethical measures. The magnitude of choice of actions can be greater in some situations compared to others. If cost evaluations were systematically published, part of the risk assessment, and documented in the pandemic response plans, we would be able to perform this analysis.

Notes

1 Van Kerkhove et al. (2013) analyzed data from twenty-seven published/unpublished studies from nineteen countries/administrative regions: Australia, Canada, China, Finland, France, Germany, Hong Kong SAR, India, Iran, Italy, Japan, the Netherlands, New Zealand, Norway, Reunion Island, Singapore, United Kingdom, United States, and Vietnam.
2 Yarmand et al. (2010) defined four levels of intervention: level 1 (disease), level 2 (vaccination), level 3 (antiviral), level 4 (self-isolation) and formulated the assumption that the effectiveness of interventions is reasonably higher in lower levels.

References

Asian Development Bank. (2003). Assessing the impact and costs of SARS in developing Asia. *Asian Development Outlook Update, Manila*, 75–92.

Barrelet, C., Bourrier, M., Burton-Jeangros, C., & Schindler, M. (2013). Unresolved issues in risk communication research: the case of the H1N1 pandemic (2009–2011). *Influenza and Other Respiratory Viruses*, 7(s2), 114–119.

Brahmbhatt, M. (2005). Avian and human pandemic influenza: Economic and social impacts. Presented at the meeting on Avian Influenza and Human Pandemic Influenza, November 7–9, 2005, WHO, Geneva. Retrieved from: www.worldbank.org/content/dam/Worldbank/document/HDN/Health/AHI-SocioImpacts.pdf.

Brender, N. (2014). *Global Risk Governance in Health*. London: Palgrave Macmillan.

Brender, N., & Gilbert, C. (2018). From emergence to emergences: a focus on pandemic influenza. In S. Morand & M. Figuié (eds) *Emergence of Infectious Diseases: Risks and Issues for Societies* (35–57). Versailles: Edition Quae.

Brouwers, L., Cakici, B., Camitz, M., Tegnell, A., & Boman, M. (2009). Economic consequences to society of pandemic H1N1 influenza 2009: preliminary results for Sweden. *Eurosurveillance*, 14(37), 1–7.

Brown, S. T., Tai, J. H., Bailey, R. R., Cooley, P. C., Wheaton, W. D., Potter, M. A., … Lee, B. Y. (2011). Would school closure for the 2009 H1N1 influenza epidemic have been worth the cost? A computational simulation of Pennsylvania. *BMC Public Health*, 11, 353–363.

Burns, A., van der Mensbrugghe, D., & Timmer, H. (2006). Evaluating the economic consequences of avian influenza. Working paper, Washington DC, The World Bank. Retrieved from: http://documents.worldbank.org/curated/en/977141468158986545/Evaluating-the-economic-consequences-of-avian-influenza.

Council of Europe, Parliamentary Assembly. (2010). Resolution 1749. Handling of the H1N1 pandemic: more transparency needed. Retrieved from: http://assembly.coe.int/nw/xml/XRef/Xref-XML2HTML-en.asp?fileid=17889&lang=en.

Dan, Y. Y., Tambyah, P. A., Sim, J., Lim, J., Hsu, L. Y., Chow, W. L., ... Ho, K. Y. (2009). Cost-effectiveness analysis of hospital infection control response to an epidemic respiratory virus threat. *Emerging Infectious Diseases, 15*(12), 1909–1916.

Durbin, A., Corallo, A. N., Wibisono, T. G., Aleman, D. M., Schwartz, B., & Coyte, P. C. (2011). A cost-effectiveness analysis of the H1N1 vaccine strategy for Ontario, Canada. *Journal of Infectious Diseases and Immunity, 3*(3), 40–49.

Ernst & Young. (2010). *Review of Switzerland's H1N1 immunization strategy. Final report.* Bern: Federal Office of Public Health.

European Commission. (2009). *Impact Assessment Guidelines.* Brussels. Retrieved from: http://ec.europa.eu/smart-regulation/impact/commission_guidelines/docs/iag_2009_en.pdf.

Federal Assembly of the Swiss Confederation. (2012). *Communicable Diseases Legislation Epidemics Act* (EpidA; RS 8918.101). Available in three Swiss national languages. Retrieved from: www.admin.ch/opc/fr/classified-compilation/20071012/index.html.

Fineberg, H. V. (2014). Pandemic preparedness and response: lessons from the H1N1 influenza of 2009. *New England Journal of Medicine, 370*(14), 1335–1342.

FOPH (Federal Office of Public Health). (2013). *Swiss Influenza Pandemic Plan* (4th edition).

FOPH (Federal Office of Public Health). (2018). *Swiss Influenza Pandemic Plan* (5th edition). Retrieved from: www.bag.admin.ch/bag/en/home/service/publikationen/broschueren/publikationen-uebertragbare-krankheiten/pandemieplan-2018.html.

González-Canudas, J., Iglesias-Chiesa, J. M., Romero-Antonio, Y., Chávez-Cortes, C., Gay-Molina, J. G., & Rivas-Ruiz, R. (2011). Cost-effectiveness in the detection of influenza H1N1: clinical data versus rapid tests. *Revista panAmericana de salud pública, 29*(1), 1–8.

Grépin, K. A. (2015). International donations to the Ebola virus outbreak: too little, too late? *British Medical Journal, 350,* h376.

Halder, N., Kelso, J. K., & Milne, G. J. (2010). Analysis of the effectiveness of interventions used during the 2009 A/H1N1 influenza pandemic. *BMC Public Health, 10,* 168–181.

Hutubessy, R., Chisholm, D., Edejer, T. T. T., & WHO-CHOICE (2003). Generalized cost-effectiveness analysis for national-level priority-setting in the health sector. *Cost Effectiveness and Resource Allocation, 1*(1), 8.

International Organization for Standardization (ISO). (2009). IEC 31010:2009 Risk management: Risk assessment techniques.

International Organization for Standardization (ISO). (2018). ISO 31000:2018 Risk management: Guidelines.

JMHW (Japan Ministry of Health, Labour and Welfare). (2010). *Report of the Review Meeting on Measures against Pandemic Influenza (A/H1N1).* Retrieved from: www.mhlw.go.jp/english/topics/influenza/dl/influenza.pdf.

JMHW (Japan Ministry of Health, Labour and Welfare), Inter-ministerial Avian Influenza Committee. (2007). *Pandemic Influenza Preparedness Action Plan of the Japanese Government.* Retrieved from: www.mhlw.go.jp/english/topics/influenza/dl/pandemic02.pdf.

Jonas, O. (2013). *Pandemic Risk.* Background Paper. World Development Report 2014 on Risk and Opportunity: Managing Risks for Development, World Bank. Retrieved from: www.worldbank.org/content/dam/Worldbank/document/ HDN/Health/WDR14_bp_Pandemic_Risk_Jonas.pdf.

Khazeni, N., Hutton, D. W., Garber, A. M., & Owens, D. K. (2009). Effectiveness and cost-effectiveness of expanded antiviral prophylaxis and adjuvanted vaccination strategies for an influenza A (H5N1) pandemic. *Annals of Internal Medicine, 151,* 840–853.

Lavelle, T. A., Uyeki, T. M., & Prosser, L. A. (2012). Cost-effectiveness of oseltamivir treatment for children with uncomplicated seasonal influenza. *The Journal of Pediatrics, 160*(1), 67–73. e6.

Lee, B. Y., McGlone, S. M., Bailey, R. R. et al. (2010). To test or to treat? An analysis of influenza testing and antiviral treatment strategies using economic computer modeling. *PLoS One,* 2010;5: e11284.

Lee, B. Y., Tai, J. H. Y., Bailey, R. R., McGlone, S. M., Wiringa, A. E., Zimmer, S. M., … Zimmerman, R. K. (2011). Economic model for emergency use authorization of intravenous peramivir. *The American Journal of Managed Care, 17*(1), e1–9.

Lugnér, A. K., & Postma, M. J. (2009). Mitigation of pandemic influenza: review of cost-effectiveness studies. *Expert Review of Pharmacoeconomics & Outcomes Research, 9*(6), 547–558.

McKibbin, W. J., & Sidorenko, A. A. (2006). *Global Macroeconomic Consequences of Pandemic Influenza.* Sydney: Lowy Institute for International Policy, The Australian National University.

McKibbin, W. J., & Sidorenko, A. A. (2007). The global costs of an influenza pandemic. *The Milken Institute Review, 9*(3), 18–27.

Medlock, J., & Galvani, A. P. (2009). Optimizing influenza vaccine distribution. *Science, 325*(5948), 1705–1708.

Murray, C. J. L., Evans, D. B., Acharya, A., & Baltussen, R. M. P. M. (2000). Development of WHO guidelines on generalized cost-effectiveness analysis. *Health Economics, 9*(s3), 235–251.

Nagase, H., Moriwaki, K., Kamae, M., Yanagisawa, S., & Kamae, I. (2009). Cost-effectiveness analysis of oseltamivir for influenza treatment considering the virus emerging resistant to the drug in Japan. *Value in Health, 12*(3), S62–S65.

OFSP (Office fédéral de la santé publique). (2009). *Plan suisse de pandémie influenza. Stratégies et mesures en préparation pour le cas d'une pandémie d'influenza.* January.

Pasquini-Descomps, H., Brender, N., & Maradan, D. (2017). Value for money in H1N1 influenza: a systematic review of the cost-effectiveness of pandemic interventions. *Value in Health, 20*(6), 819–827.

Perlroth, D. J., Glass, R. J., Davey, V. J., Cannon, D., Garber, A. M., & Owens, D. K. (2010). Health outcomes and costs of community mitigation strategies for an influenza pandemic in the United States. *Clinical Infectious Disease, 50*(2), 165–174.

Potter, C. W. (2001). A history of influenza. *Journal of Applied Microbiology, 91*(4), 572–579.

Prager, F., Wei, D., & Rose, A. (2017). Total economic consequences of an influenza outbreak in the United States. *Risk Analysis, 37*(1), 4–19.

Prosper, O., Saucedo, O., Thompson, D., Torres-Garcia, G., Wang, X., & Castillo-Chavez, C. (2011). Modeling control strategies for concurrent epidemics of seasonal and pandemic H1N1 influenza. *Mathematical Biosciences and Engineering*, *8*(1), 141–170.

Prosser, L. A., Lavelle, T. A., Fiore, A. E., Bridges, C. B., Reed, C., Jain, S., … Meltzer, M. I. (2011). Cost-effectiveness of 2009 pandemic influenza (H1N1) vaccination in the United States. *PLoS One*, *6*(7), e22308.

Renn, O. (2008). *Risk Governance: Coping with Uncertainty in a Complex World.* London: Earthscan.

Rossi, V., & Walker, J. (2005). *Assessing the Economic Impact and Costs of Flu Pandemics Originating in Asia.* Oxford: Oxford Economic Forecasting.

Sander, B., Bauch, C. T., Fisman, D., Fowler, R. A., Kwong, J. C., Maetzel, A., … Krahn, M. (2010). Is a mass immunization program for pandemic (H1N1) 2009 good value for money? Evidence from the Canadian experience. *Vaccine*, *28*(38), 6210–6220.

Stern, P. C., Fineberg, H. V., & National Research Council USA. (1996). *Understanding Risk: Informing Decisions in a Democratic Society.* Washington, DC: National Academy Press.

US GAO (United States Government Accountability Office). (2011). *Influenza Pandemic: Lessons from the H1N1 Pandemic Should Be Incorporated into Future Planning.* GAO-11-632, Washington, DC. Retrieved from: www.gao.gov/assets/330/320176. pdf.

US HHS (United States Department of Health and Human Services). (2005). *HHS Pandemic Influenza Plan.*

US HHS (United States Department of Health and Human Services). (2017). *Pandemic Influenza Plan.* Retrieved from: www.cdc.gov/flu/pandemic-resources/pdf/pan-flu-report-2017v2.pdf.

Van Kerkhove, M. D., & Ferguson, N. M. (2012). Epidemic and intervention modelling: a scientific rationale for policy decisions? Lessons from the 2009 influenza pandemic. *Bulletin of the World Health Organization*, *90*(4), 306–310.

Van Kerkhove, M. D., Hirve, S., Koukounari, A., & Mounts, A. W. (2013). Estimating age-specific cumulative incidence for the 2009 influenza pandemic: a meta-analysis of A (H1N1) pdm09 serological studies from 19 countries. *Influenza and Other Respiratory Viruses*, *7*(5), 872–886.

Viboud, C., Simonsen, L., Fuentes, R., Flores, J., Miller, M.A., & Chowell, G. (2016). Global mortality impact of the 1957–1959 influenza pandemic. *Journal of Infectious Diseases*, *213*(5), 738–745.

Wang, B., Xie, J., & Fang, P. (2012). Is a mass prevention and control program for pandemic (H1N1) 2009 good value for money? Evidence from the Chinese Experience. *Iran Journal of Public Health*, *41*(11), 34–43.

WHO (World Health Organization). (2009). *Pandemic Influenza Preparedness and Response: A WHO Guidance Document.* Retrieved from: www.who.int/influenza/resources/documents/pandemic_guidance_04_2009/en/.

WHO (World Health Organization). (2011). *Public Health Measures during the Influenza A(H1N1) 2009 Pandemic: WHO Technical Consultation, Gammarth, Tunisia, 26-28 October 2010: Meeting Report.* Geneva: WHO. Retrieved from: www.who.int/iris/handle/10665/70747.

WHO (World Health Organization). (2017). *A WHO Guide to Inform and Harmonize National and International Pandemic Preparedness and Response.* Geneva: WHO. Retrieved from: http://apps.who.int/iris/handle/10665/259893.

WHO (World Health Organization), Epidemic and Pandemic Alert and Response. (2004). *Estimating the Impact of the Next Influenza Pandemic: Enhancing Preparedness.*

Wildavsky, A., & Caiden, N. J. (1997). *The New Politics of the Budgetary Process,* third edition. New York, NY: Addison Wesley Longman.

Yarmand, H., Ivy, J. S., Roberts, S. D., Bengston, M. W., & Bengston, N. M. (2010). Cost-effectiveness analysis of vaccination and self-isolation in case of H1N1. *Proceedings of the 2010 Winter Simulation Conference.* IEEE, 2199–2210.

8 Financing the crisis

Public expenditure on the A(H1N1) influenza pandemic in Switzerland, Japan and the United States

Hélène Pasquini-Descomps, Nathalie Brender and David Maradan

Introduction

In March 2009, a new strain of influenza virus, the swine-originated A(H1N1) influenza, was detected in Mexico, and shortly after, in the United States. The World Health Organization (WHO) declared the first ever "public health emergency of international concern" under the new International Health Regulations (IHR) on April 25, soon raising the pandemic alert to Phase 4 on April 27, 2009. On June 11, since the virus had reached two continents, the WHO raised the pandemic level to Phase 6, stating simultaneously that the A(H1N1) virus's severity was mild. Nonetheless, with a quickly circulating novel virus strain and an initial estimate of fatality higher among children, developed countries had to manage the risk and propose an adequate response to concerned citizens.

This pandemic response required new budgets and funding in amounts that were in some cases subject to public criticism. However, several years later, we found little information about the total amount of public expenditure spent during the pandemic and its impact on the national budgets. Similarly, actual evidence does not indicate if there was "over-spending". The economic research post crisis mostly focused on the cost-effectiveness or cost–benefits of specific interventions, or the macro-economic impact, and we have limited data on the overall expenditure of the response. Considering an increasing scrutiny of public finances and the high public exposure of a government's actions during a health crisis, we believe that providing such evidence is critical for improving the management of future pandemics.

Our objective is to analyze the government's public expenditure for handling the 2009 A(H1N1) pandemic in three countries: Japan, the United States and Switzerland. We compare the pandemic's budgets to the regular, yearly budgets and between countries, and compute metrics to understand the required public expenditure to handle such a crisis. This cross-continent comparison of budgets is original since comparative studies tend to focus on neighboring countries. Our study, on the other hand, concerns three countries in different continents but similar in terms of their potential to handle future pandemic crises. The countries, although very different in their population's size (approx. 8, 128 and 307 million inhabitants respectively for Switzerland, Japan and the United States), are all high-income countries with a high GDP per inhabitant (World Bank, 2016; CIA, 2016), a reliable health system (IndexMundi, 2016) and the organizational ability and finances to cope efficiently with a pandemic.

We believe that this study, by looking at the finances and accounting numbers from a past pandemic crisis, can provide an additional dimension for pandemic crisis management. First, by comparing the necessary budgets, and the related expenses allocated at the time, we propose a useful set of economic data. Following the 2008 financial crisis, there is growing political pressure to limit expenses in all sectors, including health, and an increasing need for public government organizations to understand the factors that drive their expenditures. Second, there is an increasing requirement for transparency. Little or no communication on the financial part and related actions leaves the door open for controversies post fact. On the other hand, appropriate communication on the budget at the early stage of a crisis, when uncertainty and anxiety is high, may reassure the public and increase the trust required for good crisis management.

Framework and methodology

Most studies on the economic aspect of the A(H1N1) pandemic perform a cost-efficiency analysis for a specific intervention or set of interventions (for instance vaccination, social distancing, etc.) or a cost–benefit analysis for a country. Such work already exists and can provide guidance about which interventions to undertake and their cost compared to their potential benefits (Pasquini-Descomps et al., 2016), helping to solve organizational issues. Instead, this study proposes a comparative cost analysis of direct public expenditures related to A(H1N1) in three countries, using a framework inherited from corporate finance and cost accounting (Horngren et al., 2015). We look at the budgets at the national level for the expenditures of a pandemic response strategy and provide a high-level analysis of costs. Our focus is therefore on the *direct costs* of the pandemic at the federal or national level, namely the spending that can be directly attributed to the pandemic, such as supplemental budgets approved by the government specifically for this matter. We choose not to compute the indirect costs of the pandemic (for instance, proportion of work of the government's regular staff in each department that was dedicated to the pandemic). Indeed, the estimation of the indirect costs would require making numerous assumptions to compute a cost that would be incurred nonetheless. For the same reason, we did not compute the potential benefits of the strategy (such as GDP loss reduction and absenteeism avoidance), which would result in a cost–benefit analysis and take us away from our research goal.

Our study focuses on the expenditures at the federal level for the United States and Switzerland, and at the national level for Japan, as opposed to regional or local level. The countries in our study are two federal democracies, the United States (fifty states) and Switzerland (twenty-six cantons) and a unitary state, Japan, divided into forty-seven prefectures (IndexMundi, 2016). The federal/national governments coordinated the action and provided most of each country's finances for the crisis, especially by purchasing the vaccine. To complement our analysis, we reviewed a sample of regional and local budgets and activities reports in our section on regional activities.

Our main sources of data are the financial reports from the governments for fiscal years 2009 and subsequent, and especially the records of supplemental budgets dedicated to the A(H1N1) crisis, as well as activities reports, internal audit reports and accounting reports on the use of those budgets (see Annex Table 8A.1).

From the documents collected, our first step was to extract and list the items related to A(H1N1) and compute the total state/federal direct cost for the A(H1N1) response, comparing its burden with the yearly budget of the department of public health entity and the yearly public budget of the whole country. In addition, we propose a unit cost, the public expenditure per inhabitant, to understand how much the country has spent per capita to put in place a response strategy. We then compare the respective costs and percentage of the total budget, trying to identify standard costs (i.e. estimated cost of producing a service) and the cost drivers (i.e. factors that influence the expenses) in the various pandemic activities (such as vaccination, antivirals, international contribution, etc.). This analysis of past strategies and related financial data can potentially help the public authorities to anticipate their budget for future influenza pandemics.

Results

Financing process and total budget

Total of the response budgets directly related to A(H1N1)

We first analyze how the governments of the United States, Japan and Switzerland provided additional finances to handle the A(H1N1) crisis at the national level and the amounts furnished. The fiscal year (hereafter, FY) starts, for the US federal government, in September of the previous year, for Switzerland in January, and for Japan in March. Therefore, when the first signs of the A(H1N1) pandemic appeared, in March 2009, the US were already completing their second semester of FY2009 (started in October 2008), Switzerland was ending its first semester, and Japan was just starting FY2009.

The United States were among the first countries to be hit by A(H1N1), along with Mexico (GAO, 2011). The extra funding for handling A(H1N1) was provided within the Supplemental Appropriations Act "H. R. 2346" (Public Law 111–132) that was submitted to Congress in mid-May 2009 and approved and signed by the president by June 24 (US Congress, 2009). It included a "public health and social services emergency fund" item "to prepare for and respond to the influenza pandemic" in the following amounts: $1.85 billion available immediately ("immediate needs") to the Department of Health and Human Services (HHS) and a reserve fund of $5.8 billion ("contingency funds") available by request from the president to Congress (The White House, 2009a). Out of those $5.8 billion available, the president requested $4.541 billion in total: $1.825 billion on July 14 and $2.716 billion on September 2, 2009 (The White House, 2009b). As a result, the total funds appropriated were $6.391 billion. However, when the pandemic ended in August 2010, $1.983 billion remained at HHS (GAO, 2011) and could arguably be excluded from the A(H1N1) response budget. Since the remaining funds were kept by HHS but allocated to future pandemic preparedness, we decided to exclude them from the response budget. Therefore, we estimate the total federal expenditure for the response to be $4.408 billion, hereafter referred as the total response budget.

In Switzerland, the budgets to handle the A(H1N1) crisis were requested in August 2009 in the second supplementary budget (EFV, 2009a), approved by the Federal Council on September 30, 2009. The A(H1N1) items included three budgets for the Federal Office of Public Health (FOPH): CHF1 million for "A2111.0102 Enforcement measures (antivirals)"; CHF84 million for "A2111.0252 Pandemic (vaccine)"; CHF5 million for "A2310.0109 International contribution to health prevention and promotion". In addition, a budget of CHF6.8 million was allocated to the Federal Department of Defense Civil Protection and Sport (DDPS): "A2150.0102 Equipment renewal (masks)". The total budget was therefore CHF96.8 million. However, federal accounts reports in 2009 and 2010 show that only CHF79.2 million of the Pandemic (vaccine) budget were spent and only CHF5.7 million of the Equipment renewal budget (EFV, 2009b, 2009c, 2010a). The remaining budget was neither reported past FY2010, nor allocated to inter-pandemic activities. Considering the updated amount, we estimate the total response budget used for the crisis by Switzerland to be CHF90.898 million, about $61.9 million (all currency conversions hereafter are done using 2009 Purchasing Power Parity, see Table 8.1).

Table 8.1 Estimated supplemental budgets for managing the 2009 A(H1N1) crisis in Japan, the United States of America and Switzerland at national/federal level

	Japan	US	Switzerland	Mean	Stdev	Min	Max
Population (as of 2009)	127,510,000	307,006,550	7,785,806				
Health administration entity	Ministry of Health, Labour and Welfare (MHLW)	Department of Health and Human Services (HHS)	Federal Office of Public Health (FOPH)				
Fiscal year (FY) 2009 total national/federal budget	¥88,548,000,000,000	$3,107,000,000,000	CHF59,968,000,000				
Fiscal year (FY) 2009 health administration budget	¥25,156,845,724,000	$70,400,000,000	CHF2,175,242,200				
Total of supplemental budgets for A(H1N1)	**¥390,641,250,000**	**$4,408,000,000**	**CHF90,898,109**				
Purchasing Power Parity (PPP) as of 2009*	¥115.17	$1	CHF1.468				
Total of supplemental budgets for A(H1N1) in $ (PPP equivalent)	**$3,391,866,371**	**$4,408,000,000**	**$61,919,693**				
Total of supplemental budgets for A(H1N1) as percentage of the FY 2009 national/federal budget	0.44%	0.14%	**0.15%**	0.24%	0.2%	0.1%	0.4%
... as percentage of the health ministry budget	1.6%	6.3%	4.2%	4.0%	2.4%	1.6%	6.3%
Expense per inhabitant	¥3,064	$14.36	CHF11.67				
Expense per inhabitant in $ (PPP equivalent)	**$26.60**	**$14.36**	**$7.95**	$16.30	$9.48	$7.95	$26.60
Federal/national spending as percentage of total spending	83%	55%	33%				
Regional and local spending as percentage of total spending	17%	45%	67%				
Adjusted expense per inhabitant in $ (PPP equivalent)**	**$32.05**	**$26.11**	**$24.10**	$27.42	$4.13	$24.10	$32.05

Notes
* Source: imf.org, April 2018.
** Adjusted to the ratio of federal/national spending vs total spending.

In Japan, the budget for the A(H1N1) crisis was provided mainly within the FY2009 budget, but also by residual items in the FY2010 and FY2011 budgets. The domestic vaccination in Japan had a cost estimate of ¥300.28 billion ($2.6 billion), financed by the requests of the Ministry of Health, Labor and Welfare (MHLW) in the first and second FY2009 budget revisions. First, ¥127.9 billion ($1.1 billion) in April 2009 (MOF, 2009a) and ¥95 billion ($824 million) in August 2009 (MOF, 2009b) were requested for domestic vaccine development ("Supply of important medicines"[1]). Those, and immunization-related items found under "Infectious disease control costs" also extending to FY2010 (MOF, 2010a, 2010b), account for the rest of the ¥300.28 billion of the domestic vaccination. In October 2009, the Japanese government decided to buy vaccine from two foreign manufacturers in order to complement domestic production (HPM, 2010) – Found under FY2009 and FY2010 "Special chemicals accrued fee" (MOF, 2010a, 2010b). The total price negotiated was ¥112.6 billion (HPM, 2010) later reduced to ¥86.9 billion ($754.5 million), as the government reduced their order by 32 percent. To complement the domestic and foreign vaccination budgets above, the FY2009 first budget revision also included a supplementary budget for border control and immigration of ¥699 million ($6.1 million), of which ¥439 million ($3.8 million) was attributed to A(H1N1).[2] The second budget revision contained ¥1.6 billion ($13.9 million) for enhanced medical countermeasures in the regions. In addition, the Ministry of Foreign Affairs (MOFA) gave a total of ¥1.4 billion ($12.3 million) in various international aid across 2009 and 2010 for pandemic relief (MOFA, 2010). Therefore, we estimate the total response budget in Japan to have been ¥390.641 billion ($3.392 billion).

Response budget as percentage of regular budget, public expenditure per inhabitant

Overall we find that the response budgets for handling the A(H1N1) pandemic were consequential but not a major disruption to the finances. Compared to the yearly budget, the three countries approved on average an extra budget of 0.24 percent of their FY2009 budget for handling the A(H1N1) pandemic, with a maximum of 0.44 percent for Japan, 0.14 percent in the United States and 0.15 percent in Switzerland (Table 8.1). Compared to the budget of the respective health ministry, the A(H1N1) response burden accounted for 4.2 percent of the Swiss FOPH, and 6.3 percent of the US Department of Health and Human Services (HHS). In Japan, it represented about 1.6 percent of the MHLW, which is a larger entity encompassing social security and labor activities.

An interesting unit cost measure for future pandemics, the direct public expenditure per inhabitant, is obtained by dividing the total response budget by the number of inhabitants in the country. The estimated public expenditure per inhabitant was ¥3,064 or $26.60 per inhabitant in Japan,

$14.36 per inhabitant in the United States, and CHF11.67 or $7.95 per inhabitant in Switzerland, on average $16.30 per inhabitant (Table 8.1). Although it is interesting to consider the range ($7.95–$26.60) of public expenditure per habitant for these three developed countries, we must argue that there is no point in ranking the countries' expenditure on that basis. Japan has the highest public expenditure per inhabitant because it is a unitary state where the national government manages most of the budget (in Japan, overall national expenditures represent 83 percent of the total "National + Local" spending). In the United States, federal spending represents only about 55 percent of the total (Federal + States + Local) and in Switzerland, 33 percent of the total (Federal + States + Local). Adjusting the previously computed total public expenditure per inhabitant by dividing it by the percentage of spending at the federal/national level, we can compute an adjusted public expenditure per inhabitant (adjusted to 100 percent public spending). This adjustment would result in an adjusted expenditure in the range $24.10–$32.05 per inhabitant, with an average of $27.42 per inhabitant, and a lower variance (see Table 8.1). The adjusted public expenditure figure is a useful to understand the differences in the proportion of budget handled at the national/federal level, but does not represent a reality, nor does it make it possible to see if one country has spent more. The collection of all budgets at the regional and local levels would be necessary to allow a fair comparison but would be subject to a large margin of error due to differences in expenditure classification between collectivities.

The next section explores in more details the activities covered by the above budgets and each country's specific implementation and costs of similar activities.

Pandemic activities and budget

Although the WHO provided guidance to states throughout the crisis, each country ultimately had the responsibility to implement their own pandemic strategy, according to their national pandemic plan. Accordingly, there was no single answer to the pandemic. Some activities, such as intensified border control only made sense in an insular country like Japan, which travelers can only access by air or sea, and with a long tradition of border protection that was easy to activate when A(H1N1) was declared. But even activities conducted in all countries, such as vaccine purchase, were implemented differently. For instance, the United States, Switzerland and Japan had a distinct vaccination policy and ordered vaccine for a different percentage of the population, which explains some of the variations found in the budgets, as explored in the following paragraphs.

Immunization costs

Unsurprisingly, the procurement of the vaccine and the vaccination campaign accounted for the most significant costs of the A(H1N1) response budget (Table 8.2 and corresponding charts). Purchase of the vaccine itself was a significant budget in all three countries.

In the United States, over $2 billion, or 46.7 percent (Table 8.2) of the response budget was dedicated to the vaccine purchase and the vaccination campaign. Of this, $1.72 billion, or 41 percent of the response budget, was spent to supply over 190 million doses of A(H1N1) vaccine, purchased from five manufacturers (GAO, 2011). This budget also included the purchase of 200 million of related ancillary supplies, such as needles and syringes. This represents a cost of $9.05 per dose of vaccine (Table 8.3), which is in line with the standard cost of "$9 per dose based on the CDC price of injectable influenza vaccine, and ancillary supplies,

Table 8.2 Supplemental budget required by 2009 A(H1N1) crisis at national level

(a)

Japan

Population (2009)	127,510,000	
FY2009 State budget	¥88,548,000,000,000	
FY2009 Ministry of Health, Labour and Welfare (MHLW) budget	¥25,156,845,724,000	
	¥390,641,250,000	
Estimated supplemental budgets for A(H1N1)		
Budget categories		
Domestic and foreign vaccine development and immunization	¥300,280,000,000	76.9%
Foreign vaccine purchase	¥86,900,000,000	22.2%
Enhanced medical countermeasures	¥1,600,000,000	0.4%
Enhanced border control	¥439,000,000	0.1%
WHO contribution and international relief	¥1,422,250,000	0.4%
Total	**¥390,641,250,000**	**100.0%**

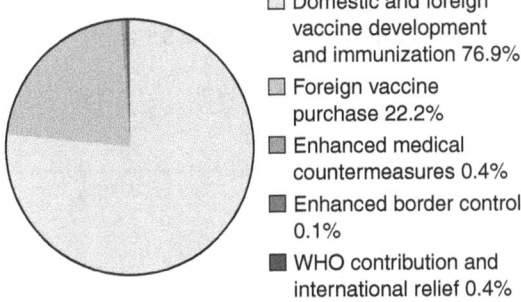

☐ Domestic and foreign vaccine development and immunization 76.9%

☐ Foreign vaccine purchase 22.2%

▨ Enhanced medical countermeasures 0.4%

■ Enhanced border control 0.1%

■ WHO contribution and international relief 0.4%

Table 8.2 Continued

(b)

USA		
Population (2009)	307,006,550	
FY2009 Federal budget	$3,107,000,000,000	
FY2009 Department of Health and Human Services (HHS) budget	$70,400,000,000	
Estimated supplemental budgets for A(H1N1)	**$4,408,000,000**	
Budget categories		
Vaccination (vaccine purchase and campaign)	$2,059,000,000	46.7%
Regions and local jurisdictions support	$1,404,000,000	31.9%
Antivirals	$231,000,000	5.2%
Disease control center activities	$199,000,000	4.5%
Research on vaccine	$95,000,000	2.2%
Hospital preparedness	$90,000,000	2.0%
International contribution	$44,000,000	1.0%
Communications	$31,000,000	0.7%
Drug licensing	$9,000,000	0.2%
Funds transferred by HHS to other departments for pandemic preparedness	$241,000,000	5.5%
Other	$5,000,000	0.1%
Total	**$4,408,000,000**	**100.0%**

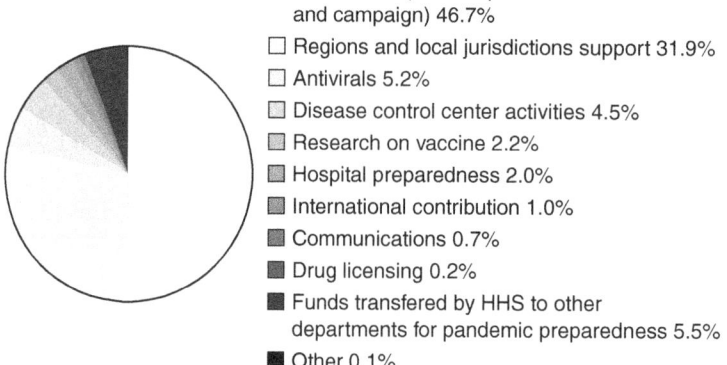

☐ Vaccination (vaccine purchase and campaign) 46.7%

☐ Regions and local jurisdictions support 31.9%

☐ Antivirals 5.2%

☐ Disease control center activities 4.5%

▨ Research on vaccine 2.2%

▨ Hospital preparedness 2.0%

▨ International contribution 1.0%

▨ Communications 0.7%

▨ Drug licensing 0.2%

■ Funds transfered by HHS to other departments for pandemic preparedness 5.5%

■ Other 0.1%

Table 8.2 Continued

(c)

Switzerland		
Population (2009)	7,785,806	
FY2009 Federal budget	CHF59,968,000,000	
FY2009 Federal Office of Public Health (FOPH) budget	CHF2,175,242,200	
Estimated supplemental budgets for A(H1N1)	**CHF90,898,109**	
Budget categories		
Vaccine purchase	CHF79,198,109	87.1%
Antivirals purchase	CHF1,000,000	1.1%
Equipment and materials for the armed forces	CHF5,700,000	6.3%
International contribution	CHF5,000,000	5.5%
Total	**CHF90,898,109**	**100.0%**

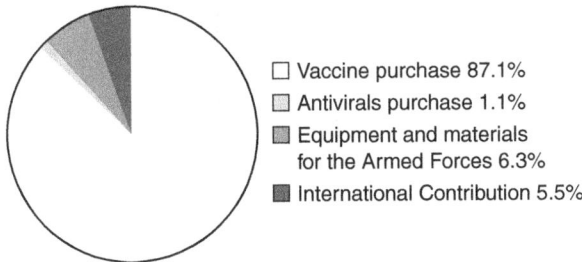

□ Vaccine purchase 87.1%

▨ Antivirals purchase 1.1%

▨ Equipment and materials for the Armed Forces 6.3%

■ International Contribution 5.5%

such as the syringe and needle, at $0.30 per dose" found in previous studies (Kansagra et al., 2012). The vaccination guideline in the United States was one shot per person, and two shots per child aged six months to nine years. Considering this, 190 million doses would represent a coverage of 58 percent of the population (Table 8.3).

In Switzerland, the purchase of the vaccine represented 87.1 percent of the budget (Table 8.2). The initial budget of CHF84 million was attributed to the FOPH to finance the purchase of vaccines from two pharmaceutical companies in July and August 2009. The first contract was a purchase of 8 million vials of Pandem-rix® (antigen only, ten-dose vials/package of fifty vials) from GSK for CHF20 million. The Confederation only bought the antigen because they already had a stock of 8 million adjuvants bought from GSK in 2006 during the H5N1 crisis (Van Tam et al., 2010; EFV, 2009a). The second contract was the purchase of 5 million doses of Celtura® (multidose vials) from Novartis for CHF62 million (Van Tam et al., 2010; EFV, 2009a). Based on this, we can compute a standard cost of the vaccine of CHF12.40 ($8.45) for Celtura® and CHF2.50 ($1.70)

Table 8.3 Estimated immunization costs, vaccine orders and intended coverage during the 2009 A(H1N1) crisis for Japan, the United States of America and Switzerland

	Population (2009)	Intended coverage (in number of inhabitants)	Intended coverage (in percentage of the population)	Initial vaccination policy	Quantity of vaccine purchased (shots)	Supplemental state budget for vaccine purchase in $ (2009 PPP)	Average cost per inhabitant ($)	Average cost per vaccine shot ($)	Average cost per covered inhabitant ($)	Remarks
Japan	127,510,000	36,900,000	29	2 shots per person	73,800,000	979,421,724	7.68	13.27	26.54	Vaccine procurement only
USA	307,006,550	177,650,000	58	1 shot per person, 2 shots for children 6m–9y (13%)	190,000,000	1,719,000,000	5.60	9.05	9.68	Includes development costs, adjuvant and 200 million ancillary kits (syringe and needle)
Switzerland	7,785,806	6,500,000	83	2 shots per person	13,000,000	57,220,708	7.35	4.40	8.80	No adjuvant bought for Pandem-rix®
							Mean 6.88	8.91	15.01	
							Sigma 0.91	3.62	8.16	

Japan

Vaccine purchase	Quantity ordered (shots)	Budget (¥)	Budget in $ (2009 PPP)	Average price per shot in ¥	Average price per shot in $	% budget
Domestic (2 shots per person)	54,000,000	25,900,000,000	224,884,953	480	4.16	23
Foreign (2 shots per person)	19,800,000	86,900,000,000	754,536,772	4,389	38.11	77
Novartis Celtura®	5,000,000					
GSK Pandem-rix®	14,800,000					
Total	**73,800,000**	**112,800,000,000**	**979,491,724**	**1,528**	**13.27**	

Switzerland

Vaccine purchase	Quantity ordered (shots)	Budget (CHF)	Budget in $ (2009 PPP)	Average price per shot in CHF	Average price per shot in $	% budget
GSK Pandem-rix®	8,000,000	20,000,000	13,623,978	2.50	1.70	24
Novartis Celtura®	5,000,000	62,000,000	42,234,332	12.40	8.45	74
"Purchase costs"		2,000,000	1,362,398			2
Total	**13,000,000**	**84,000,000**	**57,220,708**			

for the antigen only of Pandem-rix®. The total of 13 million vaccine doses purchased would cover 83 percent of the Swiss population, with two doses per person, which was the government's intended initial vaccination policy. The ancillary supplies were not specified in the budget, but an additional "purchase cost" of CHF2 million was added within this budget. The federal state also had the task of repackaging the vaccine and delivering it to pharmaceutical wholesalers for each canton (state) to pick-up, which was not itemized in the budget. The cost of transportation should indeed not be forgotten. As an estimate, the WHO report that the redeployment of the vaccine surplus donated by countries has a unit cost of $0.30 per set moved (a set equals one syringe plus an amortized portion of a safety box) (WHO, 2010).

In Japan, the strategy to secure the vaccine was to rely as much as possible on domestic manufacturers, who were to produce the vaccine for 27 million people. The vaccination policy was two shots per person, per the basic guidelines for vaccination of the novel influenza (A/H1N1) established on October 1, 2009. Four Japanese makers (Denka Seiken Co., Ltd, the Research Foundation for Microbial Diseases of Osaka University, the Kitasato Institute, and Kaketsuken-The Chemo-Sero-Therapeutic Research Institute) manufactured A(H1N1) vaccine beginning July 2009 with the intent to produce the required 54 million doses of vaccine by March 2010. To this effect, the FY2009 budget was raised twice, as mentioned above, during FY2009. Including 2010 budgets, the cost of domestic and foreign vaccination development is estimated to about ¥300.28 billion, which represents 76.9 percent of the total budget (Table 8.2).

The costs of the procurement of the domestic vaccine itself was estimated to ¥25.9 billion for 54 million doses (MLHW, 2010) representing a unit cost of $4.16 per dose (Table 8.3). In addition to the domestic vaccine, as the estimated domestic production would only cover 20 percent of the population if two doses were required, the Japanese government also reached an agreement to procure 9.9 million doses (2.5 million doses from Novartis, 7.4 million doses from GSK) of pH1N1 vaccine (HPM, 2010), at a cost of ¥112.8 billion. Considering the high cost of the foreign vaccine and its weak popularity, the Japanese government managed to later renegotiate the original contract with the vendors, lowering the amount ordered by 32 percent and saving about ¥29 billion. With this reduction, foreign vaccine procurement represented 22.2 percent of the final costs. With an initial target of 54 million shots for the domestic vaccine (with two shots per person) and 9.9 million single shots for the foreign vaccine, Japan had coverage of 29 percent of the population. If the vaccination policy were a single shot per inhabitant for the domestic vaccine, the coverage would have reached about 60 percent of the population. Including the foreign vaccine, the average unit cost per shot rises to an average of $13.27 per shot (Table 8.3).

Regional support and hospital preparedness

In the United States and Japan, parts of the supplemental budgets were dedicated to finance the regional pandemic activities. Indeed, the government would coordinate decisions and take action at the national level (such as closing the borders, tracking the first cases' contacts, vaccine purchase, etc.) but the cooperation of and implementation by regional authorities were required (for instance, local police at airports and for tracking, immunization campaigns at designated hospitals and regional centers, etc.). Other interventions are shared or duplicated by state and regional authorities (for instance, hotlines, hospital preparedness and school closure). To anticipate the division of tasks and other legal issues, Switzerland and Japan proceeded with legal modifications post the A(H1N1) crisis (OFSP, 2013; Shobayashi, 2010).

In the United States, about $1.404 billion was spent on supporting state and local jurisdictions' responses to the A(H1N1) pandemic, provided to the states through Public Health Emergency Response (PHER) grants (Table 8.2). Additionally, $90 million were dedicated to hospital preparedness. This represents in total 33.9 percent of the total budget and a public expenditure per inhabitant of $4.57 for regional support and $0.29 for hospital preparedness. The PHER grant funds were distributed in four phases beginning in August 2009, with each phase of funding targeting specific focus areas, such as vaccination, communication efforts with high-risk populations, etc. A report by the Association of State and Territorial Health Officials (ASTHO) concluded that the state and local jurisdictions could not have responded as efficiently to the A(H1N1) pandemic without the PHER grant funds, particularly given states' ongoing budgetary constraints (ASTHO, 2010). The funding process, however, was criticized because a documented budget needed to be submitted for each round and according to ASTHO, this bureaucratic procedure was time consuming and of limited efficiency. The CDC proposed to provide, for future pandemics, a template to simplify the application of this procedure.

Japan's budget also included a program submission and grant system, which was amended for greater flexibility after the pandemic (Shobayashi, 2010). In FY2009, a special increase of the budget of ¥1.6 billion was granted to MHLW for regional support of the pandemic, representing 0.4 percent of the total supplemental budget and $0.11 per inhabitant. This comparatively low budget per inhabitant may be because the actions were mainly taken and financed at the national level (85 percent of the country's spending). Another cause might be that the cost of vaccination had to be borne partially by individuals, which were to pay ¥3600 yen ($31) nationwide for receiving the vaccine via entrusted medical institutions – a price estimated to cover vaccine purchase, cost of transportation and vaccination. However, low-income, untaxed households (about 20 percent of the population) would receive the vaccine for free, the cost being shared half by the state, and a quarter each by the prefecture and municipality. In addition, the budget for stockpiling masks and handwash supplies might have been low because the high standards of personal hygiene in Japan (Takahashi, 2017) made those products widely available.

In Switzerland, the federal budget did not include any extra funding for the cantons (states), which had to manage with their existing finances. As previously mentioned, the states and local jurisdictions represent two-thirds of the country's budget, while federal spending represented only 33 percent. Although a procedure to obtain federal funding during crises exists, it was not triggered for the A(H1N1) pandemic. In order to estimate the regional costs for Switzerland nonetheless, we retrieved an estimate of the budget for the Geneva canton, which was about CHF2.3 million for a population of 453.3 thousand inhabitants. This represents a cost of CHF5.13 ($3.50) per inhabitant. The biggest cost drivers in this budget were masks, alcohol handwash and such supplies (39 percent) followed by vaccination centers (30 percent) and participation in the act of vaccination (20 percent). An important point is that the insurance companies reimbursed the canton CHF1.3 million for acts of vaccination, so the bill the canton had been required to pay up front was CHF3.6 million and not CHF2.3 million.

International contribution

The three countries in our study also contributed to help other countries through international donation. In the United States, a budget of $44 million was dedicated to CDC international response, which would cover "support for H1N1 influenza surveillance, laboratory and research projects in over 13 countries, and personnel support provided to WHO regional offices to handle H1N1 pandemic surge activities" (GAO, 2011). This international contribution represents 1.0 percent of the response budget (Table 8.2) and an expense of $0.14 per inhabitant in the United States.

Japan had an ongoing concern to fight pandemic influenza, especially in Asia, and had contributed as much as $416 million since 2005 (MOFA, 2010), including disbursements posted for the FY2010 budget. For the A(H1N1) crisis specifically, Japan's Ministry of Foreign Affairs donated over ¥1.422 billion ($12.3 million over FY2009 and 2010), representing 0.4 percent of the response budget and an expense of $0.1 per inhabitant. This amount includes an aid fund to the WHO for A(H1N1) vaccine in developing countries of ¥1.1 billion ($9.6 million), and an in-kind aid fund to Mexico estimated at ¥7.65 million, relief supplies to Mexico (¥21 million) and a donation to the Inter-American Development Bank ($2.5 million).

Switzerland also had a specific budget for international contributions of CHF5 million ($3.4 million), donated to the WHO to buy vaccine for developed countries (EFV, 2009a). This represented 5.5 percent of the overall response budget and $0.44 per inhabitant.

Following an initiative of US President Obama in October 2009, the donation of vaccine doses in kind also happened during the A(H1N1) crisis. Notably, the United States donated 25 million doses through the WHO in January 2010 (Kumar et al., 2012), and Switzerland 1.5 million in December 2009 (Van Tam et al., 2010). Although the vaccine donation initiative was intended to happen during the peak of the pandemic, only a limited vaccine became available in October 2009 and vaccine donation was delayed until the beginning of 2010. This timing and the surplus of the vaccine at the end of the pandemic that eased the decision of donating countries raises the question of equitable access to the vaccine in middle- and low-income countries (Kumar et al., 2012).

Antivirals

Another common action during an influenza pandemic is the purchase of antivirals. In Japan, due to the frequent use of antivirals for the treatment of seasonal influenza, the availability of antivirals through normal circuits was guaranteed and no additional stockpiling was required. In the United States, a budget of $231 million, representing 5.2 percent of the response budget, was allocated to supply pediatric doses of antivirals. In Switzerland, CHF1 million, or 1.1 percent of the response budget, was allocated to purchase 40,000 boxes of Tamiflu 75 mg (ten capsule boxes = one treatment), representing a cost of CHF25 per treatment. Recently, Roche published a pandemic pricing table for developed countries providing the following figures: 15 euro per pack of ten capsules for the 75 mg variety, 9 euro for the 45 mg and 6 euro for the 35 mg. The Oseltamivir Phosphate API (active pharmaceutical ingredient) was 7.7 euro per treatment. Prices did not include transport and related costs (insurance costs, taxes and tariffs) (Roche, 2016).

In the United States and Switzerland, the costs for antiviral stockpiling were low as well because the stockpile had already been high since the 2006 crisis. The strategic national stockpile coverage for antivirals covers about 25 percent of the population and contains oral formulations (Tamiflu), inhaler formulations (Relenza), and doses for pediatric patients. As early as the end of April 2009, the CDC released 11 million courses of antiviral that were rapidly allocated to the states (GAO, 2011). In Switzerland, the National Reserve stockpiles Tamiflu in various formats for about 25 percent of the population, and prophylaxis of medical staff, including, as of 2015, 145,000 treatments already in the form of ten capsule boxes. In Japan, the stockpile of antivirals covers 45 percent of the population (Berera & Zambon, 2013).

The antiviral stockpiles were not depleted during the A(H1N1) crisis. However, with unit costs of antiviral courses higher that the vaccine, the costs could have been much higher if the crisis had been more severe and/or lasted longer. For instance, prior to the A(H1N1) pandemic in

2006 , HHS had spent nearly a quarter of the supplemental funds (about $1.30 billion) on activities related to developing and stockpiling antiviral drugs, which included a purchase of 50 million treatments that were added to the stockpile (GAO, 2011).

Masks, antiseptics and protective clothing

In Switzerland, the purchase of material such as masks and antiseptics was budgeted specifically at the national level inside a budget of CHF6.8 million ($4.6 million) – of which CHF5.7 million was actually spent – for the armed forces, which contained CHF4.8 million for the purchase of respiratory masks. The CHF4.8 million represented 5.3 percent of the total response budget. In addition, while looking at the regional budget of the canton of Geneva, we found that the purchase of masks, alcohol handwash cleaning and such represented 39 percent of the Canton's response budget. Indeed, the purchase of such materials for various institutional regional levels cannot be neglected. In the United States, ASTHO also noticed that materials such as masks, handwash, garbage bags, etc. accounted for a significant amount of the state's response, which was problematic since it was not possible to budget for much of it in the above-mentioned PHER grant, in opposition to vaccination (ASTHO, 2010). In Japan as well, we found that the cost of protective clothing, masks, gloves and disinfectant was mentioned in an extra pandemic budget for the city of Kawasaki (1.5 million inhabitants). The costs of such represent about 10 percent of their regular yearly influenza budget.

Staff increase and deployment, communication and other

In the United States, there were specific budgets for deployments and for increases in activity at the CDC ($199 million) and ASPRs ($1 million), as well as for the pandemic activities of the Food and Drug Administration ($9 million) (GAO, 2011). That $209 million represented 4.7 percent of the response budget. A specific budget for communication materials and translation of $31 million (or 0.7 percent of the budget) was also available, in addition to the communication activities included in the vaccination campaign budget.

Although the Swiss federal government did not budget specifically for the increase in its activities, the FOPH reported an increase in their regular budget of about CHF2.5 million related to the pandemic's communication campaign (0.11 percent of the FOPH FY2009 budget) (EFV, 2009c).

Finally, two additional items were included in the United States' pandemic activities, but not itemized in the other countries. First, a research budget for "ongoing activities" of $95 million (2.2 percent of the budget,

$0.31 per inhabitant), including research into antivirals and monitoring of vaccine and antiviral effects on pregnant women. Second, a compensation fund for adverse effects of the various pandemic interventions was also set up, to the amount of $4 million or $0.01 per inhabitant (GAO, 2011).

Discussion

Our research question evaluates the public budget and public expenditure (per inhabitant and as a percentage of total expenditure) of the pandemic response for the A(H1N1) influenza crisis and relates it to differences in the strategies between countries, in order to improve the management of a future pandemic. Although the last pandemic turned out to be milder than expected, the pandemic plans deployed at the time considered a more severe epidemic, which makes the budget from the last pandemic relevant.

Looking at the documents and the mechanism for the approval of the budget for the pandemic, we found that the approval of those budgets faced no difficulty. Arguably this is because the budgets were relatively small and included in the regular mechanism for approval of supplemental budgets. On one hand, this is very positive, because it shows that money was not a blocking point in the decision-making process during the crisis. On the other hand, it may leave the impression that countries left aside the economic dimension in the risk management process. As we explore in Chapter 7 of this book, this is somehow true, but it is also a question of missing economic evidence.

Although we believe our research fills an important gap by providing economic evidence related to the costs of interventions in the influenza pandemic, we are nonetheless aware of the limitations of our work, such as the difficulty to collect regional and local expenditure figures, leading to a focus on the national/federal expenditure. Another important limit is the fact that we did not compute the indirect costs. Indeed, the staff of health offices across countries spent many hours working on this response, as did other offices (police, army, communication, etc.). However, since the cost of the regular staff exists regardless of the pandemic, we argue that the management of the supplemental budget is the most critical during the crisis. Governments willing to compute the indirect costs of the response can effectively use a specific percentage attributable to the pandemic over other activities for the regular staff, as is generally the case for indirect costs. As we also stated, we did not put the costs that we estimated in perspective by taking into account the potential savings of the response, as this is debatable.

Another limitation occurs because by looking at and comparing the total response budget and expenditure per inhabitant, one could make assumptions without considering the multiplicity of factors that led to the decision. For instance, as we can see in the results, vaccines are the main cost, and the vaccination policy (one or two shots, coverage intended) and the number of doses ordered directly drive this cost. Therefore, one could imagine reducing the quantity of doses to be ordered, considering the percentage of the population that was vaccinated *in fine* (Switzerland 21 percent, Japan 13 percent and the United States 15 percent). However, one must consider that the mild nature of the pandemic may have been responsible for the low demand for vaccinations and that other parameters also played a role in the quantity of vaccine purchased. Switzerland, for instance, had the highest coverage ratio (83 percent), but one must bear in mind two issues: first, the pre-existing contracts, and second, placing an order too small might have created issues in the procurement of the vaccine in a timely manner, since the manufacturers were delivering vaccine little by little due to limited production capacity. On the other hand, Switzerland, despite its high coverage and two-shots policy, had a low unit cost for the vaccine because it had some adjuvant left from the H5N1 crisis. Japan had the highest unit cost for the vaccine and spent some additional budget to enhance its national production, as part of its ongoing effort towards self-reliance.

Indeed, supply chain and the capacity to produce a certain amount of medical supplies is now a critical issue in health crises. With the globalization of viruses and suppliers, the epidemics become more frequent and countries may compete to get resources on time. During the 2009 influenza, even though the United States had ordered 190 million doses, the country did not have enough vaccine at the beginning of the season during the peak. This fear of shortage of vaccine and other drugs is a factor that drives the pandemic costs up for governments. During the Ebola crisis as well, it was hard to obtain protective equipment even if finances were available, as the demand was high and the manufacturers struggled to satisfy the orders. Such issues will hopefully be sorted out by the research to shorten the delay of vaccine manufacturing but should also be addressed by a global coordination effort with stockpiles created at the regional, or even worldwide level, as suggested by the WHO.

Conclusions

We found that the public expenditure for a pandemic for the national governments of the three countries in our studies would fall in the range $7.95–$26.60 per inhabitant, and in the range $24.10–$32.05 per inhabitant including a federal/national vs regional and local adjustment (see Table 8.1). The total public budget for the response at the national level, though important, represented less than 0.5 percent of respective national yearly budgets, at maximum, and less that 7 percent of respective health budgets.

The main expenditure for the pandemic was the vaccine costs and vaccination campaign (Table 8.2), accounting for an average of 78 percent of the response budget. This expense is directly related to the quantity of vaccine doses purchased for the country's population, and the vaccination policy and pre-existing conditions can partly explain the differences in the public expenditure per inhabitant between the countries. The reduction of expenses for vaccine procurement (Table 8.3) is not a simple topic: pre-existing contracts and supplies, limited production capabilities, eagerness for self-reliance, and the delay between the order and supply that may not be sufficient at the peak of demand are all factors which limit the ability of countries to control their costs.

The second biggest expenses are the regional activities that include the vaccination campaign at the regional level, the purchase of material such as masks and disinfectant, hospital preparedness and various staff increases. Other important expenses include the purchase of antiviral for stockpiling (which may have been low for A(H1N1) due to the previous H5N1 stockpiling), staff increases and deployment across countries, and the international contribution.

We believe that, along with the entire medical and non-medical factors that drive the decisions and risk management process, the listing of the public expenditures provided in this research might improve the management of future pandemic crises at the national level. Although we found that the 2009 A(H1N1) pandemic did not disrupt the yearly public budget, the under-supply of vaccine at the early stage of the pandemics was an issue and is problematic for mild pandemics but even more so for severe cases. The problematic of over-supply at the end of the pandemic, though difficult to anticipate, is an economic issue as well. National governments should continue working together with the industry to improve the scalability of vaccine production, as well as their purchase contract, in order to optimize production of the pandemic vaccines. The second biggest cost being the regional activities, another suggestion is to create an all-hazard fund at the regional level, funded on a yearly basis to ensure sufficient liquidity and access to finances during crises and distribute the expenditure over the years.

Annex

Table 8A.1 Documents containing information about the financing of the A(H1N1) crisis at the state/federal level

Country	Year	Type	Subject	Entity	Name	Source
USA	2009	Yearly financial report	Budget	US Government	Budget of the United States Government	www.gpo.gov/fdsys/browse/collection.action?collectionCode=BUDGET&browse=true
USA	2011	Audit	Pandemic response	Government Accountability Office	GAO-11-632 Influenza Pandemic: Lessons from the H1N1 Pandemic Should Be Incorporated into Future Planning	www.gao.gov/assets/330/320176.pdf
Japan	2009	Yearly financial reports (English)	Budget	Ministry of Finance	Highlights of the Budget for FY2009 Outline of the Second Supplementary Budget for FY2009 Summary of the Second Supplementary Budget for FY2009 Japanese Public Finance Fact Sheet 2009	www.mof.go.jp/english/budget/budget
Japan	2009	Yearly financial reports (Japanese)	Budget	Ministry of Finance	Budget for FY2009 (平成21年度一般会計予算) and FY2010 (平成22年度一般会計予算) First Supplemental Budget Revision (平成21年度一般会計補正予算(第1号)) Second Supplemental Budget Revision (平成21年度一般会計補正予算(第2号))	www.mof.go.jp/budget/budger_workflow/budget/fy2009/
Japan	2010	Audit	Pandemic response	Ministry of Health Labour and Welfare	Annual Health, Labour and Welfare Report 2009–2010 Part 2. Measures for the current political issues Chapter 1	www.mhlw.go.jp/english/wp/wp-hw4/hombun.html
Japan	2010	Summary	Pandemic response	Ministry of Health Labour and Welfare	Annual Health, Labour and Welfare Report 2009–2010, Countermeasures against Novel Influenza A Outbreak Situation of Novel Influenza (H1N1) in the World	www.mhlw.go.jp/english/wp/wp-hw4/dl/health_and_medical_services/P87.pdf

Country	Year	Type	Category	Organization	Title	URL
Japan	2010	Audit	Vaccination	Kinugasa Research Institute, Ritsumeikan University, Kyoto	Survey on Pandemic Influenza A(H1N1) Vaccine Policy in Japan	www.hpm.org/en/Surveys/Ritsumeikan_University_-_Japan/16/Pandemic_influenza_A(H1N1)_vaccine_policy_in_Japan.html
Japan	2010	Summary	International cooperation	Ministry of Foreign Affairs	MOFA: Japan's International Cooperation on Pandemic Influenza (since the end of 2005)	www.mofa.go.jp/policy/health_c/influenza/cooperation_since05.html
Japan	2009	Public communication	Vaccination	Ministry of Health Labour and Welfare	GENERAL INFORMATION: Influenza A (H1N1) Brochure	www.mhlw.go.jp/english/topics/influenza_a/index.html
Switzerland	2009	Yearly financial reports	Budget and accounting	Swiss Government	Compte d'état vol. 2B	www.efv.admin.ch/f/dokumentation/finanzberichterstattung/staatsrechnungen.php
Switzerland	2010	Audit	Vaccination	Federal Office of Public Health (by Ernst & Young)	Evaluation de la stratégie de vaccination H1N1 de la Suisse	www.bag.admin.ch/pdf_link.php?lang=fr&download=Schlussbericht+H1N1+f
Switzerland	2009	Audit	Pandemic response	Department of Finance	Rapport de la Délégation des finances aux Commissions des finances du Conseil national et du Conseil des Etats concernant la haute surveillance sur les finances de la Confédération en 2009	www.parlament.ch/fr/organe/delegations/delegation-des-finances/rapports
Switzerland	2012	Audit	Pandemic response	Commission de gestion du Conseil des Etats	Organisation de la lutte contre la pandémie de grippe	www.admin.ch/opc/fr/federal-gazette/2013/211.pdf
Switzerland	2009	Records	Pandemic response	The Federal Assembly (Swiss Parliament)		www.parlament.ch/en/suche#k=h1n1

Notes

1 Original names of budget items: Supply of important medicines (20 重要医薬品供給確保対策費); Infectious disease control costs (12 感染症対策費); Special chemicals accrued fee (5311–03 特殊薬品売 払 代); Drug approval, etc. promotion expenses (16 医薬品承認審査等推進費); Pharmaceuticals, etc. R & D Promotion expenses (21 医薬品等研究開発推進費); Immigration expenses (72 出入国管理業務); Regional health measures cost (29 地域保健対策費).
2 Estimate provided during an interview at Japan's Ministry of Health, Labor and Welfare.

References

ASTHO (Association of State and Territorial Health Officials) (2010). Pandemic Influenza | State Public Health | ASTHO. Retrieved from www.astho.org/Programs/Infectious-Disease/Pandemic-Influenza/ (accessed January 28, 2016).

Berera, D., & Zambon, M. (2013). Antivirals in the 2009 pandemic: lessons and implications for future strategies. *Influenza and Other Respiratory Viruses* 7, 72–79. doi:10.1111/irv.12172.

CIA (Central Intelligence Agency) (2016). *The World Factbook.* Retrieved from www.cia.gov/library/publications/the-world-factbook/docs/profileguide.html (accessed October 18, 2016).

EFV (Eidgenössische Finanzverwaltung) (2009a). Supplément II/2009: Suppléments. Retrieved from www.efv.admin.ch/efv/fr/home/themen/finanzberichterstattung/nachtragskredite.html (accessed July 29, 2016).

EFV (Eidgenössische Finanzverwaltung) (2009b). Tome 2A Unités administratives, Chiffres C2009: Comptes d'Etat. Retrieved from www.efv.admin.ch/f/dokumentation/finanzberichterstattung/staatsrechnungen.php (accessed January 22, 2016).

EFV (Eidgenössische Finanzverwaltung) (2009c). Tome 2B Unités administratives, Exposé des motifs C2009: Comptes d'Etat. Retrieved from www.efv.admin.ch/f/dokumentation/finanzberichterstattung/staatsrechnungen.php (accessed January 22, 2016).

EFV (Eidgenössische Finanzverwaltung) (2010). Supplément I/2010: Suppléments. Retrieved from www.efv.admin.ch/efv/fr/home/themen/finanzberichterstattung/nachtragskredite.html (accessed July 29, 2016).

GAO (United States Government Accountability Office) (2011). GAO-11-632 Influenza pandemic: Lessons from the H1N1 pandemic should be incorporated into future planning. Retrieved from www.gao.gov/assets/330/320176.pdf (accessed January 8, 2016).

Horngren, C. T., Datar, S. M., & Rajan, M. V. (2015). *Cost Accounting: A Managerial Emphasis.* Fifteenth edition. Boston, MA: Pearson.

HPM (Health Policy Monitor) (2010). HealthPolicyMonitor | Surveys | Ritsumeikan University – Japan | 16 | Pandemic influenza A(H1N1) vaccine policy in Japan. Retrieved from www.hpm.org/en/Surveys/Ritsumeikan_University_-_Japan/16/Pandemic_influenza_A(H1N1)_vaccine_policy_in_Japan.html (accessed January 14, 2016).

IndexMundi (2016). Country comparisons. Retrieved from www.indexmundi.com/factbook/compare/japan.united-states (accessed October 18, 2016); www.indexmundi.com/factbook/compare/switzerland.united-states (accessed October 18, 2016).

Kansagra, S. M., McGinty, M. D., Morgenthau, B. M., Marquez, M. L., Rosselli-Fraschilla, A., Zucker, A. R., & Farley, T. A. (2012). Cost comparison of 2 mass vaccination campaigns against influenza A H1N1 in New York City. *American Journal of Public Health* 102(7) (July), 1378–1383. doi:10.2105/AJPH.2011.300363.

Kumar, S., Quinn, S. C., Kim, K. H., & Hilyard, K. M. (2012). US public support for vaccine donation to poorer countries in the 2009 H1N1 pandemic. *PLoS ONE* 7, e33025. doi:10.1371/journal.pone.0033025.

MHLW (Ministry of Health, Labour and Welfare) (厚生労働省) (2010). 今般の新型インフルエンザ (A/H1N1) 対策の経緯について～ワクチン～ (Vaccine report, May 19, 2010). Retrieved from www.mhlw.go.jp/bunya/kenkou/kekkaku-kansenshou04/dl/infu100519-19.pdf (accessed October 21, 2016).

MOF (Ministry of Finance Japan) (財務省) (2009a). 平成 21 年度一般会計補正予算(第1 号) (2009 general account revised budget (No. 1)) Retrieved from www.bb.mof.go.jp/server/2009/dlpdf/DL200911001.pdf (accessed October 21, 2016).

MOF (Ministry of Finance Japan) (財務省) (2009b). 平成 21 年度一般会計補正予算(第 2 号) (2009 general account revised budget (No. 2)) Retrieved from www.bb.mof.go.jp/server/2009/dlpdf/DL200921002.pdf (accessed October 21, 2016).

MOF (Ministry of Finance Japan) (財務省) (2010a). 平成 22 年度一般会計予算 (2010 general account budget). Retrieved from www.bb.mof.go.jp/server/2010/dlpdf/DL201011001.pdf (accessed October 21, 2016).

MOF (Ministry of Finance Japan) (財務省) (2010b). 平成 22 年度一般会計補正予算(第1 号) (2010 general account revised budget (No. 1)). Retrieved from www.bb.mof.go.jp/server/2010/dlpdf/DL201021001.pdf (accessed October 21, 2016).

MOFA (Ministry of Foreign Affairs Japan) (2010). Japan's international cooperation on pandemic influenza (since the end of 2005). Retrieved from www.mofa.go.jp/policy/health_c/influenza/cooperation_since05.html (accessed January 15, 2016).

OFSP (Office fédéral de la santé publique) (2013). Office fédéral de la santé publique – Loi sur les épidémies. Retrieved from www.bag.admin.ch/themen/medizin/00682/15904/index.html?lang=fr. (accessed October 21, 2016).

Pasquini-Descomps, H., Brender, N., & Maradan, D. (2016). Value for money in H1N1 influenza: a systematic review of the cost-effectiveness of pandemic interventions. *Value in Health.* doi:10.1016/j.jval.2016.05.005.

Roche (2016). Roche: preparing for pandemic flu. Retrieved from www.roche.com/sustainability/for_patients/access_to_healthcare/making_innovation_accessible/tamiflu_corpres.htm (accessed February 5, 2016).

Shobayashi, T. (2010). Japan's action to combat pandemic influenza (A/H1N1). *Journal of the Japan Medical Association* 139(7), 1459–1463.

Takahashi, S., Sato, K., Kusaka, Y., & Hagihara, A. (2017). Public preventive awareness and preventive behaviors during a major influenza epidemic in Fukui. *Japan Journal of Infection and Public Health* 10(5), 637–643.

The White House (2009a). FY 2009 Emergency Designation of Contingent Funds: Department of Health and Human Services (emergency designation for $1.825 billion) to Address Critical Needs Related to the Emerging 2009-H1N1 Influenza Virus–07/16/09: Supplementals, Amendments, and Releases | The White

House. Retrieved from www.whitehouse.gov/omb/budget_09amendments (accessed July 29, 2016).

The White House (2009b). FY 2009 Emergency Designation of Contingent Funds: Department of Health and Human Services (emergency designation for $2.716 billion) to Enhance the Nation's Capability to Respond to the Potential Spread of the 2009-H1N1 Influenza Virus–09/02/09: Supplementals, Amendments, and Releases | The White House. Retrieved from www.whitehouse.gov/omb/budget_09amendments (accessed July 29, 2016).

US Congress (2009). Text – H.R.2346-111th Congress (2009–2010): Supplemental Appropriations Act, 2009 | Congress.gov | Library of Congress. Retrieved from www.congress.gov/bill/111th-congress/house-bill/2346/text (accessed July 28, 2016).

Van-Tam, J., Carrasco, P., Lambert, P.-H., Leppo, K., Tschanz, B., Sauter, C., Beck, P., & Meier, L. (2010). Évaluation de la stratégie de vaccination H1N1 de la Suisse. Retrieved from www.bag.admin.ch/pdf_link.php?lang=fr&download=Schlussbericht+H1N1+f (accessed January 14, 2016).

WHO (World Health Organization) (2010). WHO H1N1 vaccine deployment report. Retrieved from www.who.int/influenza_vaccines_plan/resources/h1n1_deployment_report.pdf (accessed October 10, 2016).

World Bank (2016). Country profiles. Retrieved from http://data.worldbank.org/data-catalog/country-profiles (accessed October 18, 2016).

9 The organizational puzzle of the Global Health System

Insights from high reliability organizations theory

Mathilde Bourrier

Introduction

This chapter aims at reflecting on some puzzling issues regarding the Global Health System that have been present throughout the collection of empirical evidence during the preparation of this book. From their specific angles, contributing authors in this volume have presented their point of view of the management of the Global Health System; they all point towards the complexity of managing such an open system. The first section of this chapter presents a characterization of the Global Health System and asks the question: under what conditions can the Global Health System actually be considered a system? Positioning the World Health Organization (WHO) within the Global Health System and analyzing its long-lasting quest for reforms will help raise issues related to governance. The second section of the chapter goes back to what appears to be one of the key features of the Global Health System, namely, the incomplete model for public health interventions during epidemics. This framework benefits from a general consensus among members of the Global Health System. However, this framework has been the subject of critique for quite some time, especially among social scientists, who have provided criticisms which seem to be regularly forgotten throughout the ranks of those responsible for global responses to epidemics. We therefore ask the question: what might be fueling this forgetfulness? However, somehow unsatisfied with this analysis, we sought out alternative frameworks. The third section of the chapter introduces what the literature on high reliability organizations (HRO) can bring to the table. Most notably, constant worries shared by the Global Health System and HRO revolve around striking a balance between prescription and autonomy, anticipation and adaptation, while retaining the necessity to cope with radical uncertainties, and the difficulties faced when organizing a highly diverse and fragmented workforce. It is hoped that the design principles of HRO might offer a fruitful path forward. Finally, the chapter concludes by arguing that, instead of continuing the calls for more structure, more control and more reforms, the Global Health System would benefit from decentralized emergency responses to health crises which rely on local expertise of all kinds, including the expertise of victims.

Characterizing the Global Health System

Can we even call it a system?

A quick look at the online *Oxford Dictionary of Sociology* (Scott & Marshall, 2015) gives the following definition of a system:

> A system is any structured or patterned relationship between any number of elements, where this system forms a whole or unity. It is assumed that a system has an environment and thus there is the requirement of boundary maintenance. There is an interchange between a system and its environment. It is further assumed that systems will tend towards an equilibrium state or homeostasis.

With this definition in mind, we find it worthwhile to consider the following question: is global health a system after all?

Undoubtedly, there are interacting pieces and interdependent components. Actors are interacting with one another in complex networks and sub-networks, forming an intricate whole, or a true lattice. This system is surrounded and influenced by a myriad of social, political, institutional, economic, ecological and geographical elements, facing "existential challenges", to borrow from Garrett (2013). It is definitely an "open system" (Scott, 1992). However, there is no easily readable structure, few common purposes, and some alignment of positions. On one hand, the "frontrunner health target is Universal Health Coverage" (Garrett, 2013, 20), formally endorsed by the UN General Assembly in December 2012. This lofty goal requires a massive reorganization in order to tackle health management and health infrastructures' financing. On the other hand, malaria, HIV/AIDS, tuberculosis and infectious diseases, which forged the historical backbone of international health and are still on the agenda, require investment and attention. No clear and definite set of rules governs its structure. There are few common processes, some shared health infrastructures (like the WHO collaborative centers), highly diverse target populations, and diverse methodologies to carry out public health interventions. However, those that are accepted are producing a strong normative order and professional doxa, derived essentially from biomedical knowledge.

If, even despite the limitations mentioned above, we choose to envision the Global Health System as a system, then the important questions pertain to Global Health System governance, including the forces driving decision-making processes. Holding this view lies possibly at the core of the permanent urge towards institutional reform, which seems to target specifically the WHO. However, if confronted with the same elements above, we reach the conclusion that the Global Health System is not a system, then the question becomes less about its governance, but rather its capacity to self-organize and self-design in order to introduce resilient strategies to achieve "better" tailored public health interventions. The answer given to the system question and its institutional design thus plays a large role in framing the type of remedies that are regularly put on the table.

The following quote from Bill Gates expresses this fundamental ambiguity:

> The problem isn't so much that the system didn't work well enough. The problem is that we hardly have a system at all ... [Global Health needs to be] coordinated by a global institution that is given enough authority and funding to be effective.
> (Bill Gates, co-chairman of Bill and Melinda Gates Foundation, in an interview given at *New York Times*, March 18, 2015)

As organizational theorists would suggest (Scott, 1992), if there is no system, centralized coordination is a long shot and has almost no chance to emerge. Furthermore, even if a system can be defined, decentralization might also be at play. Bureaucratic systems are hosts for both centralized coordination and pockets of decentralization that allow for soft adaptation of the rules (Crozier, 1963). Let us see if we can make further sense of the puzzle.

In search of "global health"

Both the A(H1N1) pandemic and 2014 Ebola epidemic revealed the complex landscape of global health actors in action. In the course of this research, we counted no less than 138 organizations or institutions. For Chabrol (2014),

> The Global Health label generally designates the diversification of the actors (particularly, private actors), the competition between the WHO and the World Bank and philanthropic foundations, as well as the technologization of interventions and health policies that are oriented toward access to medication.

In this maze-like context, some actors in global health governance obviously held more weight in the field than others (Youde, 2012). With a historical distance and an analytical lens, this story can now be told (Packard, 2016). The WHO, based in Geneva, was and continues to be composed of six regional offices[1] and representatives in 196 countries. The WHO is flanked by its World Health Assembly, hosted every May in Geneva, by an executive board, whose principal meeting is held every

January, and the institution's secretariat (Lee, 2009; Kamradt-Scott, 2010, 2011). Based in Atlanta, the American agency, the Centers for Disease Control and Prevention (CDC), represents a veritable Mecca of global public health and has offices in sixty countries. The health ministers of Member States of the WHO are also in the picture. Along with large medical NGOs, such as Doctors without Borders or Doctors of the World, a myriad of mid-size and small NGOs add support by participating in care delivery and vac-cination campaigns. Research labs, such as the network of large research institutes (like Pasteur or Koch), pharmaceutical companies which develop and devise medicinal treatments and vaccines are crucial members of the Global Health System. Large private consortiums and philanthropic founda-tions, like the Bill and Melinda Gates Foundation, the Clinton Foundation, the Global Fund to Fight AIDS, Tuberculosis and Malaria, GAVI (the Global Alliance for Vaccines and Immunization), based in Geneva, the Wellcome Trust, based in Great Britain, represent very important global health financ-ers. The World Bank is also a powerful player on this international chess-board. The various Red Cross organizations, all of which are regrouped under the International Federation of the Red Cross, based in Geneva, are also key players, especially when it comes to social mobilization. Hospitals,[2] academic research in general, and public health research institutions or epi-demiology training schools, such as the highly reputable internal training program offered by the CDC, Epidemic Intelligence Service (Thacker et al., 2001; Thacker et al., 2011) home of "Disease detectives", are key in develop-ing clinical management guidelines and sustained evidence-based research. The providers of automated tracking systems like the Canadian Global Public Health Intelligence Network (GPHIN) and powerful networks of experts, for example the Global Influenza Surveillance and Response System (GISRS), are also part of the Global Health System.

The inner functioning of some of these segments are better known than others. This is true for the CDCs (e.g. Ansell & Keller, 2014), for the WHO (e.g. Lee, 2009; Kamradt-Scott, 2011, 2016; Chorev, 2013; Brender, 2014; Abeysinghe, 2015), for Médecins Sans Frontières(MSF)/Doctors Without Borders (e.g. Fox, 1995; Redfield, 2013; Péchayre, 2014; Hofman & Au, 2017; Neuman & Weissman, 2016) and for the International Com-mittee of the Red Cross (e.g. Forsythe, 2005), to name only a few. However, other crucial parts of the system and the roles they play in global health have been less investigated so far. This is the case for the so-called Big Four accounting and audit firms – Deloitte, PricewaterhouseCoopers (PwC), Ernst & Young and KPMG – that regularly figure when money is involved. This is also true of philanthropic foundations whose budgets are scrutinized (McCoy et al., 2009) but not so much of their inner function-ing (with the notable exception of Levich, 2015).

These organizations find themselves at the interstices of a complex web where different logics tend to assert expert knowledge and evidence-based medical expertise in a landscape where they are often subjected to other factors, such as politics and diplomacy. For example, in the case of the WHO, there is some tension between operational expertise versus technical recommendations based on evidenced-based surveys. Our informants felt that their mandates were not set in stone and fluctuated depending on the situation, the context or the country affected. For example, during the 2004 Ebola virus disease technical officers at the WHO's secretariat navigated between different postures that were somewhat in opposition. Were they expected to coordinate public health interventions in affected countries or were they responsible for establishing evidenced-based guidelines for specific areas? Depending on the person we talked to, different views on such matters were offered. This observation echoes Littoz-Monnet's analysis (2017) of how international bureaucrats – "bureaucratic entrepreneurs", as WHO technical officers and members of the secretariat appeared to us – expand their expertise and forge their agency. They often relied on external experts, some of them being former employees, who are regularly invited to numerous informal consultations to advance certain issues (like risk communication or mathematical modeling).

However, this potential "mission creep" (Littoz-Monnet, 2017), or tension between their professional nature (supposedly apolitical civil servants) and the political and legal requirements of emergency decision making, regularly exposes them to criticism. This has been true for the A(H1N1) pandemic and for the 2014 Ebola virus disease. As Law scholar Heath (2016, 3) suggests when reflecting on the emergency power of the WHO: "Attempts by emergency governors to manage this tension are frequently pathological or even catastrophic, producing decisions that are neither scientifically nor politically justifiable".

At first glance, even just by briefly mentioning the actors to be considered, that their ability to coordinate common struggles is not self-evident is easily recognizable. There is not one global health but rather numerous global health agendas depending upon each player's position on the chessboard, the "causes" that they claim to support as a priority and the resources they manage to secure. This setup reveals a system of interdependencies and interwoven alliances, some of which are bureaucratic in places and flexible in others. Both inter-knowledge and self-distancing are at the same time primordial (Vardin, 2015; Saluzzo, 2011), particularly across institutions that, at least in appearance, hold contrasting positions on the global health chessboard, as is the case with the WHO versus MSF or the WHO versus the CDC.

Lakoff presents two versions of what he calls the global health regime: the "global health security" regime and the opposing "humanitarian biomedicine" regime. Both versions are complementary and represent two faces of the same coin: "the two regimes might best be understood as complementary rather than inherently contradictory facets of contemporary global health governance" (Lakoff, 2010, 75). Most scholars describe a system where humanitarians, security and capitalistic logics are all interacting, playing a bigger role than ever in the outcomes observed on the ground (Fassin & Pandolfi, 2010; Neuman & Weissman, 2016).

These actors, the most prominent of which were trained as medical doctors, benefit a priori from heightened reputational capital: not only virologists, epidemiologists, virus hunters and vaccinologists, but also humanitarian doctors, hold the upper hand (Wald, 2008; Lynteris, 2016). The Global Health System displays a profusion of strong networks of past experiences and socialization shared among some sets of experts, mainly through former medical training and former battles against deadly viruses (Saluzzo, 2011). These networks work across organizations and institutions. For many informants, there is no doubt that careers have been made thanks to past outbreaks. In addition, the Global Health System is intrinsically highly competitive vis-à-vis resources, scientific publications, legitimacy, expertise, visibility and institutional standing (Weisz et al., 2017).

Nevertheless, criticisms of the functioning of the Global Health System regularly bring to the forefront the following:

1   The turn towards reliance on funding sources per program at the end of the 1990s provoked the desertion of transversal funding opportunities for public health infrastructures (Navarro, 2004; Calain, 2007).
2   The collusion of interests between the bioterrorism agenda and the public health agenda has deepened, to the detriment of the latter, leading to what has been called the "securitization of public health", under the global health security agenda (Calain, 2007; Abraham, 2011; Calain & Sa'Da, 2015). This logic would come to favor a populations' monitoring policies in this regard, operating purely to the benefit of rich countries, rather than developing accessible treatments for poorer ones (Horton, 2014).
3   The systematic recourse to vaccines.
4   The fact that the coordination of severe events, particularly the surveillance of infectious diseases, was done via non-coercive International Health Regulations (IHR). These remained the only real means of action available to the WHO (Fidler, 2003, 2004, 2005; Fidler & Gostin, 2006; Youde, 2012).
5   The global health security agenda provided the basis for heavier weight to be given to scientific, humanitarian, safety and capitalistic logics, which were already strongly intertwined (Roemer-Mahler & Elbe, 2016) and still all too often tainted by neocolonial intervention (King, 2002).

The regular surge of coordination arenas signals also that interorganizational relationships are a constant challenge (Scoones & Forster, 2008). The creation of the health cluster, coordinated under the auspices of the WHO's secretariat, is also a tribute to the necessity to coordinate big players in sanitation and humanitarian arenas. One of our informants mentioned also the role of the Global Health Security Initiative (GHSI)

Advisory Group,[3] which in his mind failed to assume leadership in the 2004 Ebola crisis. Finally, the creation of UNMEER (United Nations Mission on Ebola Emergency Response) in this respect, in September 2014, although surprising at first, is in line with this constant uphill battle to coordinate heterogeneous actors, institutions, networks and countries (UNMEER, 2015).

Some organizational traits

The Global Health System is very fragmented; 138 organizations are listed in our project's database. It is polycentric (WHO, CDCs, GAVI, Wellcome Trust, National Institute of Health, International Federation of the Red Cross, large NGOs like MSF, etc.) and newcomers are constantly joining (especially small NGOs and civil society groups). Borrowing Perrow's concepts (1984)[4] of *tight coupling* (no pauses, substitutions, diversions or slack) and *loose coupling* (substitutions are possible, slack exists), while describing high-risk systems – like nuclear power plants, weapons systems, air traffic management and many more vital infrastructures – we also envision the Global Health System as both tightly and loosely coupled. It is tightly coupled when one considers the singularity of many types of expertise, few formal coordination mechanisms through the IHR provisions, for example, or long-established programs (like that for the surveillance of *influenza*) and strong and exclusive ties with WHO collaborative centers. And it can be considered loosely coupled when informal networks, disparate sources of funding, temporary mechanisms, and ephemeral roadmaps or initiatives are taken into account. It is also at some level uncoordinated globally despite the WHO's institutional role and its occasionally contested leadership in global health (Lee, 2009). For example, different accounts made by our informants during the 2014 Ebola epidemic revealed that it was difficult to find a legitimate arena, when hosting different organizations, to openly debate certain contentious points (e.g. Ebola treatment units versus home-base care or community care centers) that rapidly emerged during deployment operations on site.

These frictions can also be interpreted as the result of the impossible task of coordinating actors who resist coordination on the ground and at various levels. Large NGOs like MSF, most notably, cherish their independence and freedom to act on the ground. As a consequence, they tend to escape coordination mechanisms (Nunes, 2017). The same observations were made during the A(H1N1) pandemic where countries, through their ministries of health, expressed their sovereignty. However, some coordination for outbreak management exists. Formal networks of communication, based on the trading of different forms of technical expertise, embody the transboundary dimensions of the Global Health System, when responding to large outbreaks. The Global Outbreak Alert and Response Network (GOARN), created in 2000, represents one clear example of these coordination mechanisms (Ansell et al., 2012). It links 120 different organizations, ranging from labs, scientific institutions and NGOs to public health institutions. The Emergency Communication Network (ECN), analyzed in this volume by Bastide (Chapter 5), during the Ebola crisis offers yet another example.

Finally, the Global Health System has a few generic instruments, which are deemed applicable to a wide spectrum of countries, regions and problems. While some of these instruments are not all-powerful, they are nonetheless often discussed. The preparedness concept is one of these instruments, and its social history is of importance to understand how epidemics and pandemics are framed by public health actors and their institutions (Zylberman, 2013; Caduff, 2014; Lakoff, 2017; Bastide, Chapter 2). The IHR and its provisions for core capacities and components (2005, implemented in 2007) are also a way to envision progress and give meaning to achievements among diverse countries (Katz & Dowell, 2015). The Pandemic Influenza Preparedness framework (PIP, established 2011), an agreement between WHO Members States, pharmaceutical companies and other interested parties, is also an institutional space where key actors debate viruses, knowledge, vaccines and benefits sharing. PIP and IHR seem to grow in influence, alongside other permanent structures dealing with disease, epidemics and intervention.

Positioning the WHO within the Global Health System

Regarding the WHO's position, the intertwining nature of the numerous global health agendas (for example chronic illnesses, epidemics caused by emerging or re-emerging viruses, reinforcing health infrastructures, campaigns to eradicate certain diseases, maternal and child health), the struggle for financing between departments and programs within the WHO, the power of certain large philanthropic donors, like the Bill and Melinda Gates Foundation or the Clinton Foundation, the dependence on compromises between Member States, the mechanisms for the allocation of funds and resources, the savvy internal arbitrations between nations and regions of the world, the three-level structure of the organization (central, regional, national) render the WHO's functioning complex and difficult to decrypt (Lee, 2009; Kamradt-Scott, 2010, 2011; Brender, 2014; Dupras, Chapter 6). In this context, which has come to be incessantly reviewed and scrutinized, the WHO had since the 1990s been summoned upon to go through institutional reforms (Taylor, 1992; Sridhar & Gostin, 2011; Hein & Kickbusch, 2010; Clift, 2014; Horton, 2015; Kickbusch & Reddy 2015). Reports have been piling up for more than twenty years. Consequently, the WHO is constantly under reform and regularly portrayed as being in a permanent state of crisis. The literature on the WHO's twenty-year reform cycle is also abyssal. Many scholars and experts are fine connoisseurs of the WHO's shortcomings (Yamey, 2002; Sridhar & Gostin,

2011; Fidler, 2015, 2016; Sridhar et al., 2016; Cassels et al., 2017). Yet, in the end, the UN institution has managed to stay in business, so to speak. The A(H1N1) pandemic and 2014 Ebola epidemic provoked yet another round of discussions concerning urgent reforms that needed to be put in place without delay (Brender, 2014; Moon et al., 2015; Moon et al., 2017). Both crises have once again sparked criticisms and a new reassessment of the WHO's position (Gostin & Friedman, 2014; Gostin, 2015; Heath, 2016).[5] Such insistence on the WHO's reforms may be interrogated as such in the light of Nils Brunsson's arguments about administrative reforms (Brunsson, 1989a, 1989b) more generally.

First, organization theorist Brunsson sees administrative reforms as routines and argues that they are attempts to provide administrative solutions to problems. He contends that reforms can be regarded as part of organizational stability rather than of organizational change. He observes that conventional wisdom places reform under the banner of progress, and equivocates stability with backwardness. However, reforms bring further reforms because they benefit from problems: "Administrative reforms can be suggested as a remedy for almost any kind of problem such as low profitability, growing competition or bad leaders" (Brunsson, 1989b, 245). One important source of administrative problems is the tension between the way an organization is perceived by outsiders and the way it actually works. Coherence, consistency, action and control are difficult to build and align in any organization.

Brunsson's remarks are especially interesting when considering the WHO's position. One of his observations resonates in this context, particularly when he mentions that an important source of institutional problems lies in the tensions between the front organizations project for the public versus their actual inner workings. Members of the WHO that we interviewed during our study were caught in this disjunction. For example, interrogations about the issue of money during the difficult period of the summer and fall of 2014 are a marker of this kind of misalignment. According to Grépin's calculations (2015), and despite the conventional wisdom frequently heard throughout 2014, funding has never been an issue in the response to crises, whereas budget consensus and allocations of resources have been. Another example refers to the difficulty that some of our informants experienced in relation to subject matter experts in their domains, or senior experts expected to coordinate responders in the field. Another observation in Brunsson's work concerns the unsuccessful diffusion of earlier experiences, expertise and experiments as a marker of an organization being constantly under the urge to reform itself. He rationalized that reforms are eased not by learning but by forgetfulness,[6] by mechanisms that cause the organization to forget previous reforms, or at least those with a similar content. We will return to this observation when discussing the forgetfulness of anthropological and social science knowledge as being a legitimate part of a comprehensive outbreak response.

This section has helped explain why the Global Health System is not a system after all. Despite Bill Gates' urge for more structure, more leadership at the WHO and more resources, there is some doubt that this strategy might actually be fruitful. The next section turns to a feature of the Global Health System on which there seems to be more consensus and which is supported by various components on the chessboard: types of public health intervention during epidemics.

The existence of an incomplete model of public health intervention during epidemics

Interestingly, if what makes the Global Health System a system might resemble the quest for the Holy Grail, what constitutes a public health intervention itself is subject to more consensus. However, upon closer scrutiny, we realized that designing public health interventions entails a great deal of controversy. These debates not only feature normative global health experts versus the targeted populations (and their "faulty perceptions" and "resistances"), as one would spontaneously suspect. They also cut through major organizations themselves, revealing different views in the field of outbreak responses. This should not come as a surprise, since we have seen just how fragmented and diverse actors in global health are. However, this points towards designing organizational principles capable of working in such a hybrid professional milieu.

Consensus on a model

A series of apparatuses exist that most public health officers will favor, choose, know of, have been taught, or are teaching themselves. Lakoff and Collier (2008) talk about an "emergency modality of intervention". Leach and Hewlett (2010) describe a "universal rapid response". These public health interventions can be understood as repertoires of action that travel through the world. Such repertoires are normative by design, and they seem to be difficult to revise once deployed, despite the fact that deep opposition and resistance to public health measures develop at each deployment. Emergency policy making is a highly sensitive subject in any society. This comment, by Forster in the aftermath of the A(H1N1) pandemic, still resonates in the context of the 2014 Ebola virus disease:

> Universalistic, one-size-fits-all responses drawn from reductive science are therefore argued to be insufficient, and possibly misguided. Planning and response efforts must consider diverse local settings and concerns. Reductive technical framings emerging from tight, unreflexive actor networks may prevent other options from emerging, and limit response pathways.
>
> (Forster, 2012, 1)

Here again, internationally-led teams: (1) deployed isolation, containment and quarantine strategies, based on the implementation of nursing barriers techniques; (2) provided intravenous fluids; (3) organized contact tracing and surveillance of individuals suspected of having been in contact with infected individuals to identify chains of contagion; (4) put in place a "risk communication component" and (5) organized safe and dignified burials.

Many different responders, no matter to which side of the global health regime they belong (Lakoff, 2017), will favor this kind of deployment. However, critics tend to view this type of intervention as a technocratic public health dogma, top-down by nature, insensitive to context, and based on weak democratic foundations (Leach & Hewlett, 2010; Forster, 2012; Heath, 2016). It is deemed to pose great risks of rejection by targeted populations. Its generic properties also mask the fact that disparities, adaptations and controversies are in fact the norm when deploying public health interventions (Keller et al., 2012).

Consensus but controversy

Controversies were massive during the A(H1N1) pandemic and uncovered the margins of interpretation that both responders and populations showed in making sense of this episode. Despite the fact that pandemic plans were deemed too rigid and irresistibly triggered several provisions mechanically, numerous reports documented that countries, institutions and public health officers developed ad hoc strategies and soft adaptations of rigid pandemic plans. Some countries implemented school closures (France, United States, Japan). Some applied quarantine and borders controls (Japan). Antivirals were seldom used, apart from in certain severe cases or in certain countries like Japan. Some countries banned imports from Mexico, while others ordered mass killings of pigs (Egypt). Vaccine campaigns generally proved to be a fiasco almost everywhere (except in the United States or in Sweden) and shed light on possible mistrust of public institutions by large portions of the population, especially in Europe (Barrelet et al., 2013).

Fighting the Ebola outbreak also moved various actors to resort to a supposedly agreed-upon deployment doctrine, shared across organizations, members of the Global Health System and first-line responders. However, debates rapidly emerged, not only in public (between the WHO and MSF for example), but also within organizations themselves, for example within the WHO (see Cheng & Satter's inquiry, Associated Press, March 20, 2015 quoted in Lakoff, 2017, 152) and within MSF (see Nierlé, 2014). They also pertained to the applicability of emergency public health measures by non-state actors (Hofman & Au, 2017; Calain & Poncin, Chapter 11). The option of the Ebola Treatment Center progressively came to be seen as a strong choice, made early by MSF teams with no turning back. We noticed earlier (Bourrier, Chapter 3) that other available options like community care centers or home-based care were not given much consideration at first, although these alternative models were formally documented, both at the WHO and MSF. We mentioned earlier as well that recommendations regarding personal protective equipment (PPE) also triggered difficulties within MSF and within the WHO, and became also a veritable *casus belli* between these two major actors. However, no real institutional space existed to discuss other possible courses of action, in light of mounting difficulties in the field. At a later stage, pushed by some experts in various organizations who were convinced that community care centers were a valid option, such centers were deployed in Sierra Leone (UNICEF, 2015, 2016).

In this rather chaotic context, anthropologists organized themselves early through platforms (Abramowitz, 2017) to convey their decades-old message (Hewlett & Hewlett, 2008): quarantine, isolation, containment, the encircling of entire villages and manhunts inevitably provoke resistance, tensions and hostility towards Ebola responders. They organized themselves and rapidly published their observations (Fairhead, 2016; Wilkinson & Leach, 2015; Moulin, 2015; Faye, 2015; Lachenal, 2014; Le Marcis, 2015; Fribault, 2015; Laîné, 2016). They rehashed once more that mitigation strategies had to be worked on with populations and their leaders. This was of utmost importance, especially because people have prior experiences with contagious diseases and have developed precautions that can be built upon, even in the case of a novel virus (Hewlett & Hewlett, 2008; Richards, 2016).

Anthropologists' and social scientists' unheeded recommendations

Interestingly, as we mentioned earlier (Bourrier, Chapter 3), international guidelines on how best to intervene in communities when loved ones need to be taken away and/or safely buried existed (Boumandouki et al., 2005). They had been established both by anthropologists and WHO experts, locally and internationally, ten to fifteen years earlier. Anthropologists Hewlett and Hewlett noted in 2008:

> The WHO took our recommendations seriously and began to include medical anthropologists in early and multiple components of outbreak control. As a result, the WHO invited us to participate in the very early stages of an Ebola outbreak in Congo in 2003.
>
> (Hewlett & Hewlett, 2008, 61–62)

The same is true of Leach and colleagues who made the same observation and explained that during an interview they conducted with the Director of Outbreak Alert and Response Operations (WHO) in Geneva in 2008, he claimed that the anthropological integration had recently became a key pillar in response strategy – as important as isolation (Leach et al., 2010). What then happened to this "anthropological piece", as our informants in CDC called it, when 2014 Ebola struck?

By and large, these early attempts seem to have been diluted. The practical and ethical conditions under which public health interventions were possible in an Ebola context had already been reviewed (Calain et al., 2009). They needed an update, but the basic message could remain (Calain & Poncin, Chapter 11). Similarly, what anthropologists had written on hemorrhagic fevers some years ago was still valid and useful (Leach & Hewlett, 2010). However, our study shows that it had been somehow put aside and hardly transmitted at all. Why did this important piece of knowledge get lost in the past few years?

First, anthropologists and social scientists in general are not represented in the traditional ranks of outbreak response units. At the onset of the 2014 Ebola virus outbreak, WHO technical experts were openly sharing the fact that they had no solid expertise in social sciences. They felt uneasy about risk communication guidelines, for example. Second, social scientists have a simple message, urging emergency responders to deploy a comprehensive response, sensitive to context and in constant dialogue with affected persons. However, this could also certainly be interpreted as a radical critique of the off-ground intervention model proposed per se. Social scientists' publications constitute a critical reservoir, representing a constant thorn in the side, ready to question principles under which decisions are made, especially on behalf of vulnerable others. This might explain why their message, which was controversial by nature, failed to come across more strongly. However, anthropologists came to the rescue again (Abramowitz, 2017) and their essential knowledge has constantly been mentioned since then during high-level talks.

The neglecting of anthropologically informed recommendations in the case of the 2014 Ebola virus outbreak serves as an excellent case study for the challenges faced by the Global Health System to connect different bodies of knowledge, coming from various epistemic communities, each of which are developing at different paces. Designing a consensus on how to operate locally, based on rationales embodied by so many diverse and heterogeneous groups and organizations is probably beyond reach. And it should be recognized as such. This should not be seen as a defeatist attitude but as a more realistic position, from which some elements can be discussed on surer ground and decided upon.

In this section, we have seen that controversies are everywhere. Managing outbreak responses is about managing debates, not only with diverse publics, but internally within networks, professions, organizations and regions. Hence, invoking better risk communication tools will not be sufficient. Rather, designing "heedful interrelations" and nurturing the development of "mindfulness" (Weick & Roberts, 1993) seems to be key in strengthening better-tailored outbreak responses. David Nabarro, still frustrated by the difficulties encountered during the 2014 Ebola response, delivered a speech in front of global health experts in December 2015 in which he acknowledged this statement of fact.

Vignette

David Nabarro, representative for the Secretary-General of the United Nations, and unsuccessful candidate to become the WHO's Director General in the spring of 2017, made the following observations on December 2, 2015 in front of a large number of global health experts.

> More presidents, prime ministers are thinking of global health now than ever; more journalists are writing on global health than ever; there are more interests on health risks than ever; there are more actors involved than ever. Our narratives need to be acceptable to multiple actors. It is not satisfactory to say, we are the experts in every aspect; society is strong and resilient. The circus is normal life; whole of society in the norm, leadership in the circus with multiple actors is difficult; to gain in early detection, we need to listen to multiple actors; everybody has to be involved; risk assessment won't be based on public health professionals; humans are embroiled with nature: we need to be working with nature and animals; communication is two ways with trust and respect: you can't buy trust; our problem is not so much that we need more data, but rather what is done with data: ethical use; sharing; accessibility; we need to move from "health systems" to "systems for health" and much better, "systems for life, ability for function"; we need to create space, with trust and respect; others have a place and a role, and we need to create safe spaces; we need to engage in re-learning and be multi-disciplinary; we are hampered by our professions, sectoral orientation; we need to be agents of transformation, regenerative; impartiality and transparency, human rights are our principals. We are also communities, we are also games and power struggles; we need to look at our language. When we say "We are going to", who is "we". We need to be good at using power. We are all Humanitarians, we need to be careful at the way we use our institution, our uniforms; and let's stop using these terms "contact", "cases", and "irrationality", when this is about family members, friends, beloved ones.
>
> (Anticipating Emerging Infectious Disease Epidemics consultation in Geneva, Dec. 2, 2015)

This speech, reproduced in a leaflet to remember the event, triggered nourishing applause in the large room. Appearing at the end of the day, as a guest star, David Nabarro delivered a message that seemed to curtail tensions and bad feelings. In the room, many experts could easily relate to this proposed vision, and dream at least for a couple of moments that this agenda of reconciliation could be implemented once leaving the premises.

Testing the Global Health System against theories and practices of high reliability organizations (HRO)

Puzzled by the organizational complexities and challenges at stake, which inevitably impact vital operations on the ground, and aware of their recurrence throughout the history of outbreaks, we felt the need to decenter the focus. This decentralization of focus is particularly of interest, largely due to what was spelled out in the first sections of this chapter. In this section, we look for possible alternative theories and practices that might be helpful. Notably, references from high-hazard organizations models might offer new angles to complex questions that the Global Health System and its various organizations and networks encounter. In particular, problems of institutional design will be addressed.

Meeting high-reliability-seeking organizations

The central importance of high-hazard organizations (for example nuclear power plants, chemical plants, airlines, railways, air traffic control systems and critical infrastructures) operating in modern society has triggered, and continues to prompt, much scrutiny. The importance of this has also sustained a large body of research in management, sociology, political science, anthropology, public administration and psychology (Le Coze, 2016). The operations, products and services of these often fragmented networks of organizations are deemed to be both essential and risky. To cut a long story short (Bourrier, 2011), much of this literature on reliability-seeking organizations, appearing on the scene in the 1990s (La Porte & Consolini, 1991; Roberts, 1988, 1993; Rochlin, 1996; Weick & Sutcliffe, 2005), is concerned with the following set of questions, which might recast the current deadlock that one suspects in managing global epidemics (Lakoff, 2017): How and why, under challenging conditions, do some organizations do better and learn better than others? What could account for their differences and variance? What lies at the core of recurrent reliable performance? These types of organizations face a series of common challenges. High reliability theorists argue that organizations that can be described as highly reliable or as aspiring to highly reliable performance, and as showing a high degree of preoccupation with the four following problems: (1) balancing between an appropriate level of prescription and at the same time allowing for an essential autonomy in dealing with surprises in the field; (2) balancing between anticipating as much as possible while at the same time supporting adaptations when necessary; (3) coping with uncertainties and constantly seeking new perspectives on problems that organizations face; and (4) designing cooperation mechanisms to sustain frank collaboration in a highly fragmented system. As Karl Weick eloquently puts it:

> HROs are important because they provide a window on a distinctive set of processes that foster effectiveness under trying conditions ... Organizing for high reliability in the more effective HROs, is characterized by a preoccupation with failure, reluctance to simplify interpretations, sensitivity to operations, commitment to resilience, and underspecified structuring.
>
> (Weick et al., 1999, 81)

Complementary to these principles, Erik Hollnagel, leader of the resilient engineering school of thought, argues that resilience is: "The intrinsic ability of a system to adjust its functioning prior to, during, or following changes and disturbances, so that it can sustain required operations under both expected and unexpected conditions" (Hollnagel, 2012, 199).

It is our observation that the management of epidemics within the Global Health System is also concerned with the four concrete tensions mentioned above. This preoccupation with organizing meaningful resilience meets recent legal considerations about institutional design. Heath (2016, 4) articulates three principles, which in his view should guide a renewed perspective on designing global emergency power, especially the power exercised by the WHO in response to health emergencies: (1) "managed decentralization", (2) "epistemic openness" and (3) "forced dissent". In the final discussion, we will return to these propositions in the light of what we learned from the management of epidemics.

Prescription versus autonomy

Working with rules and procedures and expanding bodies of regulations is a given in most contemporary organizations (Graeber, 2015), and even more so within high-risk organizations. However, what are the implications for daily operations of having to document each and every stage of any process? At a certain level, one could consider that one of the key cultural features of these organizations, where safety is paramount, is an ever-increasing reliance on procedures that seems endless and unavoidable (Bieder & Bourrier, 2013). However, social scientists have long demonstrated that detailed prescriptions, although promoted everywhere, are not sufficient to obtain safe operations (Bourrier, 1999). Experts are operating with far greater levels of informalities and ambiguity (Wynne, 1988). Procedures are important (Gawande, 2010), but they are imperfect and sometimes counterproductive: orderly procedures to reduce errors are not foolproof barriers. Sometimes errors travel a long way and a long time in a very orderly system (Vaughan, 1997; Hofmann & Frese, 2011). As a consequence, the following crucial questions are constantly on the table: Which groups are in charge of creating and updating rules and procedures, and how is this done? How is the classic tension between prescription and autonomy organized and thought about in organizations expected to produce and deliver an outstanding level of safe performance? Furthermore, how is the coherence of diverse sets of rules both simultaneously maintained and critically questioned?

To these crucial questions, there is not one single answer. High reliability theorists argue (Roberts, 1993) that one way to mitigate this tension is always to defer to the expertise closest to the problem. Proponents of this theory argue that expertise does not necessarily derive from technical knowledge. Rather, it is something that one gains from experience with the problem at hand. This has been referred to as "migrating decision making", meaning that the expert closest to the problem is in charge of the decision. However, at the same time, the top takes responsibility for the decision, no matter what the consequences are. Along with a preoccupation with failure and a sensitivity to operations, deference to expertise ensures that the people who are directly concerned by a situation always offer their opinion and, more importantly, their solutions. Experts closest to the problems are the ones making the calls and should get all the support they need. Prescriptions designed by people directly concerned with the issues at stake are better suited to their needs.

What many observers and what our informants frequently recalled is that, too often, staff in the field were required to feed the upper level with data and information, which diverted too much of their energy and time. This was true for both pandemic flu A(H1N1) and for the 2014 Ebola epidemic. In the latter case, logistics were often talked about by our informants as being lacking or insufficient. Yet, at the same time they had to report and to log into complex IT systems in order to upload information about the response. Discrepancies were often noted between the level of sophistication of some of these interfaces deployed on the ground, and the absolute poverty of means that first-line responders experienced. This observation is not valid for MSF, which notoriously puts great emphasis on diligently supporting its staff on the ground. This is made possible also by the relative strategy of isolation that MSF Ebola treatment units put in place. As some of our informants explained, they did not want to coordinate with anybody and wanted to maintain their independence.

Anticipation versus adaptation

The second feature leads us to the cultural core of high-risk organizations, which could be summarized as a culture of anticipation that operates through planning and scheduling. Sociologist Richard Sennett (1998) once brilliantly explained why developing routine patterns was important in the workplace. He argued that employees cannot be expected to constantly respond to surprises. A minimum secure bedrock of rehearsed routines is necessary to work relatively peacefully. Furthermore, it is all the more important in hostile work environments, where risks are present and should be reduced to a minimum through careful preparation. However, how to best plan, schedule, and anticipate crucial activities, while at the same time staying alert to avoid the tragic complacency that such activities inevitably produce, is always an uphill battle. Indeed, this very culture of preparedness is also an identified obstacle to learning how to face the unexpected (Weick & Sutcliffe, 2005). The false promise of scenario planning has already been documented (Clarke, 1999) and has been constantly revisited in the light of special events and catastrophes. The A(H1N1) pandemic told a story of *excessive and inadequate* planning, which left work teams overloaded. The Fukushima-Daïchi nuclear accident told a story of *unthinkable and undone* planning, which moved work teams to decide for themselves, under very stressful conditions[7] (Guarnieri et al., 2015; Kadota, 2014). Ebola told the story of *faulty and contextually insensitive* planning. Preparing, scheduling and planning are an important component of any organization dealing with complex operational conditions. However, these tasks should not be understood as distinct phases (Keller et al., 2012), but rather as completely integral to the job and subject to adaptations. To decide upon these adaptations, high reliability theorists suggest resisting the tendency to simplify. Enriching the picture with different views, opinions, crafts and expertise, from various positions especially in a fragmented system, is of paramount importance. These theorists suggest that this multifaceted echo chamber should intentionally be designed as such and not obtained by mere chance (Rochlin, 1993; Bourrier, 2005).

How to best share ad hoc and successful adaptive strategies in order to diffuse knowledge on what works, and not only on what does not work, is an issue concerning and discussed among high reliability theorists and resilient engineering scholars (Hollnagel et al., 2006). They argue that too often management tends to focus on problems, masking improbable, yet successful, recoveries. In this line of argument, the 2014 Ebola epidemic provides another example of local mitigation strategies that have been overlooked and under supported. Emergent local knowledge, "a vibrant People's Science" in Richards' words (2016), undoubtedly helped to contain the epidemic. However, its undetermined paths of improvisation and bricolage have not been systematically recorded, leaving the question of organizational learning from crisis open once again (Keller, Chapter 1). Weick (1987) long argued that storytelling inside high-risk organizations was crucial to allow for the circulation and sharing not only of problematic events and how they unfolded, but also of inventive and resourceful options to solve tricky problems.

This commitment to resilience is often quoted as an HRO principle. The capacity to reorder, to move rapidly from normal operations to emergency conditions and in doing so to adopt a decentralized and team-based approach to problem-solving is one of the key characteristics of resilient organizations (La Porte & Consolini, 1991; Boin & Van Eeten, 2013). It obviously echoes the situation that outbreak responses encounter frequently, as we will further develop.

Coping with uncertainties

A third question that high reliability theorists have discussed at length is the following: How do actors best cope with uncertainties and risks inherent to the industrial process within a changing institutional environment while still maintaining products and services at a socially and economically reasonable cost? If risks might be recognized and taken into account, uncertainties might still remain. Hence, cultivating vigilance for unforeseen combinations of events remains a task in itself. This can only be done by challenging frameworks, norms and conventional wisdoms, which have been taken for granted, in order to question their intrinsic limitations and biases.

Some organizations have purposively designed institutional mechanisms to encourage criticism from within. The US CDC use "Team B" groups of experts and scientists to offer a new perspective on unfolding events and provide possible critiques of the core response's options. "Team B" was used for the A(H1N1) pandemic, but less so for the 2014 Ebola epidemic. High reliability theorists argue that a balance has to be established between relying too much on very compliant people, with no inclination to challenge their working environment, and encouraging hotheads, who are always ready to break rules and procedures to set their own norms of performance. HROs do not look for heroes but, rather, for questioning minds. Hence, striking a balance between compliance and improvisation is probably one of the most difficult issues in management.

One approach is to accommodate and constantly seek new perspectives on complex issues. The idea here is to organize multi-level perspectives to enrich the vision on emerging, tricky and unclear problems. The requisite variety principle has often been discussed in this context. Political scientist Paul Schulman defines the requisite variety as a conceptual slack: "a divergence in analytical perspectives among members of an organization over theories, models, or causal assumptions pertaining to its technology or production processes" (Schulman, 1993, 364). In other words, in order to deal properly with the diversity of problems the world throws at you, you need to have a repertoire of responses which is as nuanced as the problems you face. Cultivating this mix of persons with their views, idiosyncrasies and expertise is problematic in itself. In the context of this book, it could be used as a reminder to battle against the forgetfulness of disquieting or misaligned facts.

Organizing cooperation in a highly fragmented system

High-risk organizations are often the theater of complex coordination mechanisms involving highly diverse work teams, with ultra-specific expertise, hardly transferable or co-shared. In these challenging human relations contexts, how best to enable coordination among various professions, crafts, trades and companies is key. Co-working with many subcontractors and partners while avoiding the formation of clans, baronies and loss of information along the way remains a daily challenge. How best to depend on highly skilled personnel, where almost no substitution is possible among them (hence no rotating option), while not being trapped in their world views, entrenched wars and sometimes corporatist interests is a constant worry. Organization theory and sociology of organizations have long demonstrated that power relations play a huge role in the final result being delivered. As a limiting factor of power plays, scholars of crisis management and transboundary crises have already pointed out: "In fact, the research on crisis coordination suggests that 'less is more': self-organization tends to work better than imposed cooperation schemes" (Ansell et al., 2010, 199).

As Roberts and Rousseau (1998, 132) explain, taking the example of an aircraft-carrier, these work environments display a "hyper-complexity [due to] an extreme variety of components, systems, and levels and tight coupling [due to] reciprocal interdependence across many units and levels". Anyone interested in organizational design is challenged by this feature: the degree of specialization and expertise among the different units, departments, crafts and subcontractors inevitably triggers a difficulty in adequately communicating each other's concerns and needs. Work is done in silos (Perin, 2005), "structural secrecy" prevails and knowledge does not travel easily throughout the system of organizations (Vaughan, 1997). Pockets of crucial knowledge, both implicit and explicit (Broadbent et al., 1986), can stay hidden for a long time and do not travel through the hierarchical ladder easily, nor through the crucial network nodes. Vaughan has eloquently demonstrated how the culture at NASA, relying so much on hard data, supported by mathematical modeling, had not allowed other types of evidence, deemed soft or in the form of gut feelings, to be shared and acted upon. It allowed pending issues, deemed illegitimate, and hence unresolved, to strongly contribute to both the *Challenger* and *Columbia* accidents. High reliability theorists claim that paying attention to the circulation of stories about operational events and building plausible narratives explaining how they happened is a rewarding path to overcome the hurdles of "structural secrecy" (Weick, 1987).

Therefore, constantly battling against clans, entrenchment and stagnant pieces of knowledge is vital for achieving safe and reliable performances. A constant effort has to be made to navigate between experts. The same is true when dealing with widespread practices of subcontracting and delegation. Outsourcing requires a lot of reorganization at the principal level. Organizing a degree of leadership and "followship"[8] is a task in itself. The degree and extent of distributed cognition is a constant challenge that needs to be monitored. Roberts and Rousseau (1998) once coined the expression "having the bubble" to best describe this extraordinary capability to collectively co-adjust courses of action and decisions. Weick calls it "sensemaking activities". By that, he means that organizational failure and catastrophic events are best understood as the collapse of a collective sensemaking (Weick, 1993). "Mindfulness" and "heedful interrelations" are key properties to maintain collective dedication to safe performances (Weick et al., 1999). The quality of organizational attention to organizing processes is central to this discussion.

Conclusion: the place of high reliability organizations (HRO) theory in global health frameworks

The larger question remains: How can these insights and principles from other types of organizations be meaningfully translated into the context of the Global Health System that was described in the first part of this chapter? It appears to us that designing cooperation mechanisms in such a fragmented, hyper-competitive, both tightly and loosely coupled Global Health System is daunting. Yet, we can point to several examples of dedicated organizational designs aimed at addressing these challenges. First, CDC in Atlanta runs structures like the Emergency Operations Center and uses Incident Management System (IMS) theory to enable strong commitment and resource rallying from various parts of the organization in order to strengthen outbreak responses. It allows experts to work across departmental boundaries and diminish possible turf battles and bureaucratic red tape (Ansell & Keller, 2014). The IMS concept was applied in Liberia (as well as in other countries, like Nigeria, or Sierra Leone) during the Ebola epidemic (Pillai et al., 2014, 931). As Pillai and colleagues explain:

> A clearly defined chain of command and organizational structure, effective resource management, and advanced planning are important aspects of an emergency response. An IMS is a standard structure based on these principles that is used in large and small-scale incidents throughout the United States at the federal, state, and local level. CDC has adapted IMS principles in managing their responses to public health emergencies, which in addition to the command, operations, logistics, planning, and finance/administrative functions, also includes scientific/public health response roles.

Second, during the 2014 Ebola epidemic, the WHO also reorganized and experimented with diverse organizational structures to help with management of the response. First, they used the Emergency Response Framework plan at the organization level, then moved towards a regional option with the SEOCC (Sub-Regional Ebola Operations and Coordination Centre), and then finally assembled an Ebola response team at headquarters, along the lines of matrix management principles. As Dupras (Chapter 6) explains in her chapter, it was not the first time that the WHO resorted to matrix management per se. However, it is probably the first time that it used it at such a scale. Enriching the picture and trying to get everyone's expertise on the same platform were probably the intentions. However, some of our informants described the difficulty they faced when trying to be heard and respected in whatever they had to offer.

A third example of this necessity to coordinate different perspectives might also be found in the relative failure to bring anthropologists on board in the late 1990s and early 2000s. Even marginally, they were in a position to offer a different view on outbreak management. One would think that this is probably what is expected now from the "Social Science outbreak teams", which have recently been installed at WHO headquarters within the Health Emergencies Programme (Johnson & Vindrola-Padros, 2017).

Moreover, following HRO principles, it will appear altogether problematic to coordinate an outbreak response from far away. The failure of coordination that so many people reported to us and in numerous accounts points towards a failure of a certain type: one that is based on the principle that the response can be organized from the top (WHO headquarters, CDC EOC in Atlanta; MSF's operational center in Belgium) and deployed on the ground, with even a duplication of structures, mirroring the one at the top (Pillai et al., 2014). Managing outbreak responses from centrally located institutions runs the risk of favoring standardized approaches, narrowing down options and impoverishing local contexts. Major controversies in both the A(H1N1) pandemic and the 2014 Ebola epidemic erupted from a neglect of contextual realities. Many accounts report that centrally managing epidemics has never been possible and will not be in the future, as they are eternally *unprepared* (Richards, 2016; Lakoff, 2017). As Lakoff reflects:

> [I]n the case of the 2014 Ebola epidemic, it was not clear which governmental agency or body of authorities held jurisdiction over the management of epidemic response at a global scale. Who exactly comprised or spoke for "the global community"?
>
> (Lakoff, 2017, 156)

Finally, is the WHO's eternal reform mode the only way to go forward? Or rather, are these perpetual reforms a symptom of something else? What kind of problems are these reform attempts trying to solve? Is it the governance that needs to be fixed, or the kind of intervention that needs to be agreed upon? Following the path that high reliability theorists suggest, we argue the following: the type of intervention needs to be the core of the coordination; the rest cannot be centrally coordinated anyway. Therefore, the decision to combine Outbreak and Emergency Response programs into a single new "WHO Health Emergencies Programme", allowing for a trickle-down replication at the regional and country levels, might be diversely received. On the one hand, it clarifies roles and responsibilities and especially helps the headquarters level to officially gain precedence over lower levels. It also articulates a stronger command and control structure and responds to the vocal "failure in leadership" criticisms. On the other hand, it seems to ignore some HRO theoretical paths, encouraging organizations facing deep uncertainties to underspecify structure, leaving teams, units and departments to reorganize with maximum flexibility to avoid rigidity, and neglect local adaptations, which are key in epidemic management. Standardization does not help human actors in states of abnormal operation; instead, they need strong, flexible guidance.

What remains to be seen is how to inject doses of interest for resilience into the Global Health System, which has constantly been under attack, with criticisms pointing to a lack of leadership and questioning whether or not there are clear lines of command and control. Law scholar Heath urges the consideration of three principles ("managed decentralization", "epistemic openness" and "forced dissent") as being key for seriously reforming global emergency power. "Managed decentralization" echoes HRO's "migrating decision making". Management decentralization comprises two components: "(i) a preference, articulated in law or policy, for national leadership assisted by informal transnational cooperation and (ii) a focal point for debate and decision over whether to escalate to an international response" (Heath, 2016, 38). The second principle, "epistemic openness", echoes the preoccupation of HRO theorists with "system variety" and reaching out for more expertise and constituencies to be included in the process. "Such a procedure could be destabilizing in a way that shakes old habits and breaks through accepted patterns that have proved unhelpful" (Heath, 2016, 43). Finally, the principle of "forced dissent" could be paralleled with the notion of "heedful interrelations" and the encouragement of dissenting voices to prevent complacency.

The "resilient message" comes across as being at odds with the constant urge towards more structure and leadership in attempts at strengthening outbreak responses. Indeed, resiliency scholars have long argued that distributed knowledge and local expertise are crucial to capture efficiently. Hence, designing for resilience and robustness is a totally new adventure for the Global Health System. It entails starting from, learning from and relying upon the existent and not only longing for more resources, more structure, more control and more reforms.

Notes

1 These six regional offices are in: Africa, based in Brazzaville; the Eastern Mediterranean, based in Cairo; Europe, based in Copenhagen; South-East Asia, based in New Delhi; the Americas, based in Washington, DC; and the Western Pacific, based in Manila.

2 The role of university hospitals is not presented here, although they do play a notable role in the world of global health and the fight against epidemics (cf. Parfaite, Chapter 10, on the case study of the care provided to an Ebola-infected Cuban doctor evacuated from Liberia in the autumn of 2014). This does not exhaust the subject, particularly because university hospitals in Geneva, like elsewhere in Europe and in the United States, quickly took part in developing protocols for vaccine trials in the case of the Ebola virus, and they also revised care protocols for the pandemic flu, just as they did for Ebola (cf. Roemer-Mahler & Elbe, 2016; Evans et al., 2016).
3 The Global Health Security Initiative (GHSI) was launched in November 2001 by Canada, the European Commission, France, Germany, Italy, Japan, Mexico, the United Kingdom and the United States. The WHO acts as a technical advisor to the GHSI.
4 Perrow borrowing himself from Weick's theory of tight and loose coupling inside organizations (Weick, 1976).
5 For instance, the article titled "Will Ebola change the game? Ten essential reforms before the next pandemic", written by Moon and colleagues (2015), reflects the wording that one frequently encounters when reading material on reform of the WHO.
6 A similar argument is made by Mahler & Casamayou (2009).
7 The situation encountered by Fukushima-Daïchi operators and their first-line management should not be forgotten. Sometimes nothing holds, and capabilities to improvise have to be mobilized by terrified actors left in the dark, resorting to their own meager devices (Guarnieri et al., 2015; Kadota, 2014).
8 This odd expression has been used by David Nabarro, who served in 2015 as the UN Secretary-General's Special Envoy on Ebola. He was referring to the necessity that all actors, including NGOs, accept being coordinated on the ground to enhance international response.

References

Abeysinghe, S. (2015). *Pandemics, Science and Policy: H1N1 and the World Health Organisation.* Springer.
Abraham, T. (2011). The chronicle of a disease foretold: Pandemic H1N1 and the construction of a global health security threat. *Political Studies, 59*(4), 797–812.
Abramowitz, S. (2017). Epidemics (especially Ebola). *Annual Review of Anthropology, 46*, 421–445.
Ansell, C., & Keller, A. (2014). *Adapting the Incident Command Model for Knowledge-based Crises: The Case of the Centers for Disease Control and Prevention.* IBM Center for the Business of Government.
Ansell, C., Boin, A., & Keller, A. (2010). Managing transboundary crises: Identifying the building blocks of an effective response system. *Journal of Contingencies and Crisis Management, 18*(4), 195–207.
Ansell, C., Sondorp, E., & Stevens, R. H. (2012). The promise and challenge of global network governance: The Global Outbreak Alert and Response Network. *Global Governance: A Review of Multilateralism and International Organizations, 18*(3), 317–337.
Barrelet, C., Bourrier, M., Burton-Jeangros, C., & Schindler, M. (2013). Unresolved issues in risk communication research: The case of the H1N1 pandemic (2009–2011). *Influenza and Other Respiratory Viruses, 7*, 114–119.

Bieder, C., & Bourrier, M. (2013). *Trapping Safety into Rules: How Desirable or Avoidable Is Proceduralization?*. Ashgate-CRC Press.

Boin, A., & Van Eeten, M. J. (2013). The resilient organization. *Public Management Review*, 15(3), 429–445.

Boumandouki, P., Formenty, P., Epelboin, A., Campbell, P., Atsangandoko, C., Allarangar, Y., … & Salemo, A. (2005). Prise en charge des malades et des défunts lors de l'épidémie de fièvre hémorragique due au virus Ebola d'octobre à décembre 2003 au Congo. *Bulletin de la Société de Pathologie Exotique*, 98(3), 218–223.

Bourrier, M. (1999). Constructing organizational reliability: The problem of embeddedness and duality, in Misumi, J., Wilpert, B., & Miller, R. (eds), *Nuclear Safety: A Human Factors Perspective*. London, Taylor & Francis, 25–48.

Bourrier, M. (2005). The contribution of organizational design to safety. *European Management Journal*, 23(1), 98–104.

Bourrier, M. (2011). The legacy of the high reliability organization project. *Journal of Contingencies and Crisis Management*, 19(1), 9–13.

Brender, N. (2014). *Global Risk Governance in Health*. Palgrave Macmillan.

Broadbent, D. E., FitzGerald, P., & Broadbent, M. H. (1986). Implicit and explicit knowledge in the control of complex systems. *British Journal of Psychology*, 77(1), 33–50.

Brunsson, N. (1989a). Administrative reforms as routines. *Scandinavian Journal of Management*, 5(3), 219–228.

Brunsson, N. (1989b). *The Organization of Hypocrisy: Talk, Decisions and Actions in Organizations*. John Wiley & Sons.

Caduff, C. (2014). Pandemic prophecy, or how to have faith in reason. *Current Anthropology*, 55(3), 296–315.

Calain, P. (2007). Exploring the international arena of global public health surveillance. *Health Policy and Planning*, 22(1), 2–12.

Calain, P., & Sa'Da, C. A. (2015). Coincident polio and Ebola crises expose similar fault lines in the current global health regime. *Conflict and Health*, 9(29), 1–7.

Calain, P., Fiore, N., Poncin, M., & Hurst, S. A. (2009). Research ethics and international epidemic response: The case of Ebola and Marburg hemorrhagic fevers. *Public Health Ethics*, 2(1), 7–29.

Cassels, A., Kickbusch, I., Told, M., & Ghiga, I. (2017). How should the World Health Organization reform? An analysis and review of the literature, in Matlin, S., & Kickbusch, I. (eds), *Pathways to Global Health: Case Studies in Global Health Diplomacy*, volume 2. World Scientific, 39–87.

Chabrol, F. (2014). Sida: L'eldorado africain?, *La vie des idées*, December 1. www.laviedesidees.fr/Sida-l-eldorado-africain.html.

Chorev, N. (2013). Restructuring neoliberalism at the World Health Organization. *Review of International Political Economy*, 20(4), 627–666.

Clarke, L. (1999). *Mission Improbable: Using Fantasy Documents to Tame Disaster*. University of Chicago Press.

Clift, C. (2014). *What's the World Health Organization For?* London: Chatham House.

Crozier, M. (1963). *Le phénomène bureaucratique: Essai sur les tendences bureaucratiques des systèmes d'organisation modernes et sur leurs relations en France avec système social et culturel*. Éditions du Seuil.

Evans, N. G., Smith, T. C., & Majumder, M. S. (eds). (2016). *Ebola's Message: Public Health and Medicine in the Twenty-first Century*. The MIT Press.

Fairhead, J. (2016). Understanding social resistance to the Ebola response in the Forest Region of the Republic of Guinea: An anthropological perspective. *African Studies Review*, 59(3), 7–31.

Fassin, D., & Pandolfi, M. (2010). *Contemporary States of Emergency: The Politics of Military and Humanitarian Interventions.* Zone Books.

Faye, S. L. (2015). L'"exceptionnalité" d'Ebola et les "réticences" populaires en Guinée-Conakry: Réflexions à partir d'une approche d'anthropologie symétrique. *Anthropologie & santé. Revue internationale francophone d'anthropologie de la santé*, (11).

Fidler, D. P. (2003). Emerging trends in international law concerning global infectious disease control. *Emerging Infectious Diseases*, 9(3), 285–290.

Fidler, D. P. (2004). Germs, governance, and global public health in the wake of SARS. *The Journal of Clinical Investigation*, 113(6), 799–804.

Fidler, D. P. (2005). From international sanitary conventions to global health security: The new International Health Regulations. *Chinese Journal of International Law*, 4(2), 325–392.

Fidler, D. P. (2015). The Ebola outbreak and the future of global health security. *The Lancet*, 385(9980), 1888–1889.

Fidler, D. P. (2016). Global health diplomacy and the Ebola outbreak, in Halabi, S. F., Gostin, L. O., & Crowley, J. S. (eds), *Global Management of Infectious Disease after Ebola.* Oxford University Press, 133–148.

Fidler, D. P., & Gostin, L. O. (2006). The new International Health Regulations: An historic development for international law and public health. *The Journal of Law, Medicine & Ethics*, 34(1), 85–94.

Forster, P. (2012). *To Pandemic or Not: Reconfiguring Global Responses to Influenza.* STEPS Centre.

Forsythe, D. P. (2005). *The Humanitarians: The International Committee of the Red Cross.* Cambridge University Press.

Fox, R. C. (1995). Medical humanitarianism and human rights: Reflections on Doctors Without Borders and Doctors of the World. *Social Science & Medicine*, 41(12), 1607–1616.

Fribault, M. (2015). Ebola en Guinée: Violences historiques et régimes de doute. *Anthropologie & Santé. Revue internationale francophone d'anthropologie de la santé*, (11). doi:10.4000/anthropologiesante.1761.

Garrett, L. (2013). *Existential Challenges to Global Health.* Center on International Cooperation, New York University.

Gates, B. (2015). The Ebola crisis was terrible. But next time could be much worse. *New York Times*, March 18.

Gawande, A. (2010). *The Checklist Manifesto: How to Get Things Right.* Profile Books.

Gostin, L. O. (2015). Critical choices for the WHO after the Ebola epidemic. *JAMA*, 314(2), 113–114.

Gostin, L. O., & Friedman, E. (2014). Ebola: A crisis in global health leadership. *The Lancet*, 384, 1323–1325.

Graeber, D. (2015). *The Utopia of Rules: On Technology, Stupidity, and the Secret Joys of Bureaucracy.* Melville House.

Grépin, K. A. (2015). International donations to the Ebola virus outbreak: Too little, too late? *British Medical Journal*, 350, h376.

Guarnieri, F., Travadel, S., Martin, C., Portelli, A., & Afrouss, A. (2015). *L'accident de Fukushima Dai Ichi: Le récit du directeur de la centrale*, volume 1: *L'anéantissement.* Presses des Mines.

Harman, S. (2016). The Bill and Melinda Gates Foundation and legitimacy in global health governance. *Global Governance: A Review of Multilateralism and International Organizations*, 22(3), 349–368.

Heath, J. B. (2016). Global emergency power in the age of Ebola. *Harvard International Law Journal*, 57(1), 1–47.

Hein, W., & Kickbusch, I. (2010). Global health, aid effectiveness and the changing role of the WHO. *GIGA Focus* (International Edition English), no. 03, December.

Hewlett, B. S., & Hewlett, B. L. (2008). *Ebola, Culture and Politics: The Anthropology of an Emerging Disease*. Cengage Learning.

Hofman, M., & Au, S. (eds). (2017). *The Politics of Fear: Médecins Sans Frontières and the West African Ebola Epidemic*. Oxford University Press.

Hofmann, D. A., & Frese, M. (eds). (2011). *Error in Organizations*. Routledge.

Hollnagel, E. (2012). Coping with complexity: Past, present and future. *Cognition, Technology & Work*, 14(3), 199–205.

Hollnagel, E., Woods, D., & Levenson, N. (2006). *Resilience Engineering: Concepts and Precepts*. Ashgate.

Horton, R. (2014). Offline: The case against global health. *The Lancet*, 383(9930), 1705.

Horton, R. (2015). Offline: A pervasive failure to learn the lessons of Ebola, *The Lancet*, 386(9998), 1024.

Johnson, G. A., & Vindrola-Padros, C. (2017). Rapid qualitative research methods during complex health emergencies: A systematic review of the literature. *Social Science & Medicine*, 189, 63–75.

Kadota, R. (2014). *On the Brink: The Inside Story of Fukushima Daiichi*. Kurodahan Press.

Kamradt-Scott, A. (2010). The WHO Secretariat, norm entrepreneurship, and global disease outbreak control. *Journal of International Organizations Studies*, 1(1), 72–89.

Kamradt-Scott, A. (2011). The evolving WHO: Implications for global health security. *Global Public Health*, 6(8), 801–813.

Kamradt-Scott, A. (2016). WHO's to blame? The World Health Organization and the 2014 Ebola outbreak in West Africa. *Third World Quarterly*, 37(3), 401–418.

Katz, R., & Dowell, S. F. (2015). Revising the International Health Regulations: Call for a 2017 review conference. *The Lancet Global Health*, 3(7), e352–e353.

Keller, A. C., Ansell, C. K., Reingold, A. L., Bourrier, M., Hunter, M. D., Burrowes, S., & MacPhail, T. M. (2012). Improving pandemic response: A sensemaking perspective on the spring 2009 H1N1 pandemic. *Risk, Hazards & Crisis in Public Policy*, 3(2), 1–37.

Kickbusch, I., & Reddy, K. S. (2015). Global health governance: The next political revolution. *Public Health*, 129(7), 838–842.

King, N. B. (2002). Security, disease, commerce: Ideologies of postcolonial global health. *Social Studies of Science*, 32(5–6), 763–789.

La Porte, T. R., & Consolini, P. M. (1991). Working in practice but not in theory: Theoretical challenges of "high-reliability organizations". *Journal of Public Administration Research and Theory*, 1(1), 19–47.

Lachenal, G. (2014). Chronique d'un film catastrophe bien préparé. *Libération*, 19.

Laîné, M.-O. (2016). *Ailleurs en Ebola, de l'enquête ethnographique au récit de voyage*. Paris: L'Harmattan.

Lakoff, A. (2010). Two regimes of global health. *Humanity: An International Journal of Human Rights, Humanitarianism, and Development*, 1(1), 59–79.

Lakoff, A. (2017). *Unprepared: Global Health in a Time of Emergency*. University of California Press.

Lakoff, A., & Collier, S. J. (eds). (2008). *Biosecurity Interventions: Global Health and Security in Question*. Columbia University Press.

Le Coze, J. C. (2016). Vive la diversité! High Reliability Organisation (HRO) and Resilience Engineering (RE). *Safety Science*. https://doi.org/10.1016/j.ssci.2016.04.006.

Le Marcis, F. (2015). "Traiter les corps comme des fagots": Production sociale de l'indifférence en contexte Ebola (Guinée). *Anthropologie & Santé. Revue internationale francophone d'anthropologie de la santé*, (11).

Leach, M., & Hewlett, B. S. (2010). Hemorrhagic fevers: Narratives, politics and pathways, in Dry, S., & Leach, M. (eds), *Epidemics: Science, Governance and Social Justice*. Earthscan, 43–69.

Leach, M., Scoones, I., & Stirling, A. (2010). Governing epidemics in an age of complexity: Narratives, politics and pathways to sustainability. *Global Environmental Change*, 20(3), 369–377.

Lee, K. (2009). *The World Health Organization (WHO)*. Routledge.

Levich, J. (2015). The gates foundation, Ebola, and global health imperialism. *American Journal of Economics and Sociology*, 74(4), 704–742.

Littoz-Monnet, A. (2017). Expert knowledge as a strategic resource: International bureaucrats and the shaping of bioethical standards. *International Studies Quarterly*, 61(3), 584–595.

Lynteris, C. (2016). The epidemiologist as culture hero: Visualizing humanity in the age of "the next pandemic". *Visual Anthropology*, 29(1), 36–53.

Mahler, J. G., & Casamayou, M. (2009). *Organizational Learning at NASA: The Challenger and Columbia Accidents*. Georgetown University Press.

McCoy, D., Kembhavi, G., Patel, J., & Luintel, A. (2009). The Bill and Melinda Gates Foundation's grant-making programme for global health. *The Lancet*, 373(9675), 1645–1653.

Moon, S., Leigh, J., Woskie, L., Checchi, F., Dzau, V., Fallah, M., … & Katz, R. (2017). Post-Ebola reforms: Ample analysis, inadequate action. *BMJ: British Medical Journal* (Online), 356.

Moon, S., Sridhar, D., Pate, M. A., Jha, A. K., Clinton, C., Delaunay, S., … & Goosby, E. (2015). Will Ebola change the game? Ten essential reforms before the next pandemic. The report of the Harvard-LSHTM Independent Panel on the Global Response to Ebola. *The Lancet*, 386(10009), 2204–2221.

Moulin, A. M. (2015). L'anthropologie au défi de l'Ebola. *Anthropologie & Santé. Revue internationale francophone d'anthropologie de la santé*, (11).

Navarro, V. (2004). The world situation and WHO. *The Lancet*, 363(9417), 1321–1323.

Neuman, M., & Weissman, F. (eds). (2016). *Saving Lives and Staying Alive: Humanitarian Security in the Age of Risk Management*. Hurst.

Nierlé, T. (2014). Ebola: Un défi à notre identité d'humanitaire – une lettre ouverte au mouvement MSF. Letter written by nine members of MSF Swiss movement in December 2014 published February 3, 2015 in French newspaper *Libération*. www.liberation.fr/terre/2015/02/03/parfois-le-traitement-symptomatique-a-ete-neglige-voire-oublie_1194960.

Nunes, J. (2017). Doctors against borders, Médecins Sans Frontières and global health security, in Hofman, M., & Au, S. (eds), *The Politics of Fear: Médecins*

Sans Frontières and the West African Ebola Epidemic. Oxford University Press, 3–50.

Packard, R. M. (2016). *A History of Global Health: Interventions into the Lives of Other Peoples.* Johns Hopkins University Press.

Péchayre, M. (2014). Impartialité et pratiques de triage en milieu humanitaire. Le cas de Médecins Sans Frontières au Pakistan. *Les Cahiers du Centre Georges Canguilhem,* (1), 125–142.

Perin, C. (2005). *Shouldering Risks: The Culture of Control in the Nuclear Power Industry.* Princeton University Press.

Perrow, C. (1984). *Normal Accidents: Living with High-risk Technologies.* Basic Books.

Pillai, S. K., Nyenswah, T., Rouse, E., Arwady, M. A., Forrester, J. D., Hunter, J. C., ... & Poblano, L. (2014). Developing an incident management system to support Ebola response: Liberia, July–August 2014. *MMWR: Morbidity and Mortality Weekly Report,* 63(41), 930–933.

Redfield, P. (2013). *Life in Crisis: The Ethical Journey of Doctors Without Borders.* University of California Press.

Richards, P. (2016). *Ebola: How a People's Science Helped End an Epidemic.* Zed Books.

Roberts, K. (1988). Some characteristics of high reliability organizations. *Organizational Behavior and Industrial Relations.* Working Paper No. Obir-23, Berkeley Business School, University of California.

Roberts, K. (ed.) (1993). *New Challenges to Understanding Organizations.* New York: Macmillan.

Roberts, K. H., & Rousseau, D. M. (1989). Research in nearly failure-free, high-reliability organizations: Having the bubble. *IEEE Transactions on Engineering Management,* 36(2), 132–139.

Rochlin, G. I. (1993). Essential friction: Error-control in organizational behavior, in Åkerman, N. (ed.), *The Necessity of Friction.* Physica-Verlag HD, 196–232.

Rochlin, G. I. (ed.) (1996). New directions in reliable organization research. Special Issue of *The Journal of Contingencies and Crisis Management,* 4(2), 55–59.

Roemer-Mahler, A., & Elbe, S. (2016). The race for Ebola drugs: Pharmaceuticals, security and global health governance. *Third World Quarterly,* 37(3), 487–506.

Saluzzo, J.-F. (2011). *La saga des vaccins, contre les virus.* Belin.

Schulman, P. R. (1993). The negotiated order of organizational reliability. *Administration & Society,* 25(3), 353–372.

Scoones, I., & Forster, P. (2008). *The International Response to Highly Pathogenic Avian Influenza: Science, Policy, and Politics.* STEPS, Working paper 10, STEPS Center.

Scott, R. W. (1992). *Organizations: Rational, Natural, and Open Systems.* Prentice Hall.

Scott, J., & Marshall, G. (eds). (2015). *Oxford Dictionary of Sociology* [Online]. Based on Scott, J., & Marshall, G. (eds). (2009). *A Dictionary of Sociology.* Oxford University Press.

Sennett, R. (1998). *The Corrosion of Character: The Transformation of Work in Modern Capitalism.* W. W. Norton & Company.

Sridhar, D., & Gostin, L. O. (2011). Reforming the World Health Organization. *JAMA,* 305(15), 1585–1586.

Sridhar, D., Kickbusch, I., Moon, S., Dzau, V., Heymann, D., Jha, A. K., ... & Piot, P. (2016). Facing forward after Ebola: Questions for the next director general of the World Health Organization. *BMJ: British Medical Journal* (Online), 353.

Taylor, A. L. (1992). Making the World Health Organization work: A legal framework for universal access to the conditions for health. *American Journal of Law and Medicine*, 18(4), 301–346.

Thacker, S. B., Dannenberg, A. L., & Hamilton, D. H. (2001). Epidemic Intelligence Service of the Centers for Disease Control and Prevention: 50 years of training and service in applied epidemiology. *American Journal of Epidemiology*, 154(11), 985–992.

Thacker, S. B., Stroup, D. F., & Sencer, D. J. (2011). Epidemic assistance by the Centers for Disease Control and Prevention: Role of the Epidemic Intelligence Service, 1946–2005. *American Journal of Epidemiology*, 174(suppl 11), S4–S15.

UNICEF. (2015). *Community Care Centers, Communication for Development: Responding to Ebola*. Report.

UNICEF. (2016). *Ebola Community Care Centers: Lessons Learned from UNICEF 2014–2015 Experience in Sierra Leone*, Working paper. Knowledge Management and Implementation Research Unit, Health Section, Program Division.

UNMEER. (2015). *"Making a Difference": The Global Ebola Response Outlook 2015*.

Vardin, S. (2015). *Babel Epidemic: Ebola aux cent visages*. L'Harmattan.

Vaughan, D. (1997). *The Challenger Launch Decision: Risky Technology, Culture, and Deviance at NASA*. University of Chicago Press.

Wald, P. (2008). *Contagious: Cultures, Carriers, and the Outbreak Narrative*. Duke University Press.

Weick, K. E. (1976). Educational organizations as loosely coupled systems. *Administrative Science Quarterly*, 1–19.

Weick, K. E. (1987). Organizational culture as a source of high reliability. *California Management Review*, 29(2), 112–127.

Weick, K. E. (1993). The collapse of sensemaking in organizations: The Mann Gulch disaster. *Administrative Science Quarterly*, 38, 628–652.

Weick, K. E., & Roberts, K. H. (1993). Collective mind in organizations: Heedful interrelating on flight decks. *Administrative Science Quarterly*, 38, 357–381.

Weick, K. E., & Sutcliffe, W. (2005). *Managing the Unexpected: Assuring High Performance in an Age of Complexity*. John Wiley & Sons.

Weick, K. E., Sutcliffe, K. M., & Obstfeld, D. (1999). Organizing for high reliability: Processes of collective mindfulness, in Sutton, R. I. & Staw, B. M. (eds), *Research in Organizational Behavior*, vol. 21. Elsevier Science/JAI Press, 81–123.

Weisz, G., Cambrosio, A., & Cointet, J. P. (2017). Mapping global health: A network analysis of a heterogeneous publication domain, *BioSocieties*, 12(4), 520–542.

Wilkinson, A., & Leach, M. (2015). Briefing: Ebola – myths, realities, and structural violence. *African Affairs*, 114(454), 136–148.

Wynne, B. (1988). Unruly technology: Practical rules, impractical discourses and public understanding. *Social Studies of Science*, 18(1), 147–167.

Yamey, G. (2002). WHO in 2002: WHO's management: Struggling to transform a "fossilized bureaucracy". *BMJ: British Medical Journal*, 325(7373), 1170.

Youde, J. R. (2012). *Global Health Governance*. Polity.

Zylberman, P. (2013). *Tempêtes microbiennes: Essai sur la politique de sécurité sanitaire dans le monde transatlantique*. Gallimard.

Part III

Complementing views

Double standard in ethics and care

10 Scarcity in the midst of abundance

The case of the medical evacuation of the Cuban patient in Geneva, Switzerland

Aude Parfaite

Introduction

On 19 November 2014 at 10:15 p.m., the night nursing team in the intensive care unit (ICU) at Geneva University Hospitals meet in the "break room"; a deep silence reigns. A nurse manager accompanied by the head of department walks in, as usual, to announce the distribution of the patients among the nursing staff. Normally, this night shift ritual consists of leaving the register that records the nurses' names along with their patients' pathologies. But tonight, things are different. Instead, the team is given a safety briefing, reminded of the requirement for patient confidentiality, and of the heroic nature of the situation. The meeting ends with the peremptory announcement of the names of the nurses who have been randomly selected to care for the Cuban patient suffering from Ebola haemorrhagic fever, who is expected to arrive in the unit a few hours later. The scene highlights the critical nature of the event for the ICU. This patient's repatriation was the result of a series of cascading decisions,[1] which created internal tensions within a hospital that found itself at the heart of the "theatre of operations" in a major health crisis.

In addition to various studies on this global crisis (Evans, Smith & Majumder, 2016), and as a counterpoint to other chapters in this book, we aim to answer the following question: In a situation that required admitting a patient who was a potential vector of a deadly, untreatable disease that could spread in the Swiss population, what were the thinking processes that lay behind the organization and management of his care? "The work of organizing" (de Terssac, 1998) at-risk activity addresses how to plan shared resources, and how teams draw up rules to organize their actions. It highlights the tensions and trade-offs that may arise between long-term plans and reality, which requires plans to be revised. These local adaptations constitute *organizing*[2] (Weick, Sutcliffe & Obstfeld, 2008), and they leave their mark on teams. With this as a starting point, we address two aspects of safe patient care: the first concerns the contribution of the hospital to a global public health emergency; the second deals more specifically with local issues related to the reduction of available resources (bed closures, patient transfers, consolidation of human resources) that was required in order to secure and ensure comprehensive patient care in the ICU.

This chapter is based on a case study of the care of a Cuban patient in the ICU at the Geneva University Hospitals, where I work as a research assistant. My research, conducted from November 2014 to April 2015, was based on a combination of field observations and about twenty interviews with physicians (virologists, infectious disease specialists, and intensivists), specialized nurses, and safety representatives involved in the management of the patient. Two further interviews, conducted three years later, provided additional insights into how the situation was managed.

In order to deepen our understanding of the phenomena that eventually led to a chain of decisions, we attempt to decipher the organizational model of the working environment in which patient management unfolded. We will see that environmental instability led to the creation of a certain social order that trapped the actors who were the focus of regulations. The study provides an insight into how organizational deviations became the norm, and how recovery mechanisms, the adjustment variable that increases system reliability, functioned.

In this scenario, knowing where the risks lie is a fundamental question. Taking the example of an organization which relies on a system that oscillates between rules and informal regulations to address risks, this chapter attempts to demonstrate how organizational resilience[3] (Woods, 2006) can work to normalize situations that are not normal or are an exceptional situation.

Organizational resilience: the paradox of reliability

The patient was one of 165 Cuban professionals dedicated to fighting the Ebola epidemic. In order to ensure staff safety, international medical evacuations were part of a multidimensional response organized by the World Health Organization (WHO) (Rodier et al., 2007). The WHO oversaw the deployment of the Cuban healthcare teams, and was responsible for organizing their medical evacuation in the event of contamination. Thus, at the request of the WHO, and in agreement with the Swiss Federal Office of Public Health (FOPH), the patient, who had contracted the virus in Liberia, was repatriated to the Geneva University Hospitals. This was the first attempt to evacuate a foreign medical professional to a third country (i.e. he was evacuated to Switzerland rather than Cuba). The man in question was one of twenty-seven patients who were repatriated to the United States and Europe during the epidemic (Uyeki et al., 2016); he would eventually make a full recovery and leave hospital on 6 December 2014. However, not all evacuations had such a successful outcome. In September

2014, a series of organizational failures led to the contamination of two nurses at Texas Health Presbyterian Hospital, followed a few days later by the contamination of a nurse at the Carlos III Hospital in Madrid (Ibe, 2016). These secondary contaminations, which preceded the patient's evacuation to Geneva, probably played a significant role in the clinical management and protective measures that Geneva University Hospitals took to ensure the safety of their staff (Connor, 2016). More broadly, they raised questions regarding how large-scale management plans were implemented locally.

It was no coincidence that the ICU was chosen to care for the patient. Depending on the criteria used to diagnose Ebola (for example, if a person presents with symptoms in the emergency department) and the patient's stability, both the internal medicine ward and the emergency ward are able to provide care. However, the ICU has significant human resources (200 healthcare professionals) and is able to provide acute care (emergency intubation). It also has isolation rooms equipped with the safety measures needed to manage patients with viral haemorrhagic fever (supplied-air respirators, negative pressure, and laminar flow ventilation[4]). In order to understand how, and under what conditions patient care would be organized, we need to examine how the ICU constructed reliability on a day-to-day basis.

ICU organizing in nominal mode

The ICU at the Geneva University Hospitals is one of the largest units in Switzerland, with thirty-four beds and leading-edge medical care. In 2014, the unit consisted of 234 members (34 physicians, 153 nurses, 30 orderlies, and 17 administrative staff). It cared for approximately 2300 patients per year, with an average stay of 3.8 days (Annual Report of the Swiss Society of Intensive Medicine, 2014).

To ensure continuity of care, the nursing team runs three shifts over twenty-four hours (twenty-two nurses in the morning and evening, and seventeen at night). A nurse cares for up to two patients during her/his shift. With respect to clinical care, the system must be able to cope with a further six to ten patients.

The primary function of the ICU is to treat patients with life-threatening prognoses. To accomplish this, the nominal workflow consists of two main activities:[5]

1　flow management, which consists of moving patients in and out of the unit; and
2　human resource planning, which consists of organizing patient management.

The day-to-day routine is governed by a specific assignment for nurses known as "flow management",[6] which is designed to plan for incoming patients and prepare for their departure. An attending physician evaluates emergency admissions. The flow management system is used to allocate nurses[7] and orderlies, while the attending physician allocates fellows and junior doctors, or residents; the aim is to ensure, among other things, that the necessary staff and skills are available to cope with the workload.

In exceptional situations, the ICU can also be called upon to help with disaster contingency plans, such as large-scale road accidents, train derailments, or natural disasters. These contingency plans are called HOCA (HOspital CAtastrophe) or pre-HOCA plans, depending on their severity. They are triggered following an event in which there is a risk that the influx of patients may not be managed with day-to-day resources (HOCA Plan Procedure, HUG, 2017).

In this organizational model, the system must constantly adapt to disruptions in its environment, which consists of a combination of routine and unplanned activities. Regulation or adjustment modes are intended to ensure that work can continue even during disturbances. In the ICU, these adjustments take the form of, for example, stopping all non-clinical activities (tending to wounds, pain relief, logistics, etc.), in order to strengthen the patient care team. Disturbances due to absenteeism are handled by revisions to the schedule, and imply that staff who have to cover must be flexible (recall of staff on leave, non-compliance with working time directives, no breaks during working hours, hiring temporary staff, etc.). These adjustments are "standard" regulations that allow the structure to maintain its key functions, and constantly adapt to environmental contingencies. Most complex organizations are subject to these disruptions, but these are also potential sources of multiple vulnerabilities that can lead to a crisis. However, this "normalization of deviance" (Vaughan, 1996) is generally seen by the team as an acceptable way to ensure workflow.

ICU organizing in (all-too common) degraded mode

In 2014, the unit was under heavy pressure: the team's workload had increased[8] and absenteeism and turnover had reduced the number of available staff. It had proved difficult to compensate for these disturbances using the usual recovery mechanisms. Given the situation, the supervisory authority allowed work to continue in "degraded" mode, which provided mechanisms for reorganizing resources as a function of needs. Degraded mode can be defined as a compromise. A tacit agreement was reached regarding the minimum level of safety that would allow work to continue under the sub-optimal conditions to which the unit was subject. This involved establishing priorities, checking the status of essential functions, and ensuring that the minimum resources needed to operate were available. These mechanisms are intended to allow the system to continue to operate even if unexpected events occur. They are triggered when the system is faced with complex, real-life situations that the prescribed framework cannot address, notably due to a lack of resources. The process corresponds to the resilience engineering model, defined as the system's ability to anticipate, detect its own limits, and develop new organizational modalities in response to changes in activity (Hollnagel, Woods & Leveson, 2006). In November 2014, the Ebola patient's management would become a major event that blew apart an organization that was already operating in "degraded" mode. The event required the use of adjustment modes similar to those used in HOCA plans, as it required human and material resources that could not be provided by the usual means.

In this context, and in an environment marked by greater complexity than expected, how was organizing constructed?

Organizing and intergovernmental surveillance mechanisms

Epidemic management has borrowed tools from the military domain, such as scenario development, and the transition from prevention to what has been called "preparedness" for future events (Collier & Lakoff, 2008; Bastide, 2017). National plans are partly structured around the pandemic plan defined by the WHO under the International Health Regulations framework. For example, in France, each government ministry must prepare a crisis management plan that specifies key operations and the minimum number of staff needed to maintain them (given that medical personnel may themselves be sick). This situation is designated as "working in degraded mode" (Torny, 2012). However, it could be said that the ICU was already working in degraded mode, given its pre-existing lack of human resources.

From political decision to the response

In Switzerland, the epidemic management plan (FOPH, 2018) has a global dimension (WHO guidelines), a federal dimension[9] (the crisis management model is based on federal legislation on epidemics), and a national dimension (the epidemiological situation in the country). In August 2014, the WHO declared an "international public health emergency", triggering intergovernmental cooperation mechanisms. Switzerland is one of the WHO Member States involved in international health cooperation. As such, the Swiss Federal Council agreed that the country could accept patients needing medical evacuation. In this context, the FOPH, which is responsible for, among other things, fighting communicable diseases that threaten public health, had the task of coordinating the management of the Ebola crisis. At the same time, the assessment of the risk of an Ebola epidemic in Switzerland was considered highly unlikely (Internal memorandum, FOPH, 2015).

The twenty-six Swiss cantons enjoy considerable autonomy in terms of health policy – in practice, this means that they implement a local health policy. However, neither the confederation (of cantons) nor the FOPH can take the lead, which makes it difficult to focus the country's resources on certain healthcare establishments.[10] Therefore, each canton must be able to admit Ebola patients, and develop its own action plan as a function of its resources (Epidemics Act, Articles 11–12).

Preparatory measures are based on three scenarios:

- following repatriation or medical evacuation to Switzerland of a person from an at-risk area;
- following the entry into Switzerland of an asylum seeker from an affected country;
- following the entry into Switzerland of a person who has stayed in an at-risk zone.

For example, the hospitals in Geneva, Berne, Lausanne, and Zurich are equipped to receive a patient carrying the Ebola virus. A further ten healthcare institutions have the capacity to carry out investigations, i.e. to make a diagnosis and ensure patient transfers to hospitals with appropriate facilities[11] (Büro Vatter Politikforschung & -beratung, 2015).

Organizing and regulated safety

Within the context of their crisis management framework, the Geneva University Hospitals developed preparatory measures that were based on prescribed safety. This built upon procedures for the management of viral haemorrhagic fevers. In addition, a pre-epidemic crisis unit had been activated on 31 July, 2014, to handle the management of any Ebola patients. The new recommendations encompassed the various institutions and bodies whose actions needed to be coordinated[12] (Institutional Recommendations for Infection Prevention and Control for the Management of Patients Suspected to Have, or Affected by Viral Haemorrhagic Fever, HUG, 2014). They consisted of safety regulations that set out the scope for individual action, staff roles, statuses, and functions, the conditions for implementing these actions, and the organizational mode of the various stakeholders during the process of admitting the patient. They could be called "reference knowledge".

The objective was to equip professionals by setting out the possible scope of action for carrying out their work. This included, for example, drawing up procedures to standardize practices, and individual or team training with the aim of building a shared understanding of the work and the surrounding framework. These prescriptions were designed to detect certain problems and to anticipate certain situations. The regulations were governed by a strict framework that tolerated a certain degree of overload, by relying on the capacity of the structure to maintain some degree of stability (Pavard et al., 2006). During unexpected disturbances that affected the system, adjustment mechanisms relied upon the existing organizational structure and remained under the control of the actors who managed the activity (drawing up rules in ad hoc procedures, and making adjustments as a function of disturbances in the environment). A similar situation is found when, for example, schedules are modified to meet the needs of an activity, or in exceptional catastrophic situations (HOCA planning) that require a certain degree of flexibility. It is a first level of organizational reliability that relies upon the system's capacity to draw up a set of rules to address risks.

In parallel to drawing up the protocol, information sessions were held with all of the hospital's staff to inform them about the disease (symptoms, mode of contamination, the situation in West Africa). This was followed by more specialized training for different groups of staff (guidelines, procedures for putting on and taking off personal protective equipment, simulations, etc.). Training sessions that presented the donning and removing of personal protective equipment procedure were based on the buddy system,[13] which provides a cross-check: one person performs the procedure while the other reads out the different stages and checks that the actions are correctly performed. All steps are mandatory, and the procedure is similar to that used in aviation. ICU staff began their training in the summer of 2014 and the schedule intensified between September and October 2014. Each training session was attended by about fifteen members of staff, while two people carried out the procedure. This mode of knowledge transmission assumes that procedures can be learned by observing others, and can thus serve as a guide for action – also called vicarious learning (Bandura, 1965). In addition, a presentation of the main steps required to admit the patient made it possible to raise awareness among the staff in general, and avoided expensive, time-consuming training sessions. This procedure can be carried out by operators who are not highly qualified. This second level of reliability helps to reinforce safety rules, by drawing upon, for example, the standardization of complex tasks, the supervision of operators' actions, and team training (McDonald, 2006).

Together, the two levels of reliability are based on mechanisms borrowed from resilience engineering: management commitment, raising awareness, and training teams (Wreathall, 2006), and the framework they provide addressed the imperative need for staff safety. However, activity is intended to be carried out in nominal mode, i.e. it is assumed that the system has sufficient human and material resources to carry out its work. This ideal situation, which is based on standard rules and optimal resources, is rarely found in complex organizations. Therefore, we must look more closely, and expand our analysis to an environment that is more uncertain and complex than expected.

Organizing and degraded mode

Organizing emerged in the margins of this formalized activity, to the extent that organizational contingencies were taken into account in adjustment mechanisms. The ICU, which was already operating in degraded mode, was unable to implement the organizational model that was initially expected. Starting with a model based on activity in nominal mode, there was a need to rethink its use based on an activity in degraded mode. The main reorganization concerned the resources needed to manage the Ebola patient, who required three nurses per shift. This loss of resources required the closure of six of the thirty-four authorized unit beds. Moreover, the level of care had to be maintained over a twenty-four-hour period, which meant that nine nurses were unavailable for other duties. Bed closures were achieved by transferring less critical patients to other hospital wards. All non-clinical activities were cancelled to strengthen the clinical team. The heads of care units tightened planning management rules. This translated into staff drawing lots to decide who would be responsible for taking care of the Ebola patient, reminders of the requirement to respect patient confidentiality, and sanctions for unauthorized absences.

Training in the dressing and undressing procedure was intensified for three groups of staff:

- intensivists who carried out high-risk procedures (emergency intubation, resuscitation);
- nurses who had to enter the room to care for the patient; and
- supervisors of the dressing/undressing procedure, who monitored the actions carried out by staff in the patient's room.

In order to improve the reliability of the Ebola patient's care, plans were drawn up and reviewed by physicians working with nurses outside the patient's room. Strict adherence was mandatory. This was a paradigm shift in care: there was no emergency response, each action was planned before entering the room, and it was not possible to change the plan as the action was carried out.

Therefore, two types of organizations coexisted:

- An organization in the form of a structure, which relied on a framework to improve the reliability of the Ebola patient's management. This was led by the crisis unit, one of the organization's meta-structures,[14] where risk management was based on anticipating actions.
- An organization in the form of action, which relied on coping mechanisms that enabled the system to deal with unforeseen situations (Weick, 1988). This autonomous adjustment mode is based on the

operators' ability to take action to recover in highly disrupted situations.

These two types of organization constitute *organizing*, which corresponds to the processes by which collective actions are structured, what they do to be able to carry out this work, and how they adapt the work to the environment.

Organizing in a crisis?

As the Ebola patient was being cared for, in a secure, regulated context, weaknesses began to emerge in the ICU. Very quickly, the adjustment modes that were put in place proved to be unable to cope with environmental constraints (activity flows, lack of beds and nursing staff, physician rotations). They also raised questions about the idea of "distributive justice", which involves deciding who can be admitted, and who must be cared for in other units or transferred to outlying hospitals.

The increasing complexity of the unit's activities led to adjustments that required changes to the system's structure. Clinical managers had to take difficult decisions about who to transfer where. For example, bed closures required the triage of patients based on more rigid criteria. The aim was to assess the severity of the condition of patients in the unit, and decide which ones could be transferred to the hospital's other units, or to outlying hospitals. This resulted in the exclusion of the least demanding patients, and inevitably led to the situation where only the most complex cases were treated (high-dependency patients requiring acute care or specific equipment). These adjustments were made by the unit's managers in order to allow the system to continue to function. The permanent presence of these "triage" doctors was a heavy burden for themselves, and created tensions that impacted the usual, day-to-day adjustments (for example, admitting patients who did not require specific monitoring into the unit).

The complexity of the patient's management made it necessary to bring in paediatric intensive care staff with relevant training. They were seconded to support the ICU team through pre-existing agreements between the two units. To compensate for the staff shortage and increased workload, former nurses from the adult ICU were asked to return. However, most no longer held a nursing position, having moved on to managerial positions in other wards or hospital departments. As they were no longer directly involved in healthcare, they could not manage complex cases. Thus, their skills could only be applied to secondary tasks, failing to alleviate the overall workload. Furthermore, increased dressing and undressing training disrupted the shift system. The morning shift regularly extended its working hours to allow the afternoon shift staff to attend training. A delay in telling teams about the impending reorganization of the hospital was a source of concern for all caregivers; not only in the ICU, but also in the hospital's other units. For example, surgeons who were unaware of the reorganization of the ICU's resources to provide care for the Ebola patient initially expected the usual timetable to be maintained.

It could be said that the patient's arrival was an event that brought "business as usual" to an end; this one-off event blew apart an already highly fragile activity. To overcome the problem, the Cuban patient's management was considered an outside activity at the ICU and that was coordinated by the crisis unit. It relied on one actor (the safety officer, who became the operational manager), and processes that were coordinated upstream, and that made it possible to improve the reliability of the patient's management. But this activity could not be thought of as external to the usual ICU workflow, as it relied upon resources, notably nursing staff, who had a significant impact on the unit's work.

To cope with the problem, operators devised informal cooperation mechanisms that deviated from the usual operational structure, for example calling in staff from other units of the hospital that were already working in intensive care, transferring patients, requesting human resources from outlying hospitals, creating an emergency "buffer zone" with four monitored beds, gradually reopening intensive care beds.

These initiatives were self-organizing adjustment mechanisms. As the system could not continue to function, other organizational models emerged as events unfolded. They could have been at the root of a profound restructuring of how the system operated, similar to the events that surrounded the management of communications infrastructure during Hurricane Katrina (Comfort & Haase, 2006). However, such initiatives did not escape the control of the formal organization, nor resistance from other units with personnel whose cooperation was required.

Could organizational resilience be a successful bulwark for the organization?

Two organizational modes coexisted during the Cuban patient's management: on the one hand, scenarios were developed using forecasting models and, on the other, the organization had to readjust to respond to unanticipated situations. The first (the organization as a structure) is governed by rules. It is based on classical models characterized by functional stability, the search for optimal performance and maximum safety, which can be "captured" in rules that are intended to anticipate risks (Bieder & Bourrier, 2013). The second model (the organization as action) is based on organizational resilience, and is characterized by an uncertain situation, the inability to anticipate certain parameters, and the willingness of actors in the system to adapt by coping with unforeseen events (Hollnagel, Woods & Leveson, 2006).

These two modes coexist in a universe where the system continues to function, and they are an integral part of current safety models (Reason,

1997; Rasmussen & Svedung, 2000; Weick, Sutcliffe & Obstfeld, 2008) that are thought of as a combination of a formal system and "collective mind-fulness" (Weick & Sutcliffe, 2006). In other words, a system which combines rules that govern operators' actions with recovery mechanisms that ensure safe behaviour and thus reinforce the system's robustness. These two organizational modes make up a model that is used to define the situation, and forms the context for interactions. However, what seems to be important here is the multitude of interpretations that can be given to the decisions that are taken. The organizational model that is constructed as the situation unfolds represents a multidimensional reality whose understanding is ambiguous. These different interpretations are effectively black boxes, i.e. blind spots where tension and confusion can arise. The decisional and organizational system leaves room for contradictory decisions in which a part of reality remains hidden or implicit, while the remainder organizes interactions and frames actions. The question is, what happens when these situations are not shared?

We should state at the outset that the demanding requirements for the care of the Cuban patient were largely met. Procedures were put in place, resources were made available, care plans were drawn up, dressing/ undressing check-lists were prepared, cross-checks were carried out, and communication was good. Furthermore, all of the measures designed to protect personnel (in an ideal world) were taken – a situation that is rarely found in organizations. This level of safety was clearly motivated by the contamination of medical staff in other hospitals, and the presence of WHO experts who "audited" the Clinical Management department. The patient's recovery and the quality of his care became a prestigious show-case for an organization committed to fighting the epidemic. Geneva University Hospitals now has a procedure in place for the admission of patients with Ebola and, more generally, for patients with viral haemor-rhagic fever. Furthermore, the event provided an excellent research opportunity for the virology department and, finally, provided an ideal situation for training on a "real" patient. ICU staff benefitted, as the technical knowledge they acquired could be used in other care activities. However, it is far from certain that the safety requirements that were put in place when the patient was admitted could be sustained if the situation were to persist, or if there were more cases.

Paradoxically, the reliability of the patient's care degraded the organization of the already highly fragile ICU. As resources were deployed to take care of the Ebola patient, the ICU's own resources were depleted, and its organization became precarious.[15] The organization as a structure began, in some ways, to constrain or modify the practices and behaviours of its actors. At the same time, it allowed a certain level of flexibility that was expressed through the organization as action, and which was due to actors' autonomy (de Terssac, Boissières & Gaillard, 2009). The system was able to exist in the longer term because of the ability of operators to take action to recover. However, these organizational decisions were problematical for professionals, as changes to the work that was done and the conditions in which it was carried out, impacted the people who had to do it. This destabilized the system, and other alternatives could have been considered. When admitted, the patient was in a critical condition, but his situation rapidly improved. He could, for example, have been transferred to another unit when he no longer needed intensive care; similarly, staff could have been replaced when their specialist skills were no longer required. Although these alternatives may have alleviated the problems the ICU faced, they were not really explored.

Finally, in a degraded system, it should be possible for readjustment mechanisms to allow activity to continue, as actors have internalized these recovery practices. The initiatives that are implemented during this type of event rely upon a reorganization – readjustments to how actors do things and their interactions with the environment. It could therefore be said that current safety models consider that organizational resilience is constructed from the outset within the organization. It is seen as a tool of the trade, and is no longer seen as a marginal contributor to making the system work. In some way, it appears that this "acting in safety", in other words, the ability of actors to cope, becomes the expected norm. However, the analysis of the safety rules and the exploration of reliability in this health crisis raises the question of the rationale for the construction of these responses. They highlight that the same challenge can give rise to several interpretations of what safety means, and indicate which organizational decisions produce effects whose consequences are unknown. From a general point of view, the question is, how can we manage crises when organizing in nominal conditions is already based on a lack of resources that has put the system under severe strain?

Without underestimating the importance of the anticipatory measures needed to manage safety in formal frameworks, or the readjustments that support recovery in organizations, it seems to us that we must deepen our understanding of these decisions. Current risk management models are fragile. This vulnerability does not stem from an inability to develop action plans, or even to accept a certain degree of flexibility in plans to make it possible to adapt to unexpected events that occur as the action unfolds – rather it is because they are based on feedback loops that put the system under strain even when the workflow is nominal. Overload can go unnoticed, simply because it does not fall within the definition of the situation. It manifests in tensions whose effects are minimized or downplayed, and eventually became invisible, because attention is focused on an exceptional situation that is, in the end, rather unremarkable. What is at play is the combination of two activities that left little room for adjustments. The focus on the exceptional nature of the activity means that its effects are seen as having little consequence, and do not encourage organizations to review their systems. However, it also highlighted the degradation in daily activity, out of which emerged the obvious causes of scarcity in abundance.

Finally, given the unpredictable nature of hazards, does the notion of recovery, which is part of the most recent safety models – resilience engineering (Hollnagel, Woods & Leveson, 2006), organizational robustness (Boissières, 2005), and antifragility (Taleb, 2012) – condone the idea that a stable system is built in support of accepted, local weaknesses (Bourrier, 2018)?

This small "detail", found in the organization of the response at a local level, is equally valid at a global level during this health crisis: the difficulty of articulating these different levels of reality shows that the construction of reliability relies upon degrading one organization to produce safety in another. Could it be said that structures that implement organizational resilience, cloaked as collective recovery mechanisms, capture individuals who are engaged in saving safety models that have become outdated? It is possible that we have downplayed the long-term consequences of these models, given that it appears that the construction of these responses is always to the detriment of those who have to implement them.

Notes

1 Repatriations are authorized by the Swiss Federal Office of Public Health (FOPH) and the local physician who is responsible for public health.

2 *Organizing*, as defined by Weick, Sutcliffe and Obstfeld (2008) is an action. It is part of an ongoing process that lies between the formalization of rules and the redefinition of these rules in practice by group members. It therefore encompasses a set of rules that must be flexible due to changes in what happens in practice, and that are also the result of interactions and the meaning that actors give to their practices. Organizing is similar to the notion of "the work of organizing" (de Terssac, 1998), which is defined as the activity of all of the actors that contribute to organizing. The work of organizing also integrates the idea that the concepts of "work" and "organization" are relevant to both policy makers and those who carry work out ("those who organize, work" and "those who work, organize").

3 Organizational resilience is the ability of an organization to maintain or restore the essential functions of its activity despite disruptions or weaknesses. It relies on the organization's ability to adjust its behaviour in unexpected situations.

4 Laminar flow ventilation is designed to avoid environmental contamination of infectious patients with tuberculosis, severe respiratory symptoms, etc.

5 A nominal situation is defined as the normal, operational state of the system. Disturbances are possible, but they are part of the activity of complex systems.

6 This task is usually the responsibility of one of the unit's specialized nurses who is released from his/her healthcare duties to carry out administrative tasks, monitor specialized care, or train newcomers.

7 There are several levels of nursing skills in the unit: qualified, trainee, and temporary nurses.

8 The increased workload was due to several factors:

- in June 2014, an intermediate care unit was created. This four-bed unit combined the responsibilities of the ICU and the operating theatre recovery room and required redefining the ICU's work. It was staffed by two nurses and an orderly working on an hourly rotation;

- two pre-HOCA plans that involved recalling staff in order to supplement the team expected to be part of the hourly rotation in the intermediate care unit;
- unusual peaks of activity during the summer period when many nursing staff took their annual leave or time off in lieu.

9 Switzerland is structured as a federation of twenty-six cantons.
10 On 1 January, 2016, the new Epidemics Act (*Loi sur les épidémies*) came into effect. The legislation strengthens the role of the confederation in crisis management (Epidemics Act, 2012).
11 In France, for example, the response consisted of the designation of Qualified Healthcare Establishments (*Etablissements de Santé de Référence*) (Gasquet-Blanchard & Raude, 2015).
12 This concerns institutions external to the hospital: among others, the Directorate General of Health of the Canton of Geneva (DGS), the Federal Office of Public Health (FOPH), the World Health Organization (WHO), and a doctor and an ambulance service from the airport. Internally, several services and sectors are involved, such as infectious diseases, infection control, accommodation units, laboratories, the hospital's communications department, etc.
13 An operator is supervised by another who knows the procedure. The latter is responsible for ensuring that dressing and undressing is carried out safely, i.e. with no risk of contamination.
14 A meta-structure is understood here as an element of the system that supplements the existing organization, and is designed to enhance the level of safety and ensure a certain degree of stability.
15 In other words, despite the actions that were taken, the system degrades to a point where it becomes unusable. It is no longer able to carry out its missions at the expected level of performance.

References

Bandura, A. (1965). Vicarious processes: A case of no-trial learning. *Advances in Experimental Social Psychology, 2,* 1–55.
Bastide, L. (2017). Future now: "Preparedness" and scenario planning in the United States. Institut de recherches sociologique, Geneva, Working Paper, 12.
Bieder, C., & Bourrier, M. (2013). *Trapping Safety into Rules: How Desirable or Avoidable Is Proceduralization?* Ashgate.
Boissières, I. (2005). *Une approche sociologique de la robustesse organisationnelle: Le cas du travail des réparateurs sur un grand réseau de télécommunication* (Doctoral dissertation, Toulouse 2).
Bourrier, M. (2018). Safety culture and models: Regime change, in C. Gilbert, B. Journé, H. Laroche, & C. Bieder (eds), *Safety Culture and Models, Taking Stock and Moving Forward.* SpringerBriefs in Safety Management, Springer Verlag, 105–119.
Büro Vatter Politikforschung & -beratung (2015). Rapport d'évaluation des préparatifs pour Ebola dans le secteur de la santé en Suisse. Rapport final sur mandat de l'OFSP (www.buerovatter.ch/pdf/2015-Evaluation%20des%20 pr%C3%A9paratifs%20pour%20Ebola.pdf).
Collier, S. J., & Lakoff, A. (2008). Distributed preparedness: The spatial logic of domestic security in the United States. *Environment and Planning D: Society and Space, 26*(1), 7–28.

Comfort, L. K., & Haase, T. W. (2006). Communication, coherence, and collective action: The impact of Hurricane Katrina on communications infrastructure. *Public Works Management & Policy*, *10*(4), 328–343.

Connor, M. J. Jr. (2016). Clinical management of Ebola virus disease in resource-rich settings, in N. G. Evans, T. C. Smith & M. S. Majumder (eds), *Ebola's Message: Public Health and Medicine in the Twenty-first Century*. MIT Press, 31–44.

Epidemics Act (*Loi fédérale sur la lutte contre les maladies transmissibles de l'homme*). (2012). Articles 11 and 12. Repealed and replaced on 1 January 2016. Federal Assembly of the Swiss Confederation.

Evans, N. G., Smith, T. C., & Majumder, M. S. (2016). *Ebola's Message: Public Health and Medicine in the Twenty-first Century*. MIT Press.

FOPH (*Office Fédéral de la santé publique*). (2015). Einreisende aus einem EVD-Gebiet in die Schweiz, internal document, mimeo.

FOPH (*Office Fédéral de la Santé Publique*). (2018). Plan suisse de pandémie influenza. Stratégies et mesures en préparation pour le cas d'une pandémie d'influenza. Gouvernement de la Suisse (www.bag.admin.ch/bag/fr/home/service/publikationen/broschueren/publikationen-uebertragbare-krankheiten/pandemieplan-2018.html).

Gasquet-Blanchard, C., & Raude, J. (2015). L'impact du risque d'Ebola sur les représentations de soignants. L'exemple des établissements de santé de référence en France. Groupe de travail no. 34, Module interprofessionnel de santé public, EHESP.

Hollnagel, E., Woods, D. D., & Leveson, N. (2006). *Resilience Engineering: Concepts and Precepts*. Ashgate.

HUG (*Hôpitaux universitaire de Genève*) (2014). Recommandations institutionnelles de prévention et de contrôle des infections, prise en charge de patient suspect ou atteint de fièvre hémorragique virale, procedure, internal document. (https://vigigerme.hug-ge.ch/sites/vigigerme/files/documents/procedures/fhv_recommandationspreventionetcontroledesinfections.pdf).

HUG (*Hôpitaux universitaire de Genève*). (2017). HOCA/Hospital Plan Catastrophe, procedure, internal document, mimeo.

Ibe, C. (2016). Talking about Ebola: Medical journalism in an age of social media, in N. G. Evans, T. C. Smith & M. S. Majumder (eds), *Ebola's Message: Public Health and Medicine in the Twenty-first Century*. MIT Press, 129–140.

McDonald, N. (2006). Organisational resilience and industrial risk, in E. Hollnagel, D. D. Woods, & N. Leveson (eds), *Resilience Engineering: Concepts and Precepts*. Ashgate, 155–179.

Pavard, B., Dugdale, J., Saoud, N. B. B., Darcy, S., & Salembier, P. (2006). Design of robust socio-technical systems, in *Proceedings of the 2nd International Symposium on Resilience Engineering, Juan les Pins, France*, 248–257.

Rasmussen, J., & Svedung, I. (2000). *Proactive Risk Management in a Dynamic Society*. Swedish Rescue Services Agency.

Reason, J. T. (1997). *Managing the Risks of Organizational Accidents*. Ashgate.

Rodier, G., Greenspan, A. L., Hughes, J. M., & Heymann, D. L. (2007). Global public health security. *Emerging Infectious Diseases*, *13*(10), 1447–1452.

Swiss Society of Intensive Medicine. (2014). Le minimal dataset de la SGI-SSMI, Statistiques MDSI, internal document, mimeo.

Taleb, N. N. (2012). *Antifragile: Things That Gain from Disorder* (Vol. 3). Random House.

Terssac de, G. (1998). Le Travail d'Organisation comme facteur de performance. *Les cahiers du changement, 3*, 5–14.

Terssac de, G., Boissières, I., & Gaillard, I. (2009). *La sécurité en action*. Octares.

Torny, D. (2012). De la gestion des risques à la production de la sécurité. *Réseaux*, (1), 45–66.

Uyeki, T. M., Mehta, A. K., Davey Jr, R. T., Liddell, A. M., Wolf, T., Vetter, P., ... & Evans, L. (2016). Clinical management of Ebola virus disease in the United States and Europe. *New England Journal of Medicine, 374*(7), 636–646.

Vaughan, D. (1996). *The Challenger Launch Decision: Risky Technology, Culture and Deviance at NASA*. University of Chicago Press.

Weick, K. E. (1988). Enacted sensemaking in crisis situations. *Journal of Management Studies, 25*(4), 305–317.

Weick, K. E., & Sutcliffe, K. M. (2006). Mindfulness and the quality of organizational attention. *Organization Science, 17*(4), 514–524.

Weick, K. E., Sutcliffe, K. M., & Obstfeld, D. (2008). Organizing for high reliability: Processes of collective mindfulness. *Crisis Management, 3*(1), 81–123.

Woods, D. D. (2006). How to design a safety organization: Test case for resilience engineering, in E. Hollnagel, D. D. Woods, & N. Leveson (eds), *Resilience Engineering: Concepts and Precepts*. Ashgate, 315–325.

Wreathall, J. (2006). Properties of resilient organizations: An initial view, in E. Hollnagel, D. D. Woods, & N. Leveson (eds), *Resilience Engineering: Concepts and Precepts*. Ashgate, 275–285.

11 Reaching out to Ebola victims

Coercion, persuasion or an appeal for self-sacrifice?

Philippe Calain and Marc Poncin

Foreword

This chapter was conceived and written in 2014, while the West African Ebola epidemic was still uncontrolled.[1] Starting from an ethical perspective, we have examined and challenged several aspects of public health prescriptions, which were routinely imposed on individuals and communities to counter the transmission of Ebola virus in Africa. Backed by international experts and by the legitimacy of biomedical sciences, foreign medical teams conveyed a dominant public health narrative that poorly matched the views and the experience of local communities. Impacting on individual freedoms and disrupting social norms, forceful public health measures (such as quarantine, isolation, or hasty burials) were generally imposed as absolute necessities, regardless of the time or the context of the epidemic.

When violence erupted against public health teams tasked with the detection of suspect cases, medical anthropologists were deployed to help solve tensions or misconceptions. The exact role of anthropologists affiliated with foreign teams is difficult to locate between being: academic observers, advisers to public health teams, or mediators in a dialogue that inevitably entails unequal bargaining powers. Accordingly, some anthropologists have called for a symmetrical approach, whereby victims and rescuers should both become scientific objects of socio-cultural investigations, and seen as equally resourceful epistemic communities. In the same line, Richards and others have shown how local knowledge and social adjustments could already contribute to outbreak control in isolated communities, even without outside help or resources. In such contexts, social interactions count as much as cultural norms or beliefs to understand epidemic propagation. From the same point of view, local communities and international organizations mirror each other. Unlike local empirical knowledge, the authority of public health prescriptions relies on claims of scientific evidence, epidemiological inferences and expert opinions. In reality, public health measures are also the product of complex social interactions (including controversies) between epistemic communities that happen to dominate the global health landscape at a given time. This is a major theme of the book, and perhaps a point of convergence between two approaches: ethical reasoning and socio-anthropological investigations.

Introduction

It is now commonplace to say that the 2014–2015 epidemic of Ebola virus disease (EVD) in West Africa has been "unprecedented", owing to its magnitude, societal impact, regional dimension and international spread. The disarray of local health systems, the mobility of populations, the shortcomings of global health institutions and the absence of an effective regional mechanism for outbreak response are held as prominent reasons for the delayed containment of the epidemic in Guinea, Sierra Leone and Liberia. In such exceptional circumstances, conventional public health activities to control Ebola outbreaks have magnified unresolved ethical issues and exposed the complexity of tensions between individual autonomy and the common good. Front-line responders striving to implement urgent public health measures have been working in an unusually difficult context, marked by the temporary suspension of civil liberties, controversial quarantine measures, weak human rights protection, questionable public health strategies and blurred responsibilities. These conditions have made encounters between relief workers and Ebola victims ethically problematic and prone to generating moral distress (Ulrich, 2014). This chapter will examine how patients' autonomy has been sacrificed to the public health necessities imposed by the 2014–2015 Ebola epidemic. With a focus on forcible isolation, we will develop three problematic dimensions of epidemic control activities. First, we will argue that socio-political accounts of the frequent resistance of populations to public health actions have left aside ethical perspectives in general and the question of autonomy in particular. Second, we will examine how coercive measures taken during the West African epidemic have failed to meet human rights or ethical standards and how non-governmental actors have reacted to these measures. Third, we will compare the respective strengths of practical and moral reasons that might justify facility isolation with those generally put forward against quarantine. Finally, we will offer recommendations to clarify and ease the position of non-state actors towards coercive measures used in times of major epidemics.

Filovirus outbreaks: explanatory models of resistance and violence

The public health response to outbreaks of the Ebola and Marburg viruses (members of the *Filoviridae* family, henceforth called "filovirus") has essentially remained the same since the first verified occurrence of EVD in 1976. For biomedical experts, a number of public health measures are essential and generally seen as uncontroversial: centralized case-isolation (i.e. the management of confirmed cases in designated healthcare facilities with maximal biosafety procedures), case finding (through active surveillance, follow-up of rumors and contact tracing), safe burial rites, social mobilization, health promotion and the reinforcement of standard precautions. Other measures remain disputed, for example individual or mass quarantine, border closures or social distancing. Regardless of the scientific authority of public health prescriptions, collective reactions of fear, disbelief, rumor or hostility have historically been encountered by many relief and scientific teams in their approaches to communities affected by filovirus outbreaks. This was already the case in 1995 when Ebola spread to Kikwit (currently Democratic Republic of the Congo) (Garrett, 2001). In 2001–2002 during an outbreak of EVD in a remote location straddling the border between Gabon and Congo, the reluctance of villagers to collaborate with outbreak-investigation teams created security conditions that forced international members to evacuate the area twice (WHO, 2003). In 2003, health workers received death threats and suffered acts of violence when Ebola broke out again in the same rural setting of Congo (Formenty et al., 2003). Prior to the arrival of researchers, four teachers accused of spreading the disease were assassinated in the town of Kélé. Rural areas are not the only cases. Urban settings have also been the theater of hostility and violence, notably during filovirus outbreaks in Gulu (Uganda) in 2000–2001 (Hewlett & Hewlett, 2005) and in Uige (Angola) in 2005 (Roddy et al., 2007).

Unsurprisingly West Africa has experienced the same sort of reactions, whereby national and international teams tasked with public health activities have been facing recurrent and widespread hostility from many affected communities. There are frequent reports of patients in hiding or refusing to present to treatment facilities. In Sierra Leone, during the most recent period of enforced lockdown, systematic home searches found that about one third of all patients had previously not been identified by contact tracing (Sahid, 2015). In Guinea, the frequency of incidents has been monitored by Guinean authorities since November 2014 (Reliefweb, 2015) by recording the weekly number of sub-prefectures reporting *réticences*. *Réticences* (as opposed to the more politically charged "resistance") is a neutral qualifier that encompasses all instances of opposition to either contact tracing, transfer to isolation, safe burials or other public health interventions (ACAPS, 2015a). Examples given in national weekly reports include the refusal to be put in isolation, verbal violence, vandalism, death threats, the stoning of cars or physical aggression towards outreach teams. In Guinea, the geographical spread of *réticences* culminated in January 2015, with thirty-two of the 341 sub-prefectures or urban communes reporting incidents. As of April 2015 a few areas close to the capital city of Conakry remained hostile to outreach teams. Local measures taken by the Guinean authorities have generally focused on mass communication and interventions by peers, religious leaders or traditional authorities. In January 2015, the president of Guinea authorized the use of force against those opposed to Ebola control measures (Diallo, 2015). The open epidemiological category of *réticences* is misleading, as it conflates two morally distinct actions, i.e. the legitimate reluctance of individuals to comply with extreme public health measures and genuine acts of violence. On top of minor daily incidents, a number of extremely violent events have affected and delayed the work of relief organizations. On April 4, 2014 in Guinea, less than three weeks after the confirmation of the outbreak, mobs in the town of Macenta threatened Médecins Sans Frontières (MSF) teams, forcing the suspension of all Ebola control activities for one week. In September 2014 in Womey (Forest Region, Guinea) eight members of a high-ranking delegation were murdered, including three health officials. The same month, Red Cross teams collecting dead bodies were attacked in the mining town of Forecariah. In Sierra Leone, similar incidents occurred in Koidu in October 2014, leaving two dead and residents under curfew (Ruble, 2014). The incident followed an attempt by health officials to take an elderly woman to an Ebola treatment center against the will of family members. In Liberia, the township of West Point in Monrovia was the theater of major incidents in August 2014 after mobs looted an Ebola clinic. Soon after, clashes with security forces followed quarantine and curfew orders, leaving many wounded and one dead from gunshot wounds.

The political dimension of civil unrest that accompanies major Ebola outbreaks is omnipresent and complex. In West Africa, opposition to public health authorities has been interpreted as an expression of the social divisions left successively by the colonization, civil wars, and post-conflict development policies. In Guinea for example, the frequent resistance to Ebola-response activities reflects both historical and contemporary factors, themselves influenced by national and international circumstances. In the Forest Region, where the Ebola epidemic started, long-lasting secular conflicts still divide communities and generate mistrust against national authorities (Anoko, 2015). In addition, memories of coercive public health measures during the colonial era, mixed with resentment about past international clinical trials entertain rumors of an intentional origin of the disease (ACAPS, 2015b). Putting the epidemic in a broader international context, Wilkinson and Leach (2015) see local resistances to epidemic response as a consequence of the structural violence and inequalities that prevail in post-colonial Africa, exacerbated by the inevitable presence of foreign or international agencies working in support of national authorities. Examining international biomedical perspectives, Leach and Hewlett (2010) have shown how a "global outbreak" narrative pervades health policies and their interpretation of epidemic events. This narrative privileges scientific authority over local knowledge and calls for external remediation, ignoring how popular knowledge can integrate with biomedical science. In a narrow interpretation, the global outbreak narrative shifts the blame to victims, variably accused of medical superstitions, unsafe burials, consumption of infectious wild game, or the shunning of Ebola treatment centers.

Aside from political contexts, medical anthropology provides another explanatory framework. With their pioneering field work in Uganda (Hewlett & Hewlett, 2008), Congo (Formenty et al., 2003; Hewlett et al., 2005) and Gabon (Hewlett & Hewlett, 2008), anthropologists have documented how hostile reactions to public health measures reflect a divide between biomedical representations of EVD and other cultural models prevailing in African societies. For example, traditional and biomedical communities would typically diverge in their interpretations of disease, contagion and healing, in the way they conduct protective rituals, in their handling of the deceased during burial rites, or in their understanding of risk groups and sources of the disease. Anthropological approaches are essential to guide the response to filovirus epidemics through community engagement (Epelboin, 2015; Marais et al., 2015), mediation (Anoko, 2015) and flexibility in the application of biomedical models (Chandler et al., 2015). At the same time, anthropological perspectives are incomplete and run the risk of patronizing interpretations if cultural aspects of resistances are taken at face value. Cultural explanations alone discount the capacity for autonomous decision making, expected from anyone exposed to the consequences of contagion and regardless of national or cultural affiliations. In other words, reactions of disbelief or opposition to public health measures are rational and universal and would likely be felt by many of us facing the prospect of quarantine, isolation, social ostracism, suffering and possible death. Practically, communities are keen to incorporate traditional and biomedical models in a form of medical pluralism compatible with epidemic control protocols (Hewlett & Amola, 2003). Recent work establishes how rural or urban communities can naturally adjust public health necessities to their material and social constraints. For example, Richards et al. (2015) describe the rural settlement of Fogbo in Sierra Leone, and the complexity of social factors of transmission of EVD in a community sustaining itself through family help, kinship, migration and local markets. In Liberia, Abramowitz et al. (2015) analyze how urban communities managed to organize themselves to contain the outbreak, when left on their own without outside assistance. Thus, local knowledge can bring about efficient survival strategies, particularly when the state and international response are failing. When liberty-restricting measures are imposed in this context, they are bound to exacerbate pre-existing tensions, whereas trustworthiness and reciprocity should be put forward instead. Trust in local institutions (Richards et al., 2015) and hospitals (Brown & Kelly, 2014) are important for communities to seek help for EVD. Focus-group discussions conducted in Monrovia in November 2014 (Kutalek et al., 2015) revealed additional concerns. Local participants rejected an incentive scheme intended to increase the reporting of suspected cases and pointed out specific problems compromising the credibility of public health actions, e.g. food shortages for families in quarantine, communication between patients and their families, basic health services, psychosocial support for affected families and the inclusion of Ebola survivors in the teams of active case-finders and contact-tracers.

Quarantine and restrictions of freedom

Around July–August 2014, four countries (Guinea, Liberia, Nigeria and Sierra Leone) in an attempt to contain the Ebola epidemic issued emergency presidential declarations and a comprehensive list of compulsory measures. The range of legal prescriptions varied from country to country, drawing from the following categories of measures: closures of public places, compulsory leave, *cordon sanitaire*, curfews, sanitation, isolation, price control, quarantine, screening, surveillance, testing, travel restrictions and treatment (Hodge et al., 2014). Mali and Senegal – other African countries that faced the threat of Ebola propagation – also resorted to active surveillance, quarantine and isolation.

At the very least, coercive public health measures need to be based on compelling scientific evidence and framed in clear and consistent legal and ethical principles (Rothstein, 2015a). The following analysis shows that this does not seem to have been the case during Ebola epidemics, particularly in West Africa. Quarantine has so far been the most disputed issue among other public health measures prescribed and enforced by public authorities. In contrast, isolation has usually been granted as an absolute necessity in the face of acute epidemics of highly lethal communicable diseases, and it has therefore been seen as ethically unproblematic. For example, commenting on the SARS epidemic, Wynia (2007) claimed that the isolation of sick patients "tends not to provoke much concern", compared to the quarantine of healthy people. To the contrary, we contend that the isolation of EVD patients raises different but not less concerning questions than other liberty-restricting measures.

Human rights law

The remit of liberty-restricting measures in response to public health emergencies can be analyzed from at least three different angles, i.e. national laws, the human rights doctrine (embodied in international human rights law) and ethics. The enforcement of laws and treaties, including international human rights law (IHRL), is the responsibility of states. As an element of IHRL, the UN Siracusa Principles (United Nations, 1985) spell out criteria for suspending civil and political rights in case of public emergencies. These include threats to public health, as specified in Article 25:

> Public health may be invoked as a ground for limiting certain rights in order to allow a state to take measures dealing with a serious threat to

the health of the population or individual members of the population. These measures must be specifically aimed at preventing disease or injury or providing care for the sick and injured.

According to the Siracusa Principles, restrictions to civil liberties should meet the criteria of being (1) provided for and carried out in accordance with the law, (2) in the interests of a legitimate objective of general good, (3) strictly necessary in a democratic society to achieve the objective, (4) the least intrusive and restrictive means available to reach the same objective, (5) based on scientific evidence and (6) not imposed arbitrarily or in a discriminatory manner (WHO, 2007). Furthermore, exceptional measures should be of limited duration and subject to review and appeal (Rothstein et al., 2003). In this context it is important to specify the roles and responsibilities of international and non-governmental organizations. Non-governmental agencies that simultaneously provide the expertise, materials and extra human capacity needed to contain an epidemic are inevitably at risk of misperceptions about their role in the implementation of restrictive measures. This could ostensibly be the case, for example, when protection by the police is sought to reach victims or when security forces themselves need training in or protection from biohazards. Regardless of the relevance of coercive measures imposed by national states of emergency, non-governmental medical agencies have no role or legitimacy in enforcing public health measures. They are bound to respect national laws, but they cannot possibly be held accountable for the enforcement of public health law. Neither international humanitarian law nor common ethical principles would justify such powers. In addition, the fact that none of the emergency public health laws have been declared by way of proclamation (Karimova, 2015) by West African countries could invalidate the derogations to the International Covenant on Civil and Political Rights that they represent.

Ethical pragmatism

While lacking the force of law, public health ethics recognize the necessity that some collective actions should outweigh individual autonomy. Ethicists (Presidential Commission for the Study of Bioethical Issues, 2015; Rothstein, 2015b) have reached very similar conclusions to the Siracusa Principles, by enunciating ethical principles governing quarantine and other restrictive measures during public health emergencies. These ethical principles can be summarized as public necessity, demonstrated effectiveness and scientific rationale, proportionality and least infringement, reciprocity, justice and fairness. The same or similar principles derive from several public health ethics frameworks, indicating on what conditions the common good could outweigh individual autonomy in case of public health necessity (reviewed in Bensimon & Upshur, 2007). As recent epidemic crises have shown (HIV/AIDS, multidrug-resistant tuberculosis, SARS and pandemic influenza), coercive measures are highly contextual and always controversial. The Ebola crisis has precisely exposed the limits of established ethics frameworks, in their contextual and pragmatic applications. Ethical principles have remained at best distant declarations of intent, and ethics debates have largely been sidestepped in programmatic decisions. Reflecting on quarantine and isolation from different perspectives, the following considerations lead to the very concrete point of ethical tension, where the persuasions of public health meet individual autonomy.

Compelling evidence?

With their rapid developments, influenza pandemics (MacPhail, 2014) and the SARS epidemic of 2003 are cases in point for contemporary debates about quarantine. In the case of SARS, the effectiveness of quarantine – compared to isolation alone – is still debated (Day et al., 2006; Barbisch et al., 2015), and the strength of available scientific evidence depends on variable methodological or statistical assumptions (Bondy et al., 2009). Ethicists (Bensimon & Upshur, 2007) have emphasized the contingent nature of scientific evidence and the inherent risk of deriving hasty or definitive decisions about quarantine from limited scientific information. Semantic precision is also important. At first glance, definitions are clear (Presidential Commission for the Study of Bioethical Issues, 2015). Quarantine is the "separation of persons exposed to but not exhibiting symptoms of a communicable disease". Isolation is the "separation of those infected with or exhibiting symptoms of a communicable disease". Still, we are left to define (1) what "separation" means practically, (2) what kind of symptoms count and (3) what type of exposure counts. Furthermore, separation can be forcible or voluntary and entail varying degrees of social distancing. Persons infected with SARS or influenza shed viruses before becoming symptomatic. This is unlike the case of EVD, where persons infected with current filovirus strains are not contagious until they display symptoms of the illness (Racaniello, 2014). The difference is important for both practical and moral reasons. The quarantine of asymptomatic SARS and influenza contacts could plausibly limit the odds of silent transmission in a community. In the sense of being non-discriminatory, it is a genuine public health measure. The quarantine of asymptomatic Ebola contacts does not fulfill the same epidemiological rationale. Instead of primarily limiting viral spread, Ebola quarantine is a measure to control the movement of people deemed untrustworthy for reporting their symptoms. It is therefore more open to discrimination and arbitrary enforcement.

It is simply plausible that the voluntary or compulsory quarantine of household contacts may play a role in the rapid containment of filovirus outbreaks detected at their very early stage. In Nigeria (Grigg et al., 2015) and Mali (Diallo & Felix, 2014), index cases could be identified rapidly in urban settings, and quarantine measures were applied to all traceable contacts. In Nigeria group quarantine was also imposed upon a minority of contacts posing particular risks of further transmission due to their occupations or home environments. As for mass quarantine (*cordon sanitaire*), it was probably ineffective in Kikwit in 1995 (Heymann, 2014), although this claim has also been questioned (Garrett, 2014).

Quarantine in the United States and elsewhere

For persons exposed to Ebola, the 2014 interim US guidance (Centers for Disease Control and Prevention, 2014) provided some clarity by distinguishing between "active and direct monitoring", "controlled movement", "exclusion from public places" and "exclusion from the workplace". The same document gives clear definitions of risk categories, clinical criteria and derived public health actions. It addresses the case of individual persons exposed to Ebola but remains silent about collective or mass actions.

Forcible quarantine measures implemented in West African countries are qualitatively different from public health actions considered in the US public health guidance. They fall in a normative vacuum of international guidance and certainly lack compelling scientific evidence. Significantly, in West Africa the forcible quarantine of entire Ebola-exposed families or communities has dramatic consequences. Their stigmatization is one aspect. Furthermore, the temporary loss of livelihoods and basic commodities makes quarantine practically unsustainable for poor families already taxed by the loss of relatives (Kutalek et al., 2015; ACAPS, 2015a). The distribution of food supplies to quarantined households has remained a marginal solution (ACAPS, 2015a). Anecdotal evidence (Bianchi, 2015) indicates that some patients admitted to isolation wards conceal their exact address as a way to protect their families from the dire consequences of quarantine.

Issued at the end of July 2014, the West African emergency declarations did not cause much international outcry. It is troubling that forcible quarantine and isolation started to elicit reactions in Western countries only late in October 2014, when expatriate workers returning to the United States became themselves subject to liberty-restricting measures imposed by their own state jurisdictions. In the United States, the much publicized case of Ms. Kaci Hickox, an MSF volunteer returning from Sierra Leone, unfolded successively as episodes of forcible isolation, home quarantine and controlled displacements (Miles, 2015). The controversy had multiple dimensions, i.e. human rights issues, the relevance of imposed restrictions from a public health perspective, doubts about the existence of symptoms, inconsistencies between US federal, state or military prescriptions and the relative discomfort of being detained in makeshift conditions of isolation. As a trained MSF Ebola nurse, Ms. Hickox denied any unprotected exposure to the virus and objected to any restriction of movement which put her at odds with state authorities. In support to her views, scholars (Drazen et al., 2014; Koenig, 2015) and others (MSF, 2014) have put forward a number of arguments against the forcible quarantine of healthy volunteers returning from epidemic-hit countries, e.g. the fragmentation of public health agencies, the inconsistencies of public health laws between states, practical obstacles to the implementation of coercive measures, solidarity with and respect of aid workers, evidence that active monitoring and voluntary distancing are sufficient public health measures and deterring the enrolment of other volunteer workers because of unnecessarily restrictive measures.

Thus legal, ethical and pragmatic reasons for rejecting EVD quarantine are partly different for West Africa and industrialized countries. Regardless, it would be inconsistent for international organizations to oppose quarantine orders in the United States while at the same time remaining silent on forcible quarantine in West Africa. Except perhaps for the early stages of Ebola epidemics, it appears that collective and forcible quarantine actions have failed on the grounds of public necessity, demonstrated effectiveness and scientific rationale. Concerning proportionality, least infringement, reciprocity, due process and the ability to lodge legal appeals, quarantine for EVD does not meet ethical and human rights standards either in a context of national disaster and weak institutions.

Facility isolation: an onerous public health measure

So far we have examined the shortcomings of the compulsory quarantine of EVD-patient contacts. Likewise, it is legitimate to next ask how the isolation of symptomatic patients meets the conditions imposed by international human rights law and ethics, including compelling scientific evidence. Two related questions await empirical research with survivors or the families of victims. To what extent does facility isolation reflect free choice, persuasion or some sort of coercion imposed by emergency circumstances or by the absence of any alternative option? What proportion of individuals would be ready to sacrifice themselves for the sake of the common good by entering isolation units for the sole reason of protecting their households and communities from contagion? These two questions can be approached together by preliminary considerations about the current rationale for isolation and its consequences.

The meaning of isolation

There is historical and theoretical evidence that the isolation of cases is one of the most essential measures to contain EVD (Pandey et al., 2014), together with safe burial practices and contact tracing. Yet the consequences of isolation are often shrouded by emergency considerations. Even more than with quarantine, individuals subjected to facility isolation experience extraordinary limitations to their autonomy, particularly in the circumstances of mass catastrophes. Their distress is aggravated by a sudden and sometimes definitive separation from relatives or by the frequent destruction of their few belongings for disinfection. Once in isolation, patients are allegedly free to leave, although the "escape" of patients has occasionally created difficult situations, to which relief teams have felt obliged to react forcefully (Fink, 2015). More recently in Sierra Leone, "escapees" have been publicly named and shamed by national authorities (Mac Johnson & Larson, 2015). In typical Ebola management facilities (also called Ebola treatment centers or units) isolation has at least four dimensions: physical, cognitive, affective and spiritual. To avoid any risk of physical contact with patients' bodies or fluids, mainstream standards of protective equipment call for full body coverage for attending professionals. As a consequence, cultural or linguistic barriers are compounded by additional obstacles to verbal and facial communication and by the rapid rotation of care takers exposed to hyperthermia (Sprecher et al., 2015). With these conditions, patients are inevitably left in a degree of cognitive isolation by being limited in their capacity to know about their condition, their prognosis and the state of their families. As the epidemic became more manageable in West Africa, MSF and other organizations introduced architectural adjustments to facilitate contact between patients in isolation and relatives, survivors or even religious leaders. Unfortunately, cognitive, affective and spiritual isolation remain difficult to alleviate for the most incapacitated cases, particularly when they are close to death. A most distressing situation experienced by health personnel has been the isolation of children, many of whom have been orphaned by their parents' death from EVD (Zellmann, 2015; Maron, 2015). Contrary to earlier practices, current isolation protocols fail to account for different degrees of exposure in isolation zones, making the presence of relatives at the bedside generally impossible.

Isolation paradigms

The model of isolation in centralized facilities equipped with maximal biosecurity has become a norm for pragmatic and staffing reasons. From a pure public health perspective, there is no doubt that facility isolation in "treatment beds" had a major impact on the reduction of disease transmission in West Africa (Kucharski et al., 2015a). This is not to say that it has always been an absolute necessity, in particular where the social cost could have outweighed direct public health gains. Based on the epidemic parameters of 2014, projections (Merler, 2015) suggest that epidemic control could be achieved, together with other critical measures, when 70 percent of the cases become isolated either in Ebola treatment units, at home or in community settings. Smaller community care centers (CCCs) would increase the acceptance of isolation. In theory, in terms of epidemic control CCCs could be as effective as Ebola treatment units (Witty et al., 2014; Washington & Meltzer, 2015), but they require equally strict infection-control procedures (Kucharski et al., 2015b).

Home-based isolation was used in previous filovirus epidemics to offer alternative options to those unwilling to be hospitalized (Kerstiëns & Matthys, 1999; Formenty et al., 2003; Roddy et al., 2007). For example, MSF has guidelines for "home-based support and risk reduction", a procedure where a single caregiver is allowed to provide minimal care after receiving training, protective equipment and sanitary supplies (Sterk, 2008). A review of epidemiological observations in past filovirus outbreaks indicates that family attendants sharing a room with patients are at much lower risk of contamination if they are not involved in direct nursing care (Shears & O'Dempsey, 2015). One can thus assume that minimal care (e.g. handling food and drink) can safely be offered at home under reduced protective clothing and after appropriate training of designated attendants. Thus, depending on the circumstances or phases of an EVD outbreak, facility isolation does not necessarily represent the only option or is the least intrusive and restrictive means available. While we are still unsure about how much risk reduction other models might afford, the pragmatic limits of centralized facility isolation were reached in the summer of 2014 during the peak of urban transmission of Ebola in Monrovia. When response teams became overwhelmed, clear criteria for prioritizing access to facility admissions were inexistent, and urban communities were ready to become self-reliant in managing essential outbreak-control activities (Abramowitz et al., 2015).

For EVD patients, facility isolation thus represents the most onerous among currently prescribed public health measures. It is therefore not surprising that the prospect of forcible isolation has contributed to fears and hostility from many Ebola victims towards outreach teams.

Reaching out to Ebola patients: an ethical quagmire

Implicit and explicit reasons for isolation

Obviously from a medical perspective, the fact that case-isolation is imposed by law does not imply that the patients' autonomy should be disregarded. Unless outreach teams represent public health or law enforcement authorities, the use of overt coercion would be illegal and in any case ethically problematic for health professionals. This is even more so for foreign humanitarian workers, who have neither the legal authority nor an international mandate to enforce public health measures. It is also doubtful whether patients would have the possibility of legal recourse to oppose isolation orders in the event of a major Ebola epidemic outbreak in Western Africa. Leaving aside the legality and relevance of coercive measures, let us now assume for a moment that isolation is largely voluntary with patients either presenting spontaneously at the gates of treatment units or being willingly transferred from home after being notified they were a suspected case. To respect patients' dignity, their choices need to be informed by genuine reasons for isolation. These reasons are not always made explicit, consistent or clear by the health community.

As discussed earlier, a first and prominent reason to follow measures of isolation is to *limit contagion* and offer the material possibilities of being cared for at a safe distance from unprotected relatives. While the argument is compelling from a public health perspective, patients are ultimately asked to sacrifice themselves for the common good or the safety of their families.

A less altruistic but a more convincing reason to enter isolation would be to *receive better care* and to improve one's chances of survival. This argument has been increasingly emphasized in health-promotion messages. In reality there is little evidence in claiming that the current clinical management in dedicated isolation units consistently and significantly guarantees better chances of survival in Africa. Intensive care guided by basic monitoring of biological parameters certainly makes a difference in terms of survival (Lyon et al., 2014), but local capacities for such care are still inconsistent and sparse. However deplorable, this reality should be disclosed without ambiguity to all persons advised to seek care in isolation facilities. One could argue that the combined conditions of emergency and unrest would justify some degree of deception to achieve overarching public health goals and public safety. Such a position would be in any case ethically problematic – and even more questionable in the future – with the increasing availability of experimental interventions. The latter will introduce the added dimension of consent to research in this difficult context and make the obligation of veracity towards patients and communities the more pressing. Telling the truth about limited treatment capacities does not mean relinquishing hope. In this regard, the role of survivors as witnesses and trusted sources of information about the reality of isolation (USAID, 2015) is fundamental.

Aside from better clinical care and reduced transmission, there are still other reasons for patients to opt for facility isolation, for example the *pressure applied by an unsupportive or hostile community*. Infrequently, the *mental capacity* of patients could be affected by the disease. This would be an exceptionally difficult situation, if it put attendants and medical personnel at increased risk. It would, however, be inappropriate to assume that most Ebola patients suffer from impaired cognition, even at an advanced stage of the disease. Instead, they should primarily be seen as autonomous persons, capable of choice, but placed in a position of vulnerability by the severity of the disease, the circumstances and, sometimes, by the intimidating deployment of protective paraphernalia.

Ethics principles translated in action

We now come back to the critical and ethically problematic encounter, which is central to this chapter. Contact-tracers and case-finders have testified on how they often found themselves facing moral dilemmas, when public health actions to limit contagion conflicted with their obligation to respect patients' autonomy and dignity. What remained available to them was the force of persuasion and appeals to self-sacrifice, making it difficult to find the appropriate balance between persuasion and subtle coercion, or between veracity and deception. From what precedes, and combining ethical principles with pragmatic observations, we propose six practical recommendations for medical outreach teams to avoid the pitfalls of coercion when approaching suspected EVD cases (Box 12.1). These recommendations all express moral deference for individual autonomy and dignity, while specific recommendations translate obligations of trustworthiness, reciprocity and proportionality. These moral obligations seem to us the most essential ones, as they connect with the expectations of affected communities. They are likely to reinforce trust and ease tensions, and they would probably contribute to reducing community transmission by overcoming hostility, miscommunication and the hiding of victims (Melzer et al., 2014). While veracity and clarity of roles are unconditional, other actions are progressively achievable, depending on the context. For example, the acute phase of the disaster response might initially justify inflexible procedures with little space for such considerations as the provision of basic health services or the follow-up of some Ebola patients at home. Offering all possible choices, including alternatives to facility isolation might represent a trade-off between infection control and autonomy.

Box 12.1 Practical ethical guidance to outreach teams

Trustworthiness

- Veracity: openness about the exact reasons – with their burdens and benefits – for isolation
- Clarity of roles: separation from law enforcement authorities
- The inclusion of Ebola survivors in outreach teams

Reciprocity

- Material and psychological support for families
- The provision of basic health services

Proportionality and least infringement

- The offering of genuine choices: possible alternatives to facility isolation, including home-based care

We believe that this trade-off is ethically sound, and practically manageable through sensible processes of community involvement. In any case, the conduct of therapeutic trials in treatment centers cannot be ethically defensible as long as patients have not freely consented to facility isolation.

Conclusions

During the West African Ebola epidemic, the practical limits of upholding human rights and ethical principles have been put to the test for medical teams tasked with the application of public health measures. Perhaps more than others, members of outreach teams have faced practical and moral issues when tasked with identifying cases in communities and transporting them to centralized isolation facilities. This is not only due to the constant threat of contamination but also to the concurrent circumstances imposed by (1) states of emergency accompanied by forcible public health prescriptions and (2) the frequently encountered hostility of affected communities.

In this chapter we have discussed how both quarantine and isolation enforced in West Africa after declarations of states of emergency became equally problematic in the light of human rights and ethical perspectives. They deserve the same public scrutiny as the isolated cases of coercion seen in industrialized countries with home-coming humanitarian professionals. Forceful quarantine has probably contributed little to curbing the epidemic. On the other hand, facility isolation has been imposed by a clearer public health rationale but also at some moral cost and in the absence of consistent ethical guidance. We are unsure if facility isolation was an absolute and constant necessity in the course of the epidemic. The prospect of being kept in isolation may at times have created deterrence in communities and contributed to the perpetuation of the epidemic. We would thus propose a series of pragmatic recommendations aimed at easing tensions between relief workers and communities while respecting the autonomy of the victims of epidemic disasters. We recognize that some of these recommendations are progressively achievable, depending on the specific stage or setting of an outbreak. At the same time, as circumstances evolve, respect for patients' choices should prevail. With the prospect of new therapeutic or preventive interventions, new designs of containment techniques or parallel actions to support health systems, the response to filovirus outbreaks might be different in the future. Still, complex ethical challenges will inevitably be encountered when the context imposes the co-existence of disputed public health actions, coercive laws and the carrying out of research. Disastrous circumstances can happen with any public health event of national or international concern. Our recommendations are therefore generic, beyond the specific case of filovirus epidemics.

According to a dominant worldview, the West African situation is a regional exception explained by political and socio-cultural circumstances, dysfunctional health systems and weak public institutions. We to the contrary see it more as an exemplary and universal case, anticipating what would happen when epidemic disasters impose measures that are unpopular and onerous to civil liberties and communal values. Taken alone, political or socio-cultural explanations tend to play down the autonomy of affected individuals and reduce their lack of compliance with public health measures to an African singularity. An ethics analysis opens broader perspectives, recognizing the importance of autonomy and the failure of authoritarian approaches to outbreak control.

Acknowledgments

The authors thank the following colleagues for thoughtful reviews of an earlier draft of this manuscript: Caroline Abu Sa'Da, Sergio Bianchi, Iza Ciglenecki, Fernanda Falero, Satoru Ida, Anja Wolz. We are also grateful to Mireille Lador for systematic searches of press archives, and to Timothy Fox for proofreading this version.

Note

1 This chapter was first published under the same title in *Social Science & Medicine* (2015, Vol. 17, pp. 126–133). Copyright Elsevier. Reprinted with permission. www.sciencedirect.com/science/article/pii/S0277953615302021.

A second edition appeared as Chapter 6 in *Ethical Challenges for Military Health Care Personnel: Dealing with Epidemics*, edited by Daniel Messelken, University of Zurich, Switzerland and David Winkler, International Committee of Military Medicine, Switzerland. Routledge, Abingdon, UK, 2018. www.routledge.com/ Ethical-Challenges-for-Military-Health-Care-Personnel-Dealing-with-Epidemics/ Messelken-Winkler/p/book/9781472480736.

The paragraphs in italics before the Introduction were added for this republication.

References

Abramowitz, S.A., McLean, K.E., McKune, S.L., Bardosh, K.L., Fallah, M., Monger, J., et al. (2015). Community-centered responses to Ebola in urban Liberia: the view from below. *PLoS Negl Trop Dis* 9(4): e0003706. Available at: www.ncbi.nlm. nih.gov/pmc/articles/PMC4391876/.

ACAPS (2015a). Ebola outbreak in West Africa: lessons learned from quarantine – Sierra Leone and Liberia. March 19, 2015. Available at: http://acaps.org/img/ documents/t-acaps_thematic_note_ebola_west_africa_quarantine_sierra_leone_ liberia_19_march_2015.pdf.

ACAPS (2015b). Ebola in West Africa. Guinea: resistance to the Ebola response. April 24, 2015. Available at: http://acaps.org/img/documents/t-acaps_ebola_ guinea-resistance-to-ebola-response_24-april-2015.pdf.

Anoko, J. (2015). Communication with rebellious communities during an outbreak of Ebola Virus Disease in Guinea: an anthropological approach. Ebola Response Anthropology Platform. Available at: www.ebola-anthropology.net/case_studies/communication-with-rebellious-communities-during-an-outbreak-of-ebola-virus-disease-in-guinea-an-anthropological-approach/.

Barbisch, D., Koenig, K.L., & Shih, F.Y. (2015). Is there a case for quarantine? Perspectives from SARS to Ebola. *Disaster Med Public Health Prep* 9(5), 547–553.

Bensimon, C.M. & Upshur, R.E.G. (2007). Evidence and effectiveness for decision making for quarantine. *Am J Public Health* 97(suppl. 1), S44–S48. Available at: www.ncbi.nlm.nih.gov/pmc/articles/PMC1854977/pdf/0970044.pdf.

Bianchi, S. (2015). Determinants of Ebola health seeking behaviors: reflections from Freetown, Sierra Leone, MSF-UREPH. Internal report, May 2015.

Bondy, S.J., Russell, M.L., Laflèche, J.M. & Rea, E. (2009). Quantifying the impact of community quarantine on SARS transmission in Ontario: estimation of secondary case count difference and number needed to quarantine. *BMC Public Health* 9: 488. Available at: www.ncbi.nlm.nih.gov/pmc/articles/PMC2808319/.

Brown, H. & Kelly, A.H. (2014). Material proximities and hotspots: toward an anthropology of viral hemorrhagic fevers. *Med Anthropol Q* 28(2), 280–303. Available at: www.ncbi.nlm.nih.gov/pmc/articles/PMC4305216/pdf/maq0028-0280.pdf.

Centers for Disease Control and Prevention (2014). Interim U.S. guidance for monitoring and movement of persons with potential Ebola virus exposure. Updated: December 24, 2014. Available at: www.cdc.gov/vhf/ebola/exposure/monitoring-and-movement-of-persons-with-exposure.html.

Chandler, C., Fairhead, J., Kelly, A., Leach, M., Martineau, F., Mokuwa, E., et al. (2015). Ebola: limitations of correcting misinformation. *Lancet* 385, 1275–1277. Available at: www.thelancet.com/journals/lancet/article/PIIS0140-6736%2814%2962382-5/fulltext?rss=yes.

Day, T., Park, A., Madras, N., Gumel, A. & Wu, J. (2006). When is quarantine a useful control strategy for emerging infectious diseases? *Am J Epidemiol* 163(5), 479–485. Available at: http://aje.oxfordjournals.org/content/163/5/479.long.

Diallo, B. (2015). Ebola en Guinee: le Président Condé utilise l'usage de la "force" contre les réticents. *Africaguinee.com*, January 18, 2015. Available at: www.africaguinee.com/articles/2015/01/18/ebola-en-guinee-le-president-conde-autorise-l-usage-de-la-force-contre-les.

Diallo, T. & Felix, B. (2014). Mali ends last quarantines, could be Ebola-free next month. *Reuters*, December 16, 2014. Available at: www.reuters.com/article/2014/12/16/us-health-ebola-mali-idUSKBN0JU1NR20141216.

Drazen, J.M., Kanapathipillai, R., Campion, E.W., Rubin, E.J., Hammer, S.M., Morrissey, S. & Baden, L.R. (2014). Ebola and quarantine. *N Engl J Med* 371(21), 2029–2030. Available at: www.nejm.org/doi/full/10.1056/NEJMe1413139.

Epelboin, A. (2015). Approche anthropologique de l'épidémie de FHV Ebola en Guinée Conakry. March 18, 2015. Available at: http://memsic.ccsd.cnrs.fr/hal-01090291/document.

Fink, S. (2015). Outbreak (documentary). Frontline. Public Broadcasting Service.

Formenty, P., Libama, F., Epelboin, A., Allarangar, Y., Leroy, E., Moudzeo, H., et al. (2003). L'épidemie de fièvre hémorragique à virus Ebola en République du Congo, 2003: une nouvelle stratégie? *Méd Trop (Mars)* 63, 291–295.

Garrett, L. (2001). Landa-landa. In: *Betrayal of Trust: The Collapse of Global Public Health*. New York: Hyperion.

Garrett, L. (2014). Heartless but effective: I have seen "cordon sanitaire" work against Ebola. *The New Republic*, August 14, 2014. Available at: www.newrepublic. com/article/119085/ebola-cordon-sanitaire-when-it-worked-congo-1995.

Grigg, C., Waziri, N.E., Olayinka, A.T. & Vertefeuille, J.F. (2015). Use of group quarantine in Ebola control – Nigeria, 2014. *MMWR* 64(5), 124. Available at: www.cdc.gov/mmwr/preview/mmwrhtml/mm6405a3.htm.

Hewlett, B.S. & Amola, R.P. (2003). Cultural contexts of Ebola in Northern Uganda. *Emerg Infect Dis* 9(10), 1242–1248. Available at: http://wwwnc.cdc.gov/eid/article/9/10/02-0493_article.

Hewlett, B.L. & Hewlett, B.S. (2005). Providing care and facing death: nursing during Ebola outbreaks in central Africa. *J Transcult Nurs* 16(4), 289–297.

Hewlett, B.S. & Hewlett, B.L. (2008). *Ebola, Culture and Politics: The Anthropology of an Emerging Disease*. Belmont, CA: Thomson Wadsworth.

Hewlett, B.S., Epelboin, A., Hewlett, B.L. & Formenty, P. (2005). Medical anthropology and Ebola in Congo: cultural models and humanistic care. *Bull Soc Pathol Exot* 98(3), 230–236.

Heymann, D.L. (2014). Ebola: learn from the past. *Nature* 514(7522), 299–300.

Hodge, J.G. Jr, Barraza, L., Measer, G. & Agrawal, A. (2014). Global emergency legal responses to the 2014 Ebola outbreak: public health and the law. *J Law Med Ethics* 42(4), 595–601.

Karimova, T. (2015). Derogation from human rights treaties in situations of emergencies. RULAC project. Geneva Academy of International and Humanitarian Law. Geneva, Switzerland. Available at: http://atlalix.com/project-rulac/issues/derogation-from-human-rights-treaties-in-situations-of-emergency/.

Kerstiëns, B. & Matthys, F. (1999). Interventions to control virus transmission during an outbreak of Ebola hemorrhagic fever: experience from Kikwit, Democratic Republic of the Congo, 1995. *J Infect Dis* 179(suppl. 1), S263–S267. Available at: http://jid.oxfordjournals.org/content/179/Supplement_1/S263.abstract?sid=2d2d0bd8-3faf-4264-bf50-9e549124d08c.

Koenig, K.L. (2015). Health care worker quarantine for Ebola: to eradicate the virus or alleviate fear? *Ann Emerg Med* 65(3), 330–331. Available at: www.annemergmed.com/article/S0196-0644%2814%2901571-6/pdf.

Kucharski, A.J., Camacho, A., Flasche, S., Glover, R.E., Edmunds, J. & Funk, S. (2015a). Measuring the impact of Ebola control measures in Sierra Leone. *Proc Natl Acad Sci USA*, published ahead of print. Available from: www.pnas.org/content/early/2015/10/07/1508814112.full.pdf?sid=1c78de2e-28e4-497d-9984-223608277f11.

Kucharski, A.J., Camacho, A., Checchi, F., Waldman, R., Grais, R.F., Cabrol, J.C., et al. (2015b). Evaluation of the benefits and risks of introducing Ebola community care centers, Sierra Leone. *Emerg Infect Dis* 21(3), 393–399.

Kutalek, R., Wang, S., Fallah, M., Wesseh, C.S. & Gilbert, J. (2015). Ebola interventions: listen to communities. *Lancet* 3, e131. Available at: www.thelancet.com/pdfs/journals/langlo/PIIS2214-109X%2815%2970010-0.pdf.

Leach, M. & Hewlett, B.S. (2010). Haemorrhagic fevers: narratives, politics and pathways. In: Dry, S. and Leach, M. (eds), *Epidemics: Science, Governance and Social Justice*. London: Earthscan, 43–69.

Lyon, G.M., Mehta, A.K., Varkey, J.B., Brantly, K., Plyler, L., McElroy, A.K., et al. (2014). Clinical care of two patients with Ebola virus disease in the United States. *N Engl J Med* 371(25), 2402–2409. Available at: www.nejm.org/doi/full/10.1056/NEJMoa1409838.

Mac Johnson, R. & Larson, N. (2015). Sierra Leone berates Ebola quarantine escapees as cases surge. *Agence France Presse*, May 20, 2015. Available at: http://reliefweb.int/report/sierra-leone/sierra-leone-berates-ebola-quarantine-escapees-cases-surge.

MacPhail, T. (2014). Quarantine, epidemiological knowledge, and infectious disease research in Hong Kong. In: *The Viral Network: A Pathography of the H1N1 Influenza Pandemic*. Ithaca, NY and London: Cornell University Press, 75–107.

Marais, F., Minkler, M., Gibson, N., Mwau, B., Mehtar, S., Ogunsola, F., et al. (2015). A community-engaged infection prevention and control approach to Ebola. *Health Promot Int* 1–10. Available at: http://heapro.oxfordjournals.org/content/early/2015/02/12/heapro.dav003.full.pdf+html.

Maron, D.F. (2015). The most memorable moments of the Ebola response. *Sci Am*, March 24, 2015. Available at: www.youtube.com/watch?feature=player_embedded&v=vLJPJYy1oN4.

Meltzer, M.I., Atkins, C.Y., Santibanez, S., et al. (2014). Estimating the future number of cases in the Ebola epidemic – Liberia and Sierra Leone, 2014–2015. *MMWR* suppl. 63(3), 1–14. Available at: www.cdc.gov/mmwr/pdf/other/su6303.pdf.

Merler, S., Ajelli, M., Fumanelli, L., Gomes, M.F.C., Piontti, A.P., Rossi, L., et al. (2015). Spatiotemporal spread of the 2014 outbreak of Ebola virus disease in Liberia and the effectiveness of non-pharmaceutical interventions: a computational modelling analysis. *Lancet Infect Dis* 15(2), 204–211. Available at: www.thelancet.com/pdfs/journals/laninf/PIIS1473-3099%2814%2971074-6.pdf.

Miles, S.U. (2015). Kaci Hickox: public health and the politics of fear. *Am J Bioethics* 15(4), 17–19.

MSF (2014). Ebola: Quarantine can undermine efforts to curb epidemic. Press release, October 27, 2014. Available at: www.msf.org/article/ebola-quarantine-can-undermine-efforts-curb-epidemic.

Pandey, A., Atkins, K., Medlock, J., Wenzel, N., Townsend, J.P., Childs, J.E., et al. (2014). Strategies for containing Ebola in West Africa. *Science* 346(6212), 991–995. Available at: www.sciencemag.org/content/346/6212/991.full.

Presidential Commission for the Study of Bioethical Issues (2015). Ethics and Ebola: Public health planning and response. February 2015. Available at: http://bioethics.gov/node/4637.

Racaniello, V. (2014). Nobel laureates and Ebola virus quarantine. *Virology Blog*, November 4, 2014. Available at: www.virology.ws/2014/11/04/nobel-laureates-and-ebola-virus-quarantine/.

Reliefweb (2015). République de Guinée et Organisation Mondiale de la Santé. Rapport de la situation epidémiologique maladie a virus Ebola en Guinée. Available at: http://reliefweb.int/updates?search=Rapport%20de%20la%20Situation%20Epid%C3%A9miologique%20Maladie%20a%20Virus%20Ebola%20en%20Guin%C3%A9e&page=1#content.

Richards, P., Amara, J., Ferme, M.C., Kamara, P., Mokuwa, E., Sheriff, A.I., et al. (2015). Social pathways for Ebola virus disease in rural Sierra Leone, and some implications for containment. *PLoS Negl Trop Dis* 9(4), e0003567. Available at: http://journals.plos.org/plosntds/article?id=10.1371/journal.pntd.0003567.

Roddy, P., Weatherill, D., Jeffs, B., Abaakouk, Z., Dorion, C., Rodriguez-Martinez, J., et al. (2007). The Médecins Sans Frontières intervention in the Marburg hemorrhagic fever epidemic, Uige, Angola, 2005. II. Lessons learned in the community. *J Infect Dis* 196(suppl. 2), S162–S167. Available at: http://jid.oxford-journals.org/content/196/Supplement_2/S162.long.

Rothstein, M.A. (2015a). Ebola, quarantine, and the law. *Hastings Cent Rep* 45(1), 5–6. Available at: http://onlinelibrary.wiley.com/doi/10.1002/hast.411/pdf.

Rothstein, M.A. (2015b). From SARS to Ebola: legal and ethical considerations for modern quarantine. *Indiana Health Law Rev* 12(1), 227–280.

Rothstein, M.A., Alcalde, G.M., Elster, N.R., Majumder, M.A., Palmer, L.I., Stone, H.T., et al. (2003). Quarantine and isolation: lessons learned from SARS. A report to the Centers for Disease Control and Prevention. Institute for Bioethics, Health Policy and Law, University of Louisville School of Medicine. November 2003. Available at: http://biotech.law.lsu.edu/blaw/cdc/SARS_REPORT.pdf.

Ruble, K. (2014). Ebola riots in Sierra Leone highlight marginalized youth population. *Vice News*. October 23, 2014. Available at: https://news.vice.com/article/ebola-riots-in-sierra-leone-highlight-marginalized-youth-population.

Sahid, J.S. (2015). Pros and cons of Sierra Leone's Ebola lockdowns. *IRIN*, April 9, 2015. Available at: www.irinnews.org/report/101346/ebola-lockdowns-anything-to-get-to-zero.

Shears, P. & O'Dempsey, T.J.D. (2015). Ebola virus disease in Africa: epidemiology and nosocomial transmission. *J Hosp Infect* 90(1), 1–9. Available at: www.journalofhospitalinfection.com/article/S0195-6701%2815%2900046-8/pdf.

Sprecher, A.G, Caluwaerts, A., Draper, M., Feldmann, H., Frey, C.P., Funk, R.H., et al., (2015). Personal protective equipment for filovirus epidemics: a call for better evidence. *J Infect Dis* 212(suppl. 2), S98–S100. Available at: http://jid.oxfordjournals.org/content/early/2015/03/26/infdis.jiv153.long.

Sterk, E. (2008). Filovirus haemorrhagic fever guideline. Médecins Sans Frontières.

Ulrich, C. (2014). Ebola is causing moral distress among African health care workers. *Brit Med J* 349, g6672. Available at: www.bmj.com/content/349/bmj.g6672.

United Nations (1985). Siracusa Principles. Human Rights Library. University of Minnesota. Available at: www1.umn.edu/humanrts/instree/siracusaprinciples.html.

USAID (2015). Community perspectives about Ebola in Bong, Lofa and Montserrado counties of Liberia: results of a qualitative study. Final report, January 2015. Available at: http://ebolacommunicationnetwork.org/ebolacomresource/community-perspectives-about-ebola-in-bong-lofa-and-montserrado-counties-of-liberia/.

Washington, M.L. & Meltzer, M.L. (2015). Effectiveness of Ebola treatment units and community care centers – Liberia, September 23–October 31, 2014. *MMWR* 63(3), 67–69. Available at: www.cdc.gov/mmwr/preview/mmwrhtml/mm6403a6.htm.

Wilkinson, A. & Leach, M. (2015). Briefing: Ebola – myths, realities and structural violence. *Afr Aff (London)* 114(454), 136–148. Available at: http://afraf.oxfordjournals.org/content/114/454/136.

Witty, C.J.M., Farrar, J., Ferguson, M., Edmunds, W.J., Piot, P., Leach, M. & Davies, S.C. (2014). Infectious disease: tough choices to reduce Ebola transmission. *Nature* 515(7526), 192–194. Available at: www.nature.com/polopoly_fs/1.16298!/menu/main/topColumns/topLeftColumn/pdf/515192a.pdf.

World Health Organization (2003). Outbreak(s) of Ebola haemorrhagic fever, Congo and Gabon, October 2001–July 2002. *Wkly Epidemiol Rec* 26, 217–224. Available at: www.who.int/wer/2003/en/wer7826.pdf.

World Health Organization (2007). WHO guidance on human rights and involuntary detention for xdr-tb control. January 24, 2007. Available at: www.who.int/tb/features_archive/involuntary_treatment/en/.

Wynia, M.K. (2007). Ethics and public health emergencies: restrictions on liberty. *Am J Bioeth* 7(2), 1–5.

Zellmann, H. (2015). Counseling through the fence. *TAG* 39, 23. Internal journal, MSF Switzerland.

Conclusion

Global health revisited

*Claudine Burton-Jeangros, Mathilde Bourrier
and Nathalie Brender*

This collective volume offers a further contribution to the growing literature on responses provided to re-emerging infectious diseases under the global health framework. Our social science perspective, fueled by a range of disciplines covering sociology, anthropology, economics, political science and risk management, is directly articulated with the input of public health professionals, through the fieldwork we conducted inside a range of institutions but also through their contributions with the preparation of chapters included in this book. As shown by others, infectious diseases outbreaks and their associated responses always take place in specific social, cultural, geographical, economic and political environments. Their progression, as well as the measures taken to limit their spread, are impacted by local circumstances. Compliance with public health interventions and reactions towards institutional actions are also locally shaped and therefore diverse.

The different chapters assess how the international responses provided to control the A(H1N1) pandemic and the 2014 Ebola epidemic both reflect recent developments in global health and challenge some of the assumptions of this new field. The scope of analysis was focused on these two crises, which, despite their specificities, reflect recurrent controversies that we would like to discuss in this conclusion. Beyond the analysis of a large range of documents prepared before, during and after the crises, our conclusions stem from empirical work conducted across institutions and countries. This allows us to shed light on the experience of front-line professionals, to document the difficulties they encountered in the application of the normative preparedness framework and also to report on their frustrations when exposed to contradictory injunctions and criticisms. We suggest that giving more weight to social science knowledge, before, during and after an outbreak might reduce some of the controversies.

Ebola again

As we are finishing this book, a new Ebola outbreak is declared. On May 8 2018, the World Health Organization (WHO) was notified by the Ministry of Health of the Democratic Republic of the Congo of two confirmed cases of Ebola virus disease occurring in the Bikoro health zone, Equateur Province. As of May 18, forty-six suspected, probable and confirmed Ebola cases and twenty-six deaths have been reported. Most of the cases come from a remote rural town, while four confirmed cases are in Mbandaka, the provincial capital with a population of over 1 million people, rendering the initial containment plan irrelevant. Three different chains of transmission have already been identified. It looks like patients have been brought to town to be treated, despite the risk of faster contagion highlighted during the management of previous outbreaks.

The outbreak being serious, the WHO started forming a broad response, with numerous partners, organized around the implementation of a vaccination campaign. An Emergency Operations Center to coordinate the response has been activated by local authorities and supported by WHO experts. As expected, US$1 million have been released from the WHO contingency fund for emergencies to support the response. At this stage, however, cost does not appear to be a constraint and money is expected to follow. The WHO is providing technical and operational support to the Ministry of Health and also it is said to support "Partners in the activation of multi-partner multi-agency Emergency Operations Centre to coordinate the response at all levels" (WHO website, May 9, 2018). The presentation of the outbreak response seems familiar: Médecins Sans Frontières is setting up a treatment center for the management of cases in the Bikoro health zone; the WHO has shared risk communication materials in French and Lingala with WHO country offices. The Wellcome Trust is providing 2 million pounds sterling, US and African CDCs are there too, along with the Global Outbreak Alert and Response Network (GOARN) and the Global Alliance for Vaccines and Immunization (GAVI), and UN organizations like the World Food Programme and UNICEF have been mobilized too.

A press release (Jourdan, May 23, 2018, *Tribune de Genève*) reports a few elements, which also seem familiar: "On the ground medical teams are facing unexpected reactions that increase the risk of contagion. MSF revealed that 3 contaminated patients escaped from the hospital where they had been quarantined, probably afraid of being vaccinated". Consequently, African health authorities, more specifically CDC Atlanta, "are sending anthropologists in order to facilitate the vaccination campaign against Ebola", because "If we do not manage adequately our communication, the vaccination program might suffer", explains John Nkengasong, Head of CDC Africa (our translation). Anthropologists and their mediating skills along with proper risk communication tools are once again called to the rescue to help with the response – a response essentially organized around a vaccination campaign whose cost does not seem to be an issue.

This new outbreak shows that governing global epidemics is likely to continue occupying international and national public health agencies in the future.

A sense of biological vulnerability

The turn of the twenty-first century has been associated with the extending view that biological vulnerability represents a major threat to the modern world. The globalization of risks, transcending national borders and national regulation bodies, has been emphasized by a range of bodies, such as the OECD with its report on "emerging systemic risks" (OECD, 2003) or the World Economic Forum yearly report on "global risks" (World Economic Forum, 2016). Such denominations keep highlighting the highly connected nature of systems but also stress the catastrophic potential of disruptions. Renewed preoccupations with infectious diseases emerged at the same time (Washer, 2010). While the progress of medicine was for a while thought sufficient to eradicate infections, HIV/AIDS in the 1980s and the succession of epidemics that followed progressively raised an international sense of alarm regarding the limits of science and medicine to actually control those threats. In connection with a range of globalization trends, including increasing travel, deregulation of trade, migration and demographic patterns, environmental degradation, etc., the scientific and policy framework of (re-)emerging infectious diseases gained momentum (Lakoff & Collier, 2008; Bastide, Chapter 2). While Ulrich Beck in his notorious book on the risk society (Beck, 1992) emphasized the technological vulnerability of modern societies, the success of "re-emerging infectious diseases" and its extension under the biosecurity agenda highlight a renewed sense of biological vulnerability (Caduff, 2014; Zylberman, 2013).

Globalization is associated with deregulation and faster connections, bringing together objects and individuals from distant regions thus reinforcing potential channels of contamination. The increased proximity with low- and middle-income countries, often perceived as sources of risks for infectious diseases, created new anxieties. The accumulation of outbreaks further exacerbated such fears towards peripheral countries, perceived as reservoirs of exotic viruses (Caduff, 2014). Developments in preparedness thinking (Bastide, Chapter 2) made expected outbreaks seem more real and imminent. Warnings were already present in the context of the avian influenza H5N1 threat: "it's a bird disease – and affects people's livelihoods"; "human–human spread is the real risk, and could be catastrophic"; and "a major economic and humanitarian disaster is around the corner and we must be prepared" (Scoones & Forster, 2008, 12). Adopting a worst-case scenario approach, the common motto became "not if, but when", suggesting that major epidemics were inevitable. The new International Health Regulations (IHR) also reinforced such assumptions, promoting a "global outbreak narrative" (Wald, 2008; Seetoh et al., 2012). Developments in communication technologies and their potential for early detection through syndromic surveillance mechanisms further contributed to the alert imperative (Fearnley, 2008). Finally, such fears have been exploited by the cultural industry, especially in the United States, through the alarmist predictions of media reports, books and movies depicting apocalyptic futures (Wald, 2008; Keränen, 2011). As a result, such representations of biological vulnerability and imminent catastrophe are nowadays not only limited to a circumscribed circle of institutions and experts, but rather have been disseminated throughout the whole of society.

Global health in action

Next to this overall sense of vulnerability, the A(H1N1) pandemic and 2014 Ebola epidemic tested the global health system capacity to adequately respond to such biological threats. The connection between human health and (bio)terrorism (Scoones & Forster, 2008; Zylberman, 2013), particularly due to the new status of smallpox as a biological weapon, the ever-closer link between human and animal health together with the potential economic and trade disruptions contributed to give national administrations and international organizations such as the WHO a sense of urgency to act (Brender & Gilbert, 2018). As was shown in several chapters, both crises presented different characteristics and thus generated specific measures. Both offered concrete opportunities to apply the preparedness guidance, largely equipped with plans, guidelines and norms developed to tackle such events. In the continuation of risk management activities that had expanded over the last decades, this normative framework aimed at the early anticipation of the onset of an epidemic in order to control its spread and limit fatalities. However, next to this normative apparatus, both viruses did not develop as expected, thus challenging the value of anticipation and prediction (Keller, Chapter 1). We showed above how this gap between expectations or even the urge for global health action and the actual course of the disease has been very challenging for front-line public health professionals. Over a few years, the WHO and CDC staff, i.e. those involved in the two crises, were first accused of over-response and then not long after, of under-response. This can be considered a result of the attention dedicated to risk and more recently uncertainty, promoting a sense of human agency towards the future. Global health developments have directly encouraged such impulse to act, even in the absence of complete evidence. In such a context, it is no surprise that global health leadership had to make difficult decisions between two uncomfortable alternatives, i.e. acting early with limited evidence or waiting to observe the actual unfolding of an outbreak. Next to scientific and technical decisions, public interpretations over the chosen course of action have ranged from undue scaremongering in the A(H1N1) pandemic case to voluntary covering-up in the 2014 Ebola epidemic context.

Several chapters of the book addressed the difficulties associated with the prediction of events to come. As recalled by some interviewees, the A(H1N1) pandemic called for action, based on the scientific authority of models estimating potentially huge damage and high associated costs. Furthermore, with the sustained anticipation over the previous years of an inevitable pandemic, front-line professionals decided to act to avoid any regret. Having been prepared to do so following recurrent references to the precautionary approach and to worst-case scenarios, the alarm went off when a new flu virus was identified. Besides this, it is important to emphasize that despite the anticipation mode and the accumulation of plans, both epidemics overloaded the capacities of organizations. From the burden imposed on one intensive care unit service in Switzerland taking care of an evacuated Ebola-infected patient (Parfaite, Chapter 10) to the difficulties encountered by the Ebola response team within the WHO (Dupras, Chapter 6), it is clear that available resources were stretched, creating tensions with staff providing routine activities. In the context of communication, demands of 24/7 media across the globe exceeded the capacity of the CDC's and WHO's well-developed headquarters communication activities (Burton-Jeangros, Chapter 4). In the Ebola context, activities in the affected countries proved difficult if not impossible to achieve due to the limited information available to deployees (Bastide, Chapter 5) or the clash of normative and cultural frameworks (Calain & Poncin, Chapter 11). As discussed by Bourrier (Chapter 3), global health organizations, in particular the WHO, struggled to put in practice the normative framework and strived to adapt to pressing demands. Finally, it is worth noting how little economic arguments were taken into account. In the context of high-income countries' responses to the A(H1N1) pandemic, money considerations were not crucial (Brender et al., Chapter 7) and indeed the actual cost of the pandemic was minimal compared to overall health budgets (Pasquini-Descomps et al., Chapter 8). In itself, this observation should call for a reconsideration of the actual extent of the crisis.

Global health and local contexts

Responses prompted by the global health framework took place in local environments, characterized by specific social, cultural, political and geographical contexts. Historically, infectious diseases have always been associated with blame mechanisms, attributing the onset of misfortune to other social groups, as described for syphilis, cholera or tuberculosis (Joffe, 1999). Anthropological and sociological research documents similar social reactions towards re-emerging infectious diseases over the last decades. Cultural and geographical distance are typically used to establish borders between a safe inside community and a dangerous outside environment (Douglas & Wildawsky, 1983). The importance of boundaries has been made explicit through the contrast between a relative indifference to the Ebola outbreak as long as it was confined to African countries and the outrage generated by the presence of infected health professionals in Spain and the United States. In the recent 2014 Ebola epidemic, difficulties to control the outbreak were attributed to the inadequate cultural practices of local populations (in particularly burial rituals and bushmeat practices), considered not only "exotic" but also dangerous behaviors from a public health point of view. In public health, this interpretation of culture as an obstacle is frequent: "culture itself is reconstituted as a 'risk factor' for infection in light of assumptions about African 'Otherness'" (Jones, 2011, 2).

Our analyses of recent experiences in global health responses to infectious diseases suggest that such views are still prevalent. While the difficulties associated with cultural beliefs in Africa have long been debated, it is surprising how little the issue has been discussed in the context of the A(H1N1) pandemic. The only explicit mention of such differences was made in the United States, when the post-pandemic report acknowledged difficulties in reaching minority groups (Burton-Jeangros, Chapter 4). However, resistance to flu vaccination reflects the presence of sociocultural views questioning the dominant public health perspective on immunization. Furthermore, the fact that front-line professionals deployed in Africa were surprised by the local beliefs and practices is worth mentioning. Sociological and anthropological knowledge on health and illness has accumulated over the last decades and anthropologists had been specifically integrated into earlier Ebola responses. However, these were initially not mobilized in 2014. The recent inclusion of "Social science outbreak teams" in the WHO risk communication team might hopefully help overcome such forgetfulness (Bourrier, Chapter 9) and help document how culture can offer alternative solutions (Calain & Poncin, Chapter 11). Another issue discussed across the volume relates to the tension between individual autonomy and its associated responsibility towards health, very much valued in the western context, and collective interests in the name of which public health might override individual freedom. Aside from differences across countries, Calain & Poncin (Chapter 11) addressed the issue under the lens of ethics to emphasize the importance of weighing individual rights and the common good. In that respect, the absence of evidence about systematic cost–benefit evaluations during the A(H1N1) pandemic or Ebola 2014 epidemic crises also raises ethical issues, such as depleting the financial resources left to handle other risks or health issues (Brender et al., Chapter 7).

A social science perspective thus inevitably questions the value of an approach unilaterally based on epidemiological evidence and biomedical practices while remaining almost blind to cultural diversity and economic dimensions. This gap has been observed, often inadvertently, by the front-line professionals we interviewed, such as when they reported being surprised by the political nature of outbreaks, impinging on their technical work (Bastide, Chapter 5). They did not understand being blamed while they were doing their best to contain dangerous viruses, and on top of that at a reasonable cost for A(H1N1). Their surprise reflects their own embedding in a global health perspective dominated by a medical agenda focused on individual cases to identify, to protect or to treat, but oblivious to the social and economic context.

The role of social sciences in global health

Global health developed as an interdisciplinary field of expertise, calling for the integration of a range of disciplines providing what are considered relevant insights about health issues. From our journey in this project, we however conclude that the role of social sciences in this domain remains ambivalent, torn between unmet expectations and limited acknowledgment.

Public health and global health are both normative domains, promoting the improvement of conditions for health across a range of population groups, at the national or international levels. Such an approach is for example unequivocally formulated in a paper, associating global health with the normative framework of human rights and equity (Wernli et al., 2016). Such a value-laden orientation often conflicts with the aims of social scientists whose goal is to describe the range of existing norms, to analyze tensions across groups of actors, to contrast specific worldviews as embedded in specific social locations and to document constraints affecting action. Furthermore, the temporality of social science research tends to be resistant to the emergency paradigm that has become commonplace in global health.

Social sciences are typically called in when public health is confronted with "cultural problems" that cannot be solved by technical solutions. This was clearly the case in the early days of the HIV/AIDS epidemic, a time when the contribution of social science to prevention activities was considered crucial. In the context of Ebola again, the importance of anthropological expertise has been emphasized with expectations for identifying the barriers and obstacles to be alleviated in order to rapidly modify problematic behaviors. However, an understanding of the complex actions developed by global health to respond to outbreaks necessitates an extension of the research agenda, typically focused on a better understanding of "problematic audiences" towards an analysis of the work of experts themselves, including their interpretations of risks and their handling of organizational, human and financial resources constraints. A distinction has long been made between an instrumental role of the social sciences in applied projects and their critical role equated with questioning the way issues are framed and analyzing power relationships in specific settings (Gilbert & Henry, 2009). Global health would gain from acknowledging such a larger contribution of the social sciences, including analyses of the power relationships inherent to collaborative work across the disciplines engaged in global health activities.

Our original project started on the assumption that organizing, communicating and costing, three major pillars of global health responses, were too often addressed separately. This volume has confirmed that these dimensions are rarely considered together. On top of that, our work suggests that they tend to remain outside the perimeter of global health action. In other words, from a global health perspective, organizations, communications and money are not central issues. Organizations are taken for granted, with ongoing reforms that seem to divert the attention from emergency situations. Communication is still perceived as an issue of providing the bare "facts" to the public who will then adopt proper behaviors while little attention is given to the considerable challenge of communication across institutions and to alternative narratives that will necessarily develop in epidemic contexts. Costing is out of the radar of public health decisions since delaying or challenging the implementation of the response according to its cost-effectiveness is ethically and politically problematic when human lives are at stake. Furthermore, money is not a constraint. Emergency funds are committed and drawn upon quickly, with little upfront discussion, and almost no control over the nature and extent of expenses. Outside of global health, these three pillars are, however, crucial. They provide measures of the accountability of experts and institutions in their governing of global epidemics.

References

Beck, U. (1992). *Risk Society: Towards a New Modernity*. London: Sage.

Brender, N. & Gilbert, C. (2018). From emergence to emergences: A focus on pandemic influenza, in Morand, S. & Figuié, M. (eds), *Emergence of Infectious Diseases: Risks and Issues for Societies*. Versailles: Editions Quae, 35–51.

Caduff, C. (2014). On the verge of death: Visions of biological vulnerability. *Annual Review of Anthropology*, *43*(1), 105–121. https://doi.org/10.1146/annurev-anthro-102313-030341.

Douglas, M. & Wildawsky, A. (1983). *Risk and Culture: An Essay on the Selection of Technological and Environmental Dangers*. Berkeley, CA: University of California Press.

Fearnley, L. (2008). Redesigning syndromic surveillance for biosecurity, in Lakoff, A. & Collier, S. (eds), *Biosecurity Interventions: Global Health Security in Question*. New York, NY: Columbia University Press.

Gilbert, C. & Henry, E. (2009). *Comment se construisent les problèmes de santé publique*. Paris: La Découverte.

Joffe, H. (1999). *Risk and "the Other"*. Cambridge and New York, NY: Cambridge University Press.

Jones, J. (2011). Ebola, emerging: The limitations of culturalist epidemiology. *Journal of Global Health, 1*(1), 1–5.

Keränen, L. (2011). Concocting viral apocalypse: Catastrophic risk and the production of bio(in)security. *Western Journal of Communication, 75*(5), 451–472. https://doi.org/10.1080/10570314.2011.614507.

Lakoff, A. & Collier, S. J. (eds). (2008). *Biosecurity Interventions: Global Health and Security in Question.* New York, NY: Columbia University Press.

OECD. (2003). Emerging Risks in the 21st Century: An Agenda for Action. OECD, Paris.

Scoones, I. & Forster, P. (2008). *The International Response to Highly Pathogenic Avian Influenza: Science, Policy, and Politics.* STEPS, Working Paper 10. Brighton, STEPS Center.

Seetoh, T., Liverani, M., & Coker, R. (2012). Framing risk in pandemic influenza policy and control. *Global Public Health, 7*(7), 717–730. https://doi.org/10.1080/17441692.2012.699541.

Wald, P. (2008). *Contagious: Cultures, Carriers, and the Outbreak Narrative.* Durham, NC: Duke University Press.

Washer, P. (2010). *Emerging Infectious Diseases and Society.* New York, NY: Palgrave Macmillan.

Wernli, D., Tanner, M., Kickbusch, I., Escher, G., Paccaud, F., & Flahault, A. (2016). Moving global health forward in academic institutions. *Journal of Global Health, 6*(1), 010409.

World Economic Forum. (2016). The Global Risks Report 2016. WEF, Geneva.

Zylberman, P. (2013). *Tempêtes microbiennes: Essai sur la politique de sécurité sanitaire dans le monde transatlantique.* Paris: Gallimard.

Index

Page numbers in **bold** denote tables.